# PATIENT EDUCATION
# AND HEALTH PROMOTION
# IN MEDICAL CARE

# The Authors

**Wendy D. Squyres, Ph.D.**, Senior Author and Editor
Director, Center for Professional Development and Training
Centers for Disease Control, Atlanta, Ga.

**Barbara Christianson, M.P.H.**
Health Educator
Kaiser-Permanente Medical Center, Oakland, Calif.

**Maureen L. Dion, M.P.H.**
Health Education Coordinator
Total Health Care Project
Kaiser-Permanente Medical Center, Oakland, Calif.

**Enid Fallick Hunkeler, M.A.**
Regional Program Evaluation Coordinator
Medical Methods Research
Permanente Medical Group, Oakland, Calif.

**Pamela Jean Larson, M.P.H.**
Health Education Coordinator
Kaiser-Permanente Medical Center, Oakland, Calif.

**Catherine Regan, B.A.**
Health Educator
Kaiser-Permanente Medical Center, San Francisco, Calif.

**M. Cecilia Runkle, A.C.S.W., M.P.H.**
Regional Health Promotion Specialist
Northern California Kaiser-Permanente Medical Care Program,
Oakland, Calif.

# PATIENT EDUCATION AND HEALTH PROMOTION IN MEDICAL CARE

Wendy D. Squyres and Associates

MAYFIELD PUBLISHING COMPANY
Palo Alto and London

Library of Congress Catalog Card Number: 84-060883

International Standard Book Number: 0-87484-553-X

Manufactured in the United States of America

10 9 8 7 6 5 4 3 2 1

Mayfield Publishing Company
285 Hamilton Avenue
Palo Alto, California 94301

*Sponsoring editor:* C. Lansing Hays
*Manuscript editor:* Linda Purrington
*Managing editor:* Pat Herbst
*Art director:* Nancy Sears
*Designer (interior and cover):* Richard Kharibian
*Illustrator:* Unicorn Graphic Design
*Production manager:* Cathy Willkie
*Compositor:* Graphic Typesetting Service
*Printer and binder:* Bookcrafters

This book was written by Dr. Squyres in her private capacity. No
official support or endorsement by the Centers for Disease
Control of the U.S. Public Health Service is intended or should
be inferred.

This book is dedicated to all the health care workers and administrators we have worked and struggled with in developing health education programs and to all the health educators who are struggling to define their roles in medical care.

We especially wish to thank the following individuals who have inspired, encouraged, and supported our professional and personal travels:

- Lou Squyres, Anne Allport, Jeffrey Allport, and Beryl Cummings
- Anne Kmetovic, Robert Christianson, and Mark Clapham
- Celia and Robert Dion and Edward Perry
- Toby and David Fallick, Krikor Soghikian, and S. Leonard Syme
- Kenneth and Dorothy Larson
- Timothy D. Regan, Jr., Timothy D. Regan III, and Monica P. Regan
- Catherine Regan, Jack Nowicki, Lonnie Snowden, Martha Runkle, Mel Mordaunt, M. J. Stedry, Terri Combs-Orme, Wayne Duehn, and Wendy Squyres

# Contents

# Preface

THIS BOOK IS intended for undergraduate and graduate students in the health sciences who are preparing for careers that will allow them to practice health education in medical care settings—hospitals, clinics, home health, HMOs, nursing homes, employee health services. It is also for health professionals who currently practice health education in medical care settings and for professionals from a variety of training backgrounds who have earned titles such as health educator, health education coordinator, and education director without the benefit of formal training in health education.

We, the authors, are health education practitioners in medical care. Some of us have formal health education training; some do not. Some of us coordinate patient education and health promotion programs; some are managers; some work directly with clients. We all are involved in one or more aspects of health education assessment, planning, implementation, or evaluation.

Several of us are preceptors for undergraduate or graduate students in health education, nursing, medicine, pharmacy, social work, health administration, or health psychology. These students come to us after taking most of their required and elective coursework. After following us around for a day or two, they exclaim, "Why didn't we learn about these issues in our classes at school? Can't we take one or more courses to prepare us for the day-to-day, in-the-trenches operations of a health education program?" We'd like to say "yes" to this question. That is why we wrote *Patient Education and Health Promotion in Medical Care*.

Our field placement students—and hundreds more students around the country who have the opportunity to learn health education practice by doing defined tasks under professional supervision—are lucky. When graduates who are fresh out of school land their first job, they are rarely prepared for the complexities, subtleties, or politics of practicing health education in a medical care setting. After a few years in practice, however, and after sustaining a few bumps and bruises, they are better equipped to handle the challenges of working in the medical care system. Unfortunately, though, it is during this painful initiation period that we lose our best and brightest young health educators. Individuals who feel intimidated and isolated drop out.

To counter this no-win situation, our aim in this book is to provide structure as well as practical guidance for health education students and new practitioners. Medical care has a culture of its own. It has a social class system and its own vocabulary and jargon. It is characterized by one crisis after another. People both in the community and in medical care settings have tremendous expectations of the medical care system. People who intend to enter professions that take them into hospitals, clinics, or medical offices must be prepared with specific strategies that will help them understand the culture and that will reduce barriers to their acceptance as valuable members of the medical care team. This book is an effort to meet that need.

Health professionals have provided patient education and health promotion services in medical care settings for decades. The appearance of the health education *specialist* in medical care is more recent; only larger organizations have been able to afford specialists who coordinate and manage the health education function systemwide. For instance, five years ago, one multi-institutional prepaid group practice serving 1.8 million people had three health education coordinators; today, it has sixteen. The job potential for health education specialists in medical care continues to be promising. It is important, however, to be aware that prerequisites for a health education job often include specific coursework preparing specialists for medical care settings, supervised preceptorships in these settings, as well as volunteer or paid work experience in hospitals or clinics.

*Patient Education and Health Promotion in Medical Care* is an action-oriented text. It is meant to accompany books that provide the theoretical basis for the practice of health education, such as *Theory and Practice in Health Education* (Ross and Mico, 1980), and in-depth treatment of the health education planning process, such as *Health Education Planning: A Diagnostic Approach* (Green et al., 1980). The chapters were reviewed and field-tested by health professionals and workers with a variety of backgrounds and academic specialties. All described ways in which the book represents the scope of their involvement in health education. Many wished they had coursework that covered the topics presented here. The practitioners felt that the text realistically sets forth the essentials of well-designed patient education and health promotion programs. Professors in colleges and universities were excited to have a text that is practical without being simplistic.

This book is unique. None of the examples herein is hypothetical. Each one represents a real situation in a hospital, clinic, or other medical care setting. We have drawn upon our personal experiences—both successes and failures. Journals and professional magazines typically describe successful health education efforts. They rarely describe programs that didn't work. The examples and cases in this book do both, and they also advocate strategies to prevent failure. The best way to use this book is to actually work through the exercises. They represent situations that each health educator will face on the job.

We have sometimes gone out on a limb regarding standards for practice. For instance, chapters list go/no go checklists, the minimum makeup of committees, the ingredients of effective proposals. These lists are guidelines that readers can follow in their own work. We believe that, in a field of professional practice currently noted for lack of standards, someone must take a stand.

We assert these guidelines and base them on our professional training and on our collective sixty years of practice in the field of health education in medical care. We are neither theorists nor academicians; yet we have applied theoretical models, empirical tests, and peer review. Our experience in a rich variety of clinical settings has given us many opportunities to work and rework our approaches to assessment, planning, implementation, and evaluation.

The primary authors for each chapter are as follows:

Chapter 1: Wendy D. Squyres, Ph.D.

Chapter 2: Wendy D. Squyres

Chapter 3: Barbara Christianson, M.P.H., and Pamela Jean Larson, M.P.H.

Chapter 4: Wendy D. Squyres

Chapter 5: Wendy D. Squyres

Chapter 6: Wendy D. Squyres

Chapter 7: Enid Fallick Hunkeler, M.A.

Chapter 8: Maureen L. Dion, M.P.H.

Chapter 9: Maureen L. Dion

Chapter 10: M. Cecilia Runkle, A.C.S.W., M.P.H.

Chapter 11:  M. Cecilia Runkle and Catherine Regan, B.A.

Chapter 12:  Catherine Regan and M. Cecilia Runkle

Chapter 13:  Wendy D. Squyres

We have done more than simply describe "how we did it." Each reader is treated as a preceptor who is working along with us. Through the exercises at the end of each chapter, readers will have an opportunity to build their own cases and to apply to their own thinking and work experiences the guidelines that we have suggested. Our goal has been to challenge prospective and working practitioners to rise above the typical feeling of being victimized by limited resources and complex priorities and to believe that individual health educators *can* make a difference.

# Acknowledgments

Many thanks are extended to Lansing Hays for envisioning this project and encouraging us to gather our thoughts and write about our experiences. Special thanks are extended to Carol D'Onofrio, Dr.P.H., for the contribution she made to the way this book is organized. Her creativity and vision were immensely helpful in the early stages of the project. We are grateful for the professional assistance of our editors, Linda Purrington and Pat Herbst. Special mention is also given to Beryl Cummings for her help in typing numerous versions of the manuscript.

The following reviewers of a preliminary draft of the text made suggestions and comments that helped us fine-tune the final draft: Edward E. Bartlett, School of Public Health, University of Alabama in Birmingham; Joy D. Calkin, School of Nursing, University of Wisconsin in Madison; and Elizabeth Lee, Director, Center for Health Promotion, American Hospital Association.

In addition, each of us would like to make the following personal acknowledgments for assistance with the writing of individual chapters:

- Chapter 1: A Model for Patient Education and Health Promotion Programming
  Author: Wendy D. Squyres

  The author is grateful to Joan Wolle, Sigrid Deeds, and Barbara Hebert for their seminal work—on behalf of the Public Health Education Section of the American Public Health Association—that led to the model presented in this chapter.

- Chapter 3: The Health Educator's Roles in Medical Care
  Authors: Barbara Christianson and Pamela Jean Larson

The authors would like to thank Eileen Babbitt, Lorinda Sheets, and Mary Kyriopoulous for their comments, and Maureen Dion and Deborah Larson for agreeing to be interviewed for the case studies.

- Chapter 4: Setting Up a Program
  Author: Wendy D. Squyres

  The author wishes to thank Ray Fong and Robert Bodine of the Kaiser-Permanente Medical Care Program's Regional Audio-Visual Department for creating the original versions of some of the illustrations in this and other chapters. Thanks to Bonnie Clarke, M.P.H., and Marjorie Stocks, M.P.H., for their support and contributions to earlier drafts of this chapter. Many thanks also to Cecilia Runkle for her professional review of this chapter.

- Chapter 7: Evaluating Educational Services
  Author: Enid Fallick Hunkeler

  The author wishes to thank Michael Polen, S. Leonard Syme, Ph.D., Tom Vogt, M.D., and Bruce Fireman for editorial assistance. She would also like to acknowledge Caren Quay, M.S., Pamela Larson, M.P.H., Temple Harrup, and Bruce Hansen, Ph.D., for earlier help in developing the data-gathering instruments that appear in the appendices of this chapter.

- Chapter 8: Educational Assessment as Intervention
  Author: Maureen L. Dion

  The author wishes to thank Sarah Di Berto, M.P.H., Lawrence Gelb, D.M.H., Julie Howard, M.P.H., and Carol Weed, M.D., for their peer review of this chapter.

- Chapter 9: Risk Assessment and Health Improvement
  Author: Maureen L. Dion

  The author wishes to thank Eileen Babbitt, M.P.H., Louise Graf, M.P.H., and David Sobel, M.D., for their peer review of this chapter.

- Chapter 10: Techniques for Making Decisions and Commitments
  Author: M. Cecilia Runkle

  The author wishes to acknowledge the careful reading and critical comments given by Norman Cobb, Mel Mordaunt, and Lorinda Sheets to earlier drafts of this chapter.

- Chapter 11: The Role of Self-Care in Medical Care
  Authors: M. Cecilia Runkle and Catherine Regan

  The authors wish to thank Jim Perkins, Ph.D., and Mary Gorth, M.P.H., for their peer review of this chapter.

# About the Authors

**Wendy D. Squyres**
Wendy Squyres was initiated into the world of the medical care delivery system twenty years ago when she was working her way through college as a clerk on the youth ward at Children's Hospital in San Francisco. Then she taught health, science, and social science in secondary schools for five years, on assignment in Turkey, Germany, and England. At this point, a tobogganing accident put Squyres in the hospital with several fractured vertebrae. Although she received technically excellent care, she was struck by how frightening and isolating hospitals can be. Thus Squyres decided to help make hospitals better places in which to recuperate and work.

While she was taking health education classes as a nonmatriculated graduate student at the University of Utah, Squyres was encouraged to enter the Ph.D. program in health sciences. After several years of university teaching, she chose to return to medical care. For the past ten years, she has brought her formal training as an educator and health educator, her personal experiences, and her work experiences to the administration of health education services in academic medical centers and health maintenance organizations. Her special areas of interest are health education policy, quality assurance for health education practice, and evaluation of health education services. She is currently director of the Center for Professional Development and Training of the Centers for Disease Control in Atlanta, Georgia.

---

**Barbara Christianson**
Barbara Christianson is a health educator in a large medical center. She currently helps coordinate more than forty health education programs.

She received her bachelor's degree in genetics from the University of California at Berkeley and her master's degree in public health from San Jose State University. Christianson worked for two years as a biologist in a research laboratory, where she first became interested in health education, especially the area of occupational health. She has also worked as a health counselor, group facilitator, and patient advocate at a student health center and at a community women's clinic.

**Maureen L. Dion**
Maureen Dion was initially attracted to the field of health education as an undergraduate because of its practicality and its potential to enhance her own growth and development. She found health education to be an important vehicle for organizational and social changes to promote health. She received her M.P.H. in public health education from the University of California at Berkeley and has practiced health education in a medical care setting for seven years. Dion is currently employed by the Kaiser-Permanente Medical Care Program in Oakland, California, and is president of the Northern California Chapter of the Society for Public Health Education.

**Enid Fallick Hunkeler**
Enid Hunkeler received a master's degree in social anthropology and has had a long research interest in social science as applied to medicine, epidemiology, and health education. Before she joined the Kaiser-Permanente Medical Group in 1976, Hunkeler served as director of the Alameda County Hypertension Council. In that capacity she conducted studies of hypertension control, including community needs assessment, treatment practices, use of paramedical personnel, and screening for hypertension in the black community. She organized a referral service to community hypertension control programs, a multimedia education campaign, and screening programs in the local high schools.

Hunkeler now serves as a Kaiser-Permanente Northern California regional consultant for evaluation of patient education and health promotion programs, and she supervises the staff of the Division of Health Services Research. She has served as a co-investigator in several studies in health services research and epidemiology. She has coordinated and consulted on evaluations of smoking cessation, hypertension education, stress reduction, diabetes education, and paramedical personnel programs, as well as of various medical departments.

Hunkeler employs a wide variety of research techniques but says that her ideal job would be to do in-depth personal interviews seven days a week. She enjoys coordinating evaluations of health education programs because she believes such studies require ingenuity, encourage the development of more creative programs, and raise interesting issues in logistics, ethics, methodology, and philosophy.

### Pamela Jean Larson
Pamela Jean Larson is the coordinator of health education and health library services for the Kaiser-Permanente Medical Center in Oakland, California. While attending graduate school, she worked as a membership clerk for Kaiser-Permanente and as an assistant health educator. Her interest in health education motivated her to pursue advancement within the system. She was instrumental in bringing full department status to the health education program at her medical center and therefore was promoted to her current position. Larson is an active member of the Society for Public Health Education and in 1982 received the American Hospital Association's Leadership Award for Outstanding Management of Hospital-wide Patient Education.

### Catherine Regan
Catherine Regan discovered the field of health education as a reentry student. Her experience of raising a family in an urban environment led her to seek a profession that would support families' and individuals' search for improved quality of life. To her this support meant two things: (1) providing alternatives to commercial views of what constitutes the good life and (2) helping to make tools and resources accessible to people in transition who want to improve their health and well-being. For the past four years Regan has been working in a large urban HMO to define and establish a coordinated program of patient education, health promotion, and health information services for members. The rewards are in seeing providers' growing recognition of the role health education plays in the delivery of care, the gradual integration of these services with the medical services, and the delight and satisfaction of health plan members as they become more active in their own health care.

### M. Cecilia Runkle
Cecilia Runkle worked for several years as a medical social worker. Because she was often faced with clients who were experiencing the adverse effects of acute and chronic illness, she began looking for alternative ways in which individuals could better meet or avoid the dire consequences of illness. Learning skills in preventing disease and promoting health offered promise. Her professional training expanded to the field of health education and to advanced skills in decision making, social learning theory, and self-care. Runkle is now doing what she set out to do: designing and implementing health promotion programs for people at their places of work. She finds pleasure in teaching people skills that help them to become more self-directed in health-related concerns.

# PATIENT EDUCATION AND HEALTH PROMOTION IN MEDICAL CARE

# Introduction

THIS BOOK IS based on experiences in our lives and the lives of our colleagues around the country that highlight issues, dilemmas, and challenges to the field. By working through the many opportunities for self-analysis, simulation, and practice in each chapter, you will discover for yourself the links between health education theory and practice in practical, realistic ways.

We should now clarify some terms that are used repeatedly throughout the book. We use the word *client* to describe people who receive educational service, health care, or medical care in a hospital, clinic, health maintenance organization (HMO), employee health service, or nursing home. Clients can be residents of the community, employees of the hospital, or health professionals. *Participants* are clients who are in formal educational services. The word *patient* is reserved for clients who are recovering from or managing an illness or are preparing for a medical procedure. *Providers* is a general term for any caregiver in the medical care delivery system. *Instructor* usually denotes the provider of formal, planned educational services that complement, and are in addition to, the regular encounter between patient and provider. *Services* connotes the broad spectrum of education that is available in medical care—from one-to-one educational counseling to groups, support groups, evening lecture series, health fairs, outreach efforts, continuing education programs, organization development, consultations, and consumer awareness campaigns. *Programs* are specific educational services for a defined population with a set content, list of objectives, protocol, and plan—such as diabetes education or stress management.

We have made every effort to capture the realistic, practical aspects of health education practice in medical care without oversimplifying the work that needs to be done. This book will provide a contemporary introduction to the field. When you begin your careers in medical care, or if you are currently working but are just beginning to offer formal health education services, various sections of the book will serve you as resource guides and quick references, time and time again. This book is designed to speed up the orientation period for people who are beginning their health education efforts, regardless of where they are in their careers. The net effect of this type of support is that you will feel more confident and up to date.

Nevertheless, further research, new technologies, revised methods, and novel theories emerge all the time. One challenge you will always face as an educator in medical care is the need for further professional development and support over time. Professional organizations and peer networks can help. The Resources section (at the end of this introduction) includes a sample of organizations with which you may wish to affiliate. And newsletters such as *Patient Education Newsletter* (available from University of Alabama, 930 S. Twentieth Street, Birmingham, AL 35294) can keep you informed of national conferences and continuing education opportunities.

We think health education in medical care is an exciting, rewarding career. We hope that this book helps you get in touch with your own strengths and career objectives.

# RESOURCES

The following professional organizations provide resources and support for health educators in medical care settings. Feel free to write to them concerning membership rights and responsibilities.

- Society for Public Health Education, Inc.
  693 Sutter Street, 4th floor
  San Francisco, California 94102

- American Public Health Association
  Public Health Education Section
  1015 Fifteenth Street, N.W.
  Washington, D.C. 20036

- American Society for Health Manpower, Education and Training
  American Hospital Association
  840 North Lake Shore Drive
  Chicago, Illinois 60611

- American College Health Association
  Health Education Section
  2807 Central Street
  Evanston, Illinois 60201

- National Center for Health Education
  30 E. 29th Street
  New York, New York 10016

- Association for the Advancement of Health Education
  1201 Sixteenth Street, N.W.
  Washington, D.C. 20036

- International Union for Health Education
  3 Rue DeVrollier
  Geneva, Switzerland

- American Group Practice Association
  20 South Quaker Lane
  Alexandria, Virginia 22314

- American College of Preventive Medicine
  801 Old Lancaster Road
  Bryn Mawr, Pennsylvania 19010

- American Nurses Association
  2420 Pershing Road
  Kansas City, Missouri 64108

- American Psychological Association
  Health Psychology Section
  1200 Seventeenth Street, N.W.
  Washington, D.C. 20036

- The Society of Behavioral Medicine
  P.O. Box 8530
  University Station
  Knoxville, Tennessee 37996

# PART ONE

# FOUNDATIONS OF PATIENT EDUCATION AND HEALTH PROMOTION

# 1

---

# A model for patient education and health promotion programming

DURING THE 1950s, at least once a month our parents would lead the kids into the car and take off into the suburbs on a Sunday afternoon to look at model homes. At first we didn't understand why they were dragging us around to other people's houses. We knew we weren't going to move. But if our parents weren't going to buy one of those homes with all the lovely decorator touches, why did they spend so much time looking at them?

In those days, model homes were furnished by interior decorators—down to the appliances in the kitchen and the china on the dining room table. Our parents visited them to get ideas for how they could decorate their own house or apartment. They returned home each time with ideas about how to rearrange the furniture, allow more sunlight in, or make the best use of the available space.

The places we visited were models because something about the way they were set up allowed every visitor—regardless of taste or housing situation—to leave with a new idea. In this book, we present many models. Each of them provides a foundation upon which you can build your own health education practice. The models we have selected have the greatest utility for the practice of patient education and health promotion in medical care settings. They are somewhat like children's coloring books. Outlines are given, but it is up to each individual to fill in the colors. If twenty children are given the same page in a coloring book, why do some renderings look appealing or artistic, while others seem mundane or unattractive? The difference comes from each child's sense of color, of shading, and of interpretation. Each picture may communicate different messages or emotions because of the touches that the child adds. In the same way, the models in this book provide a foundation on which you can build your own practice. You will apply these models in ways that are unique to your personal style, to the setting in which you work, and to the people you serve.

A model worth staking your reputation and job satisfaction on must guide you according to the highest standards of the field and must be flexible enough so that you can modify it to fit your specific situation.

The programming model that follows integrates the key principles of patient education and health promotion planning and programming. We believe that it is an appropriate conceptual framework on which health educators can build their practice in medical care settings. Not only do we present this model to you as the foundation for your work, but we have also used it as the integrating theme of the subsequent chapters.

## ORGANIZING CONCEPTS

Two organizing concepts are built into our programming model. The first is the idea that health education services are the products of a planning process. The second is the idea that patient education and health promotion services can be organized by level of service.

Four stages of program development are built into the model: (1) assessment, (2) planning, (3) implementation, and (4) evaluation. As tempting as it is to jump right into providing the health education services that you know your clients need, it is critical that you take the time to accomplish these steps in the proper sequence. The chapters in Part Two treat the steps in detail. Moreover, we will be discussing patient education and health promotion programs in terms of three levels of service: (1) institution-wide, (2) programmatic, and (3) client. As you work through the chapters, you will have many opportunities to put these guides to work. For now, though, think through this scenario: The chief of the department of medicine has asked you to plan a back care program for clients with chronic low back pain. How would you begin? Whom would you contact? How would you ensure the program's success? The programming model will guide you. You will quickly see how important administrative support, interdepartmental cooperation, and a systematic educational diagnosis are during all steps of the program development process. These are just some of the considerations you would handle if you were planning a new back care class.

## THE MODEL

The model itself appears as Table 1.1 (see p. 10). Its strength derives from the way it integrates the two organizing concepts and three levels of service into a practical, easy-to-use schema for developing health education programs.

After you have read the model, go to the exercises at the end of this chapter. Take the time to work through these exercises before proceeding, because they will help you get the most out of this book.

# EXERCISES

1. Using the schema presented in the programming model as a guide, develop an interview schedule that you might use to interview key decision makers in a hospital, ambulatory care center, nursing home, clinic, or medical office. (The interview schedule is a list of the key questions you will ask. The schedule is your "script," so that each interview covers the same questions.) The data you collect from the interview will be the basis of making recommendations regarding the organization's need for patient education and health promotion services.

2. Using the schema presented in the programming model as a guide, prepare a time line for the implementation of a stop-smoking program that is to be offered in a university student health service. Your time line should include a list of *what* needs to be done, by *whom*, and by *when*. Make sure the chronology makes sense. Each step needs to naturally follow the one before it.

3. Using the schema presented in the programming model as a guide, list the key people you would involve in the planning of an out-patient cardiac rehabilitation program that will be offered in a clinic. In what specific activities or operations would you involve these people so that they have meaningful participation in the planning of the program?

**Table 1.1  A model for health education program development at three organizational levels**

| Program development stage | Level of organization | | |
|---|---|---|---|
| | Institutional (Institution-wide system) | Programmatic (Selected target groups) | Client (Individual client or client group) |
| I. Assessment | | | |
| A. Objectives | To determine need for policy | To generate specific client group and disease profiles | To determine knowledge, attitudes, and skill of patients and family |
| B. Outcome | Facility profile (educational needs and programs) | Priority needs for program development | Learning needs |
| C. Topics for baseline questions | • Policy statement for patient education in the facility?<br>• Support for patient education?<br>• Perceptions of utility and effectiveness of patient education?<br>• What organizational units are involved in patient education? Coordination mechanism? Administrative focus for education? Support for creating one? | • What are disease characteristics? prevalence? incidence? clusters?<br>• Who are the clients? (Demographic, psychosocial, physician levels, family configurations)<br>• Climate for change? (Staff readiness and capability)<br>• Are staff knowledge, attitudes, skills sufficient? | • Course of disease, stage, and impact on individual patients?<br>• Individual client and family psychosocial and cultural background?<br>• Readiness of client for learning?<br>• Client's level of functioning—physical, mental, etc.?<br>• Level of client-provider interaction? |

| | | | |
|---|---|---|---|
| | capacity, staff, funds, etc. Management of resources? Potential for coordinating consolidation? • Present status of quality of care: morbidity, mortality, disability, etc.? | characteristics? (Number of clients, average length of stay, total hours, number of contacts, space, records system) • Resources available? (Manpower, space, equipment, dollars) | available, adequate, used? |
| D. Participants | Multidisciplinary task force | • Health team members • Representatives of community agencies • Representative clients and family members | • Client • Family • Provider or team |
| E. Decision makers | • Administration • Board of trustees • Chiefs of services | • Chiefs of services, or section chiefs • Medical advisory committee, or equivalent | • Client • Family • Provider or team |
| II. Planning | | | |
| A. Objectives | To develop facility-wide plan for patient education and health promotion • Formulation of policy statement | To develop program plans for priority needs | To identify individual client learning objectives or contract |
| B. Outcomes | | • Standard protocols • Staff training | • Individual teaching plan for clients and family |

(Continued)

SOURCE: S. G. Deeds, B. J. Hebert, and J. M. Wolle, *A Model for Patient Education Programming* (Washington, D.C.: American Public Health Association, 1979), pp. 22–26. Reprinted with the permission of the American Public Health Association.

**Table 1.1 (continued)**

| Program development stage | Level of organization | | |
| --- | --- | --- | --- |
| | Institutional (Institution-wide system) | Programmatic (Selected target groups) | Client (Individual client or client group) |
| B. Outcomes (cont.) | • Development of goals and strategies<br>• Development of organizational structure<br>• Identification and establishment of internal and external linkage systems<br>• Establishment of data and communication systems | • Educational methods and materials<br>• Records and evaluation systems<br>• Communication channels | • Plan for follow-up and referral<br>• Documentation method |
| C. Participants | Multidisciplinary task force | • Health team members<br>• Representatives of community agencies<br>• Representatives of clients and family members | • Client<br>• Family<br>• Provider or team |
| D. Decision makers | • Administration<br>• Board of trustees<br>• Chief of services | • Chief of services, or section chiefs<br>• Medical advisory committee, or equivalent | • Client<br>• Family<br>• Provider or team |

| III. Implementation | | | |
|---|---|---|---|
| A. Objectives | • To carry out plan<br>• To test, revise<br>• To use information gained through implementation to refine and improve program | Same | Same |
| B. Processes | • Testing goals and strategies and adapting as necessary<br>• Monitoring: data and communications systems, policies and procedures | Monitoring program delivery in terms of utility and acceptance of procedures, training, materials, methods, communication patterns, record systems | Monitoring client learning in terms of utility; acceptance of methods and materials, client-provider interaction, referral mechanisms, documentation systems, staff communications |
| C. Communication mechanisms | Progress reports, staff meetings, etc. | Documentation in medical records, team conferences, etc. | Medical record notes, team conferences, etc. |
| D. Time frame | Annual | Monthly | Daily or weekly |
| E. Participants | Multidisciplinary task force | • Health team members<br>• Representatives of community agencies<br>• Representatives of clients and family members | • Client<br>• Family<br>• Provider or team |
| F. Decision makers | • Administration<br>• Board of trustees<br>• Chief of services | • Chief of services, or section chiefs<br>• Medical advisory committee, or equivalent | • Client<br>• Family<br>• Provider or team |

*(Continued)*

**Table 1.1** (continued)

|  | Level of organization | | |
| --- | --- | --- | --- |
| Program development stage | Institutional (Institution-wide system) | Programmatic (Selected target groups) | Client (Individual client or client group) |
| IV. Evaluation | | | |
| A. Focus | To guide policy formulation and administrative management and resource allocation decisions | To guide changes in program design and implementation | To identify alternative approaches and methods for communication |
| B. Outcomes | Reductions in sickness, death, disability | Improved health status related to client behaviors, especially use (composite indicators/aggregate data) of health sources, acceptance of best medical alternatives, lifestyle changes | Client demonstration of self-management, monitoring, reporting side effects and symptoms, problem-solving ability, appointment keeping |
| 1. Effectiveness | Client, staff, and community satisfaction | Client, staff, and community satisfaction | Client, staff, and community satisfaction |
| 2. Efficiency | Appropriate allocation resources to site/population/ community | • Appropriate use of resources—money, staff, materials, etc.<br>• Accomplishment of staff training goals | Staff-demonstrated competency in interpersonal skills, teaching, problem solving |

14

| | | | |
|---|---|---|---|
| C. Time frame | 3–5 years (with interim progress reporting and decision making) | Yearly or at completion of specific program | At time of discharge and/or subsequent follow-up visit |
| D. Participants | Multidisciplinary task force | • Health team members<br>• Representatives of community agencies<br>• Representatives of client and family members | • Client<br>• Family<br>• Provider or team |
| E. Decision makers | • Administration<br>• Board of trustees<br>• Chief of services | • Chief of services, or section chiefs<br>• Medical advisory committee, or equivalent | • Client<br>• Family<br>• Provider or team |

# RESOURCES

Deeds, S. G., Hebert, B. J., and Wolle, J. M. *A Model for Patient Education Programming*. Washington, D.C.: American Public Health Association, Public Health Education Section, February 1979.

This monograph provides easy-to-read guidelines for conducting the steps of health education planning (assessment, planning, implementation, and evaluation) at the institutional, programmatic, and client levels. Most of the guidelines are presented in terms of critical questions that health educators should answer during the planning process.

Martin, E. D. *A Guide to Health Education in Ambulatory Care Settings*. Washington, D.C.: U.S. Department of Health, Education and Welfare, Health Services Administration, Bureau of Community Health Services, 1977.

This report outlines ways in which health education strategies can be developed in ambulatory care centers to make sure that they are as effective and as efficient as possible. The report begins with a description of a program-planning model. The planning model includes nine steps: (1) development of support for health education, (2) designation of one individual responsible for the program, (3) identification of major health problems, (4) behavioral diagnosis, (5) setting priorities, (6) development of goals and objectives, (7) development of the program strategy, (8) implementation, and (9) evaluation. The rest of the report is devoted to applying the program-planning model to (1) recruitment of clients into the ambulatory care center, (2) proper use of the center's resources, (3) prevention of illness, and (4) treatment of illness.

Mullen, P. D., and Zapka, J. G. *Guidelines for Health Promotion and Education Services in HMO's*. Sponsored by U.S. Department of Health and Human Services, Public Health Service. U.S. G.P.O. no. 0-365-843/481. Washington, D.C.: U.S. Government Printing Office, 1982.

This document was written to help answer the questions being asked by HMO administrators, medical directors, and boards of trustees: What exactly are the definition and scope of health education and promotion? How effective are these services? How are programs best organized? What are the administrative issues that must be taken into account? And, how is the quality of an HMO's health education and promotion programs assessed? The model for program planning offered in this monograph includes five steps: (1) needs assessment, (2) establishment of priorities, (3) program design, (4) administrative support, and (5) quality assessment. The authors apply their program development model to the same levels that we do in this book: (1) organization-wide or system level, (2) programmatic level, and (3) individual patient level.

Sullivan, D. *Educating the Public About Health: A Planning Guide.* Sponsored by U.S. Department of Health, Education, and Welfare, Public Health Service Health Resources Administration, Bureau of Health Planning and Resources Development. DHEW Publication no. (HRA) 78-14004. Washington, D.C.: U.S. Government Printing Office, 1977.

This guide is the sixth publication in the Health Planning Methods and Technology Series, sponsored by the Bureau of Health Planning and Resources Development. This guide was developed to assist health planning agencies and others in planning and developing health education activities designed to influence the behavior of individuals and institutions in ways which lead to improved health of the population. However, it is also applicable to medical care settings. The guide introduces a planning model that includes five steps: (1) set goals, (2) define problems, (3) design plans, (4) conduct activities, and (5) evaluate results.

# 2

# Developing a philosophy
# and a rationale

YOU HAVE CHOSEN to be an advocate for patient education and health promotion. Because of your commitment, role, and visibility in your organization, you will often need to defend your decisions and to request support and resources on behalf of health education. This chapter surveys the ground that you should cover in order to be prepared as well as persuasive—both in talking and in writing. This survey of national policy, as well as professional, organizational, and personal philosophies, prepares you with a foundation for developing a sound rationale for patient education and health promotion programs. As shifts occur in public policy, in social ideologies, and in organizational cultures, you will experience occasional incongruities with your own personal values and beliefs. This chapter gives you the opportunity to think these issues through and to take a position on key issues in the practice of health education. Such an exercise is valuable not only to professionals who are entering the field but also to veteran health educators.

If your orientation is primarily focused on the client, this chapter will help broaden your horizons. In order to successfully apply the model presented in Chapter 1, you will have to start thinking in terms of the larger organization, of your community and of national health policy. This chapter and the next provide the foundation for your health education practice. The chapter guides you through a national perspective and through an organizational perspective, back to your personal values and beliefs.

## NATIONAL HEALTH OBJECTIVES

What did the Surgeon General mean in 1979 when he said that his report *Healthy People* was designed to encourage a *second* public health revolution in the United States? Has the nation's health strategy as outlined a few years ago affected the underlying philosophy and rationale for health education in medical care? What are your values and beliefs in regard to health and education?

The object of the *first* public health revolution was the fight against infectious diseases. In 1900, the leading causes of death were influenza, diphtheria, pneumonia, tuberculosis, and gastrointestinal infections. The annual death rate was 580 for every 100,000 people. Today fewer than 30 people per 100,000 die each year from these communicable diseases. Gains have occurred because of improved sanitation, effective vaccines and mass immunization, better nutrition, and the pasteurization of milk. Therefore a shift has taken place, from the major acute infectious diseases to major chronic diseases such as heart disease, cancer, and strokes.

The remarkable progress in the health status of people in developed countries has occurred because of efforts to eradicate communicable diseases via prevention. For example, if all the attention had been drawn to the cure of smallpox, rather than to the prevention of smallpox, the first public health revolution would not have been accomplished.

In the same ways, the second public health revolution is designed to reduce the sickness and disability of chronic disease through prevention and health promotion. This revolution is about preventive actions such as improving personal health practices (stopping smoking, wearing seat belts, drinking alcohol in moderation, eating nutritiously, and getting regular exercise) and health promotion strategies such as improving working conditions, promoting work site safety for employees, cleaning up the environment, and providing services to aid the poor, the powerless, and the disadvantaged in our society.

In spite of the fact that Americans spend more money every year on health, we still lag behind several other industrial nations in terms of life expectancy and infant mortality, which are standard indications of a country's health status. We can still learn much about causes and cures for the major degenerative diseases; nevertheless, scientists have identified some major risk factors responsible for many of the premature diseases and deaths that characterize our country's health problems. Risk factors such as smoking, occupational hazards, alcohol and drug abuse, and injuries due to automobile accidents all represent preventable health problems. The message of the current public health revolution is that the health of this country's citizens can be greatly improved through (1) actions people take for themselves, (2) actions decision makers in the

public and private sectors take to promote safer and healthier environments, and (3) the help of supportive family, friends, and community
networks.

   Stressing the value of individual actions that prevent injury or disease does not suggest that people have complete control over, or are
totally responsible for, their own health status. For instance, socioeconomic factors are powerful determinants of health, yet individuals have
limited control of these factors. People can be aware of the environmental
risks they are exposed to, but they are often at the mercy of elected and
appointed officials and others in power to reduce environmental hazards. At the same time, individuals continue to make personal decisions
that affect their health under the influence of extremely sophisticated
and powerful advertising. To make matters worse, our society supports
industries that produce unhealthful products (such as subsidies to tobacco
farmers), has ambiguous interpretations of laws against offenses (such
as drunk driving), and puts limited funds into the public support of
scientific research on disease prevention and health promotion.


## PARADOXES IN HEALTH EDUCATION

National goals for health promotion and disease prevention for the next
several years are a clear example of the ways the federal government
hopes to pay attention to the social, environmental, and behavioral factors that influence the health of the American people. A sample of these
goals (developed by the Secretary for Health and Human Services, the
Surgeon General, and the U.S. Public Health Service) includes the
following:

1. Improve infant health
   a. Increase prenatal care, improve nutrition for pregnant women,
      assist women to quit smoking, etc.
   b. Reduce environmental hazards, increase genetic screening,
      ensure rubella vaccination for mothers prior to pregnancy,
      reduce exposure to drugs and alcohol during pregnancy
2. Improve child health
   a. Increase good nutrition, prevent child abuse and neglect
   b. Reduce childhood accidents and injuries
   c. Increase childhood immunizations and advance dental health
3. Improve adult health
   a. Modify and decrease risk factors for heart attacks (smoking,
      high blood pressure, diabetes, overweight, physical inactiv-
      ity, stress, and oral contraceptive use)

      b. Reduce death from cancers through modifying risk factors (smoking, alcohol, dietary patterns, radiation, sunlight, occupational hazards, water and air pollutants) and screening and early detection

      c. Reduce alcohol abuse

      d. Provide mental health services

      e. Reduce periodontal disease

   **4.** Improve health and quality of life for older adults

      a. Increase health and social system support

      b. Reduce social isolation

      c. Develop outreach programs to help the sick and disabled

      d. Reduce premature death from influenza and pneumonia

We need to draw on our discussion of public health policy as a way to better understand and probe the philosophical basis of health education. Here are a few issues you must face as you prepare for a professional career in health education.

## The role of consumers

If we are going to emphasize prevention and health promotion in a meaningful way in medical care, we must expect the consumer, the patient, or the citizen to play a larger role in health care, both within and outside the system. In order for this role to be meaningful, individual citizens need to take responsibility not only for changing their lifestyles but also for their participation in making policy, in caring for themselves, in affecting the environment. The paradox here is that the more we convey the message of individual responsibility, the greater we run the risk of blaming the victim. The most important health goals for the nation demand that individual action be combined with changes in the environment, legislation, health and social services delivery, working conditions, research priorities, and the distribution of power in living groups, working groups, and communities.

## Who is to benefit?

Prevention and health promotion are often touted as providing a much needed answer to the escalating costs of health and medical care. For example, the foreword to the proceedings of the National Conference on Health Promotion Programs in Occupational Settings reflects this hope: "In an effort to reduce the costs of health benefits, many industries and labor organizations are seeking new approaches in health care that will improve the health and well-being of employees. Business firms and labor unions have initiated health promotion programs at the work site with the objective of reducing health benefit costs, and are discovering additional benefits of these programs such as decreased absenteeism and increased productivity" (U.S. Department of Health, Education and Welfare, Public Health Service, Office of the Assistant Secretary for Health, 1979, p. 13). We need to beware of suggesting to our constituents and our supervisors that health education is a tool of the establishment. If people get the idea that health education's main function is to save money for the system, regardless of the public's good, we have failed to convey the basis on which health education practice is built.

## The limits of behavior

The emphasis in this book is on health behavior—actions that people take individually and collectively to protect or improve their health. Behavior is a necessary step between learning and health improvement. In Chapter 5 we introduce a health education planning process that acknowledges that health problems are influenced by behavioral as well as nonbehavioral factors. Nonbehavioral factors include genetic factors, one's economic base, occupation, and environmental isolation. Generally speaking, strategies other than health education must be developed to influence nonbehavioral factors that contribute to the health problem. Behavior is one major determinant of health care that we can influence directly by health education. The two most important objective criteria for selecting crucial behavioral targets for health education are (1) evidence that the behavioral change will help reduce the health problem and (2) evidence that the behavior can be changed voluntarily (Green et al., 1978). The dilemma for health education occurs when people are led to believe that we think that the *only* influence on health is behavior, and that the only interpretation we give to behavior is lifestyle. If we limit our attention to problems of overeating, lack of physical exercise, and smoking, for instance, we are neglecting the many other activities people engage in each day that help or hurt their health.

In the introduction to their article "Health Education: Can the Reformers Be Reformed?" Brown and Margo (1978) accuse, "Health educators have created a new professional role that emphasizes the changing of individuals rather than the conditions." The article shows how historical roots, ideological perspectives, and structural constraints have combined to create an ambiguous, generally conservative role for the health education profession.

They go on to charge that, by focusing on behavior itself, health educators do not deal with the social relations and structures that may underlie and contribute to the behavior patterns they find objectionable and to diseases they wish to prevent. Brown and Margo believe that health education programs often rely on techniques that manipulate behavior rather than help people—as individuals or in groups—to influence and control their physical, social, and economic environments. The best way to avoid this emphasis on manipulation is to focus more clearly on clients in the context of their day-to-day lives.

## REALITY-BASED PHILOSOPHY

We are challenged to be advocates on behalf of our clients, who are consumers of medical care services. As advocates, we all need to beware of jumping into the content of the educational services without giving careful thought to how we and our clients are going to work toward their goal. We need to think of health behavior as actions our clients take that are directed at the medical care system and at the environment, too. Health behavior is collective behavior or social action that people must exercise to influence the health care system or to guard themselves against environmental risks. Behavior can and should influence health directly through preventive activities and through self-care. An activated, concerned, and knowledgeable public can participate more effectively in the decisions that are made by doctors, nurses, and politicians concerning personal and community health issues (Green, 1978).

One way to prevent being set up for idealistic expectations that may sabotage your efforts in medical care, and to prepare yourself to engage in the kind of constructive dialogue that is conducive to teamwork, is to begin now to become familiar with the realities of working in the medical care setting. The following example, based on the experiences of health educators in a health maintenance organization, is instructive. It is very relevant to all health educators in medical care, and it can be generalized to fee-for-service practice in hospitals, clinics, nursing homes, and other medical care settings. The example is a challenge for reality-based training; in addition, it describes skills that all health educators in medical care settings should have. How does this example challenge your thinking regarding your philosophy of your role and how you could justify your role as a health educator in a hospital or clinic?

At present sixteen professionally trained health educators work in the Northern California Kaiser-Permanente Medical Care Program.* All have had coursework in one form or another, broadly preparing them

*This discussion is adapted from W. D. Squyres, The Professional Health Educator in HMO's: Implications for Training and Our Future in Medical Care, *Health Education Quarterly,* 9(1), Spring 1982:74–77. Copyright © 1982 by Human Sciences Press, Inc.

for their positions. Yet their performance on the job varies greatly in efficiency and effectiveness, as do their satisfaction with their work and the demands of their position. Each of the health educators has the potential to be more effective and more satisfied. It is possible that throughout the professional preparation period, concepts—rather than skills—were taught; the ideal rather than the real was emphasized. Some did not have field placements in HMO's or medical care settings, thus were lacking practical experience under supervision that dealt with day-to-day issues and problems. Some professional preparation programs teach their students the skills required to cope effectively with the inherent limitations of HMO's; other programs teach their students how to engage in activities geared to changing the medical care system to better meet the health needs of the people they serve.

People do not agree on which approach best prepares students for jobs in medical care. Several health educators in practice in HMO's reviewed the following list of skills, which we developed. Most felt compelled to, as a short-term goal, learn or strengthen the skills necessary to be effective in the current system. At the same time they were also committed to, as a long-term goal, pursuing either a change in their role as it is currently specified, or a change in the system in which they currently work. The list is presented to stimulate discussion about the appropriate arena and framework for reality-based training for health educators in medical care settings. It also illustrates the continuous tension inherent in health education practice.

Skill 1. *To work effectively in a hierarchy where many of the deliverers of patient care are at the pinnacle of power and decision making.* Professional training programs do a disservice to potential health educators when they lead students to believe that those in power are the "enemy." Rather, students should be taught how to gain credibility and how to have a positive influence on decision makers in medical care. In the short term, the health educator must be effective in the hierarchy; in the long term, the health educator may operate as a catalyst for (1) the redefining of approaches to decision making and (2) a reallocation of power. The health educator, however, cannot be a catalyst in a vacuum; the organization needs to be ready for and capable of change. To be an effective change agent, the health educator must work with other organizational managers.

Skill 2. *To be an effective consultant; to operate effectively within a staff function when line functions tend to get the most attention.* Line functions have a direct relationship to the primary function of the organization; for example, hospital departments and medical services. Staff functions exist to serve these line departments. For example, nurses provide a line function in the hospital when they do direct nursing care. The hospital accounting office and the housekeeping departments provide staff functions. In the short term, health educators need to operate effectively as consultants; however, in the long term, health education may be so well integrated into all the primary functions of the organization that it will be seen and treated as a line function. The HMO emphasis on preventive services is especially conducive to this long-range goal.

Skill 3. *To take on a great deal of responsibility with little or no authority as internal consultants.* Health education specialists work with all medical center departments and specialties. They advise administration on matters relating to health education. Their ability to get things done, however, is often subject to the commitment to health education or to the goodwill of these many departments. If health educators wish their programs to be an integral part of patient and health care, then they need to sharpen their abilities to build a strong rationale for health education and to generate commitment for health education. This commitment requires earned credibility and political sophistication. Health education programs that have earned a reputation for quality services have demanded and received increased responsibility, authority, and accountability for education functions. For example, in one Kaiser-Permanente medical center, four years ago, there was only a half-time health educator. Her job was to establish a comprehensive, medical center-wide health education service for inpatient and outpatient clients. She reported directly to the medical center administrator. Through the years she worked closely with the management team, the department heads, and providers. Her educational programs were well planned, were visible throughout the community, and contributed to the goals of the organization. Clients were highly satisfied with the health education services; most participants today are referred to educational programs by former participants. Today the health educator is a department manager in her own right. She coordinates forty formal health education programs, as well as a health education center and a closed-circuit television system. She supervises seven employees and advises forty to fifty health professionals who are instructors. The health educator's budget has tripled in four years.

Skill 4. *To provide direct service; to realize that the system rewards the direct delivery of service to clients.* Many health education specialists wish to be strictly planners and managers of educational services, rather than to be involved in the actual delivery of health education services. In this age of cost consciousness and control, however, many administrators find that health educators who operate solely as coordinators are a luxury that the system cannot afford. They prefer instead to recruit health educators who have substantial health care experience and are willing to deliver educational services to members (such as smoking cessation or stress management). New health education departments usually require that the health educator operate primarily as a coordinator and consultant for a while, especially in departments where there is only one health educator. However, as the health education department becomes more established, many health educators have found it tremendously rewarding to work directly with clients in at least one program as a way to keep in touch with clients and to maintain professional relationships with other providers and instructors.

Skill 5. *To be an effective team member.* Health education specialists need to know how to encourage team building and need to be seen as valued members of the health care team. New health educators often meet ambivalence or hostility. Some providers do not believe that there is room for more players on the team. Others do not believe that a team exists. But medical care systems are open to team approaches to health care, and health educators must learn how to offer skills that will be valued as a special contribution to a team effort.

Skill 6. *To be able to set high professional standards for the delivery of health education services, and to not allow these principles to be diluted or overlooked.* If a provider feels strongly that health education is simply the dissemination of health information, the health educator must be able to explain to the provider the principles of sound health education practice and of health behavior change. The health educator must be able to maintain high standards and must be able to disagree with providers or administrators without putting others on the defensive. In addition, the health educator needs to model these principles in her or his own work, as well as to keep abreast of current theory and empirical research, in order to be effective with decision makers.

Skill 7. *To tolerate ambiguity.* HMO's have many incentives for providing preventive and health education services, yet the policies and practices of the individual organization may not be conducive to the actual delivery of effective services. Some decision makers in medical care feel that health education services are a "bottomless pit," that there is no end to the demand for such programs for both the well and the sick. This prospect leads to skepticism and to fiscal conservatism. After all, a limitless demand for any services could cause havoc with budgets. Matching the expectations of the organization to the resources allocated is difficult for health educators in all medical care settings. In order to deal effectively with this ambiguity in the short term, the health educator needs patience and optimism. At the same time, he or she must work steadfastly to persuade other health providers to focus greater attention on and investment in prevention and health promotion. As a result, health education departments with, for example, eight to ten years' history in medical care have made strides toward gaining credibility and greater support. Strong health education leadership and willingness to rigorously evaluate program effectiveness have contributed to the growth of acceptance for these programs.

Skill 8. *To work with the skeptics and individuals who feel threatened by or are hostile toward health education.* Some professionals believe health education has little or no merit in medical care and work actively to remove it. Health educators need to know how to justify their services on the basis of organizational and consumer need. Even in the long run, not everyone on staff can be converted to wholehearted supporters, but the ability to be a strong defender of health education without being defensive will prove to be a powerful long-term strategy.

Skill 9. *To have a vision of the positive marriage of patient care and health care with health education.* Health educators must be able to see the value of a symbiotic relationship, to prefer such a relationship to an adversarial one, and be willing to work toward the longevity of this marriage. Some health educators enter the work force with set beliefs that health promotion is better than patient education (that is, education for the well is better than education for the sick), or that work in the community is better than work in a health care delivery system. These judgments often lead to conflicts in loyalty and to early loss of job satisfaction. Health educators need to be able to see the potential for educational service to people on all points of the continuum, well to sick. They need to see that health care delivery systems are a form of community and to see the vast potential for integrating health care, community, and individual concerns toward a healthier society.

Skill 10. *To know the medical culture: to be conversant with medical terminology and to be able to think critically in the same frame of reference as those trained in the biomedical sciences.* Health educators need to be able to communicate with a variety of health professionals, using as little health education jargon as possible. They need to be able to judge the relative merits of current health education technologies and approaches. And they need to resist new, untested educational approaches that are still not a part of behavior science theory, let alone accepted by the medical sciences. In the long term, other health professionals will eventually feel at ease with educational concepts and terms, and health educators will feel at home with common medical and health-related concepts and terms.

Skill 11. *To generate social support: to be able to generate a network of supporters (professional and personal) both within and outside the organization.* Working as the only health educator in a medical care setting can be lonely work at times. Health educators need to find other health educators in the community for the purpose of support, resource sharing, and validation (Squyres, 1982, pp. 73–77).

In order to compose your own philosophy of health education practice, you must honestly assess your own skills and beliefs. We have reviewed eleven skill areas; for each area, you could now inventory your current abilities. Just as your skills are enhanced through coursework, reading, practice, and experience, so are your professional beliefs and ideologies.

## THE MEDICAL CARE SYSTEM: FRIEND OR FOE?

In the past, some of the health education literature separated the concepts of medical care, disease prevention, and health promotion as if they represented competing ideologies. Medical care has been stereotyped as the segment of the health care conglomerate that begins with the sick, works to keep the sick alive, makes them well, or minimizes their disability. Disease prevention has been stereotyped as the segment of the health care conglomerate that begins with some threat to health—a disease or environmental hazard—and seeks to protect as many people as possible from the consequences of that threat. Health promotion has been stereotyped as the newcomer to health care that begins with people who are basically healthy and seeks to develop community and individual measures that will help such people maintain and enhance their health.

These definitions not only foster categorization and separation of services or target populations but also tempt us to polarize them. Health care services are constantly shifting to meet the rapid technological advances as well as the changing social and cultural expectations of both providers and clients. Usually, health educators wish to participate as agents of change in these shifts in definition or thrust—as long as the changes continue to move toward more humanization of care, greater quality of care, and increased access to care. If these changes don't occur quickly enough, some health educators judge that the medical care system is in an adversarial relationship to health education and to consumers of health care services.

That impatience seems to come with the territory for health educators practicing in medical care, and now is a good time to brace yourself against it. As you are probably already aware, disease prevention and health promotion are being increasingly emphasized within medical care. As a health educator in practice in the medical care system, you will be working actively to increase the awareness of clients, health care providers, and administrators regarding the value of disease prevention and health promotion strategies. It does not serve our purposes to minimize the relationship among medical care, disease prevention, and health promotion.

As an example of the type of cooperative dialogue that can be stimulated on behalf of these goals, in 1981 the Kellogg Foundation sponsored a conference of people who were clinically active in the practice of primary care medicine and dentistry. The conference was designed to produce an outline of realistic expectations for the future involvement of medical and dental practitioners in the field of health promotion and the prevention of disease. Appendix 2.1 (at the end of this chapter) summarizes the essential elements recommended by the conference delegates for an expanded practice of clinical primary prevention (De Frieze et al., 1981). These recommendations show how interested health professionals stated their philosophy and developed an articulate rationale for patient education and health promotion in medical care. By the time you complete this chapter, you should be able to describe your own personal and professional position.

## DEVELOPING A RATIONALE

One way that you can begin thinking about your own rationale for patient education and health promotion is to examine policies, position papers, and statements of rationale created by other organizations. Appendices 2.2 through 2.5 are examples of policies that have been formulated by trade organizations representing hospitals and physicians.

Health educators can win support by integrating professional, accreditation, and legal statements supporting health education in medical care into rationale and proposals soliciting support. Appendix 2.6 is a compilation of statements provided by the American Hospital Association (1978) for this purpose.

It is also useful to know what the health education profession's position is and how that rationale has been made available as a matter of policy. The Society for Public Health Education published, in its professional journal, a synopsis of a position paper that was submitted by a Task Force on Patient Education. This paper is now public record and can be integrated into a statement of rationale. Appendix 2.7 is a synopsis of the position paper (Task Force on Patient Education, President's Committee on Health Education, 1974).

Once you have reviewed the professional, legal, and accreditation statements on patient education and health promotion in medical care, you will have one piece of the foundation on which to design a rationale for health education services within your organization. Ultimately, you want to be able to describe why you are making the decisions you are on programs and priorities. Figure 2.1 illustrates the other components of a sound framework for developing a rationale.

A clear rationale is needed at several developmental points in the natural history of a health education program. One such point is at the onset of a new health education program. The rationale provides decision makers with strong philosophical, factual, and anecdotal arguments in favor of a proposal. If the rationale is compelling, clear, and consistent with other goals, needs, and priorities, the chances of getting the proposal accepted are greatly enhanced. The rationale should also accompany proposals to initiate specific educational services for a target population. Sometimes budget requests, proposals for increases in staff, and requests for space or other resources require strong rationales.

As you prepare to write your rationale, you may want to answer the questions listed in Table 2.1.

Once you have prepared your case in terms of external and internal support, you have one more step to take before you can actually prepare your rationale for submission: you must understand your own values, beliefs, feelings, and assumptions about the health education service you

**Figure 2.1   Foundation for a health education rationale**

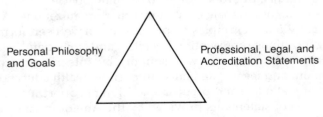

Personal Philosophy
and Goals

Professional, Legal, and
Accreditation Statements

Organizational Philosophy and Goals

**Table 2.1   Questions to ask when preparing a rationale to support health education services**

1. How does my proposal reflect existing policy? Are there internal documents, policies or procedures, goals and objectives, or mission statements that I can cite to support my case?

2. Have I documented the need (from the client, provider, and administrator points of view)? Have I demonstrated that this need is not fulfilled elsewhere in the organization?

3. Have I listed all the other departments in the organization that are joining our department in the effort? Do I have letters of support or other tangible evidence of their involvement?

4. Have I documented the costs of the proposed service? Have I documented the benefits?

5. Are the purposes of the proposed service clearly delineated? Are the measures for assuring quality and evaluating success identified?

6. Have I identified all the key people? Have they given input to the rationale, critiqued it, and thrown their support behind it?

7. Is the timing right for the organization, for the decision makers, and for me to embark on this project?

are proposing. Are the statements of organizational or professional philosophy consistent with your own? Are you comfortable with the strategies, examples, and relationships that you have proposed? Could you be an advocate of the proposal on the basis of your own convictions? Could you gain the support of others through your own commitment to the proposal?

Over time, you will notice that your experience in conducting or coordinating educational services influences your convictions and beliefs; conversely, your personal and professional beliefs will affect the way you conduct or coordinate educational services. This dynamic process is healthy and provides part of the satisfaction of being involved in health education practice. Notice, however, that Figure 2.1 suggests that all three components of the foundation for a health education rationale complement each other. How can you prepare yourself for those occasions when your personal philosophy, bolstered by professional assumptions acquired during your training, come into face-to-face conflict with the philosophy and goals of the organization? How far are you willing to go to modify an educationally sound proposal in order to get your foot in the door with a department, decision maker, or administrator? To what extent will you be tempted to make hopeful claims about the potential of a program in the absence of any real data, or in the face of research that yields no result? There are no right answers to these dilemmas.

In one hospital, a health educator was faced with a tough decision. She had to choose between developing a support group for cancer patients (advised by the patient education committee) or producing an orientation program for newly admitted patients that would be shown on the bedside televisions. The cancer support group was a high priority as expressed by clients and providers. The closed-circuit television media program was a high priority of the administrator. She had the staff and resources for only one of the programs. She decided to do the television production because she already had two cancer education programs underway (as distinct from support groups). The social services department was willing to continue to refer cancer patients to community support groups until the hospital could sponsor its own program. Although the orientation program was a major investment that would have minimal impact on client health status, satisfaction, or on hospital operations, the investment proved its worth. The administrators were so pleased to be able to communicate their messages (such as hospital visiting hours and checking in valuables) that they gave back twofold the resources to the health education department in the next year's budget. The health educator earned the reputation of being responsive and committed to the administration's goals. After she produced the orientation program, she went on to establish a cancer support group in the hospital.

Experienced health educators acknowledge that over the years they have been able to compromise their zealousness without compromising program impact or quality. In fact, the most politically astute will make tempered, reserved claims, with the hopes of making small, but significant inroads, rather than glamorous, miraculous claims that are geared to failure. The challenge is to be prepared. Do your homework—know the literature, support your claims with expert sources, understand the organization, be aware of who your friends and foes are, and know yourself.

Once you have read the appendices for this chapter, proceed to the exercises. They give you an opportunity to express your philosophy of patient education and health promotion and an opportunity to justify a health education program. Your ability to express your professional and personal position will come in handy when you must negotiate for resources. The need for effective negotiation skills is discussed in Chapters 3 and 4. If you have mastered this chapter, the material and exercises in the chapters to come will be of greater value to you.

# APPENDIX 2.1

## Strategies for the Stimulation of Clinical Primary Prevention in Medicine and Dentistry (Recommended by the University of North Carolina at Chapel Hill)

If practicing physicians and dentists in primary care specialties were to devote a greater degree of concern to prevention and health promotion, people could expect them to (in the following order of priority):

**1.** Take an interest in understanding how health promotion and disease prevention might fit into their everyday practices of primary care.

**2.** Use every reasonable means of persuasion to encourage health-promoting behaviors among their patients, because these behaviors are directly related to the management of the medical or dental problem for which their patients have come to see the clinician, or because these behaviors may relate to particular problems or health risks at the pre-symptomatic level at the time of the encounter. This is part of "good medical or dental practice." Physicians or dentists who fail to thoroughly educate their patients with respect to the consequences of existing lifestyles, insofar as such lifestyles affect the course of the problem brought to the clinician's attention, are not properly caring for these patients. Some patient education should be part of every medical practice.

**3.** Practice with basic packages of primary and secondary health protection services, including standardized measures of health risk ("life quantity") and wellness ("life quality"). As part of the effort to deal with "wellness" concerns, physicians should be encouraged to learn how to take a more thorough social, psychological, and (some would advocate) spiritual history as part of the data base for patient care. In addition to health hazard appraisal, many practitioners are using instruments that measure the effects of critical "life events" as important predictive indicators in the data base for their primary care patients (for example, see Holmes and Rahe, 1967). Other available "tools" should be explored and considered for adoption in primary care.

**4.** Seek to develop personal patterns of health behavior for themselves as models of self-care for their patients. This kind of commitment will carry over as an influence on the nature of medical or dental practice. Such an orientation to personal health practices among health professionals should begin in the course of professional education.

**5.** Develop a minimum basic set of health knowledge (in certain areas of medicine and dentistry) that the public should have. The NIH [National Institute of Health]-supported "consensus conference" approach might be used to identify those clusters of health knowledge that should be part of the public's general education, much as we might find in the curricula for self-care courses already in existence.

**6.** Recognize and incorporate the role of other resources and programs in the larger community into the practice of clinical primary prevention. Physicians and dentists need to know about and understand the capabilities of family counseling agencies, visiting nurse agencies, the local health department, the public schools, community mental health centers, and so on. An understanding of the alternative resources available in the community with which to handle health-related problems should be part of the education of the primary care physician or dentist. In addition, such curricula should contain information about the knowledge and capacity of allied health professionals in other disciplines.

**7.** Recognize and incorporate the role of the midlevel practitioner (nurse practitioner, physician's assistant, dental auxiliary) in health promotion and disease prevention as a first-echelon medical or dental care provider. Physicians and dentists make a mistake by assuming that they should shoulder the total additional burden of a concern for prevention in primary care practice. These midlevel personnel have ample training to undertake a substantial portion of the work required to implement an expanded agenda in health promotion in primary care practice. In this same direction, considerable potential can be realized from the use of local clergy as a referral source related to patient problems that require some form of counseling and nonmedical advice.

**8.** Take an active interest in and seek to mobilize public concern and action in their communities (and monitor implementation) for social and economic problems affecting the health of the population they serve. It is likely that an informed and educated citizenry with respect to public health risks (such as air and water pollution, epidemics, social problems) will have a greater total capacity for dealing with problems that pose serious health risks to the general population. A physician who sees many people in his or her office suffering from emphysema or chronic pulmonary disease acquired as a result of years of employment in a dust-contaminated textile factory may view professional intervention in the field of industrial health differently from a person who practices in a large urban area among a white-collar population of patients. Likewise, the problem of motor vehicle accidents among young males may not personally affect the practice of some physicians, although the problem may be recognized as a serious public health problem. Physicians and dentists can affect public discussion of the importance of intervention with respect to problems that affect the health status of the community. As part of an overall commitment to health promotion goals, health professionals should be willing to contribute to these discussions at the community level. Once action has been taken at the community level (such as fluoridation of public water), some form of monitoring must take place, to ensure that the change continues to be implemented as planned. As an extension of these activities, health professionals should volunteer to serve where their expertise is appropriate as community resource persons and should develop some facility in working with the lay press and other communication media.

Several strategies might be taken to reach the goal of increasing the involvement of practicing physicians and dentists in clinical primary prevention. Some of the strategies might be appropriate for more than a single element of clinical primary prevention. A review of the eight elements just enumerated suggests that the first four deal mainly with aspects of medical or dental practice under the control of the physician or dentist; they do not involve either other kinds of providers of care or a consideration of the self-knowledge of the patient with respect to health or its promotion. The fifth of these elements involves the capacity for client self-management of common health problems and the establishment of the knowledge requirements for self-care. The last three elements involve the use of health-related services and allied professional personnel in the community as an adjunct to the primary care practice.

Conference delegates also made the following recommendations with respect to the content and structure of medical and dental practice:

*Recommendation 1.* Health promotion and disease prevention should become an integral part of undergraduate medical and dental curricula, as well as the curricula for physician and dental extender personnel, including an emphasis on the personal lifestyle of health professionals.

*Recommendation 2.* Health promotion and disease prevention should be part of residency training in the primary care specialties of medicine and dentistry.

*Recommendation 3.* Health promotion and disease prevention should become an integral part of the continuing education (CE) offerings of all mandated CE and recertification programs in primary care specialties in medicine and dentistry. It is suggested that these curricula stress new and practical concepts in the office-based practice of clinical primary prevention and the "team" concept of primary care practice. Certifying bodies responsible for setting the minimum number of continuing education requirements for a profession or subdiscipline in a primary care specialty should specify a prescribed number of required credits in health promotion and disease prevention as well as foster the establishment of committees of experts to approve the content of these courses offered for credit.

*Recommendation 4.* Experimentation needs to take place with respect to various mechanisms for paying providers of medical and dental services for health promotion services. Third-party insurers should be encouraged to enter into experimental/demonstration projects that test the value of differential premium rates for persons who participate in health promotion programs. The very existence of a reimbursement arrangement will act to elevate the importance of prevention in primary care practice.

*Recommendation 5.* The general public needs to be educated to expect a concern for health promotion and disease prevention from their health care providers. Health professionals are responsive to pressures brought to bear on them by their clients and/or patients. An informed public will create its own demand for this level of care.

*Recommendation 6.* A library of health promotion "tools" applicable in primary care office practice should be developed. Some organizations need to function as information, consultation, and demonstration "clearinghouses" with respect to techniques that have proven effective in clinical primary prevention applications. This clearinghouse function would include quantitative measures of health risk, audiovisual technologies for data storage and retrieval, programmed learning packages for patient education, and continuing education materials for health professionals. Such a clearinghouse might operate training programs where entire office practice "teams" might go for directed instruction in the management of health promotion and disease prevention aspects of their respective practice settings. Co-professionals should be allowed and encouraged to contribute to the development of the content of these programs.

*Recommendation 7.* A peer review and practice audit procedure should be developed for assessing the adequacy of health promotion and disease prevention in primary care practices. The seven-year recertification procedures of the American Board of Family Practice might include such a practice audit. Individual practitioners might use the audit procedure as a means of periodic quality self-assessment in their own practices. The JCAH [Joint Commission on Accreditation of Hospitals] standards for group practices, clinics, and hospitals should be modified to reflect a concern with prevention and health promotion.

*Recommendation 8.* National professional associations need to take the lead in the development of model approaches to the integration of health promotion and disease prevention into primary care practices. These models should be evaluated with respect to cost-effectiveness and cost-benefit. These models should include risk assessment and wellness-oriented components as well as conventional screening procedures, all of which should be evaluated in terms of their presumed benefits and effects.

*Recommendation 9.* A series of "consensus workshops" needs to be organized, under some appropriate sponsorship, for the purpose of defining, for different practice settings and different target audiences, the elements, tasks, or skills that constitute the practice of clinical primary prevention. To some degree this is what was undertaken by the Canadian Task Force (of the Canadian National Health Service) on the Periodic Physical Examination. Within primary care specialties, this same sort of approach might yield the kind of consensual agreement that would provide the basis for both professional education and clinical practice of primary prevention.

*Recommendation 10.* Some form of career encouragement and guidance needs to be developed for young health professionals who show an interest in and willingness to experiment with clinical primary prevention in their own practices. Perhaps such a source of professional advice could be organized in combination with a "clearinghouse" activity, as just mentioned in Recommendation 6.

# APPENDIX 2.2

American Hospital Association Policy and
Statement on the Hospital's Responsibility for
Patient Education Services (Approved by House
of Delegates, September 1, 1981)*

## POLICY

The hospital has a responsibility to provide patient education services as
an integral part of high-quality, cost-effective care. Patient education services should enable patients, and their families and friends, when appropriate, to make informed decisions about their health; to manage their
illnesses; and to implement follow-up care at home. Effective and efficient patient education services require planning and coordination, and
responsibility for such planning and coordination should be assigned.
The hospital also should provide the necessary staff and financial resources.

## STATEMENT

### Terms

*Health education* is the use of the education process to assist individuals
to voluntarily adopt or alter behaviors that will improve or maintain their
health.

*Patient education* is used when the health education is directed to
persons, and their families and friends, when appropriate, who are either
awaiting or undergoing medical treatment.

*Planned patient education* uses a process that includes conducting a
needs assessment, setting objectives, and developing an action plan and
the implementation, documentation, and evaluation of that action plan.

*Patient education services* include a variety of services developed to
respond to the education needs of patients and families. These services
should include planned activities designed to inform patients about how
to use various health care services, to prepare patients for medical procedures, to assist patients to manage their diseases or to use a medical
device after discharge, and to modify their behavior in order to promote

*Reprinted, with permission, from *Implementing Patient Education in the Hospital*, published
by American Hospital Publishing, Inc., copyright 1981.

better health and prevent diseases. These services can incorporate one or a combination of one-to-one instruction, group sessions, a series of classes, and support groups.

## Rationale

Hospitals have always provided health information to patients and their families. However, with pressures on hospitals to contain costs while responding to the increased need for patient education services, it is important that hospitals plan and coordinate their patient education services. Planning and coordination allow hospitals to make decisions about patient education services that are appropriate for their patients and resources.

Experience and research have identified several benefits of planned patient education services both to the hospital and to the patients.

For the patient, planned patient education services can reduce anxiety, increase ability to make health decisions, and reduce readmissions for chronic diseases.

For the hospital, planned and coordinated patient education can enhance efficient use of hospital services, promote efficient use of education resources, increase physician support through the collaborative development of accurate teaching program content, increase staff satisfaction, increase patient satisfaction with patient services, and increase community support for the hospital.

In addition, the provision of planned and coordinated patient education services assists the hospital to respond to pressures of accreditation standards for patient education, requirements for informed consent, need for cost-efficient use of resources, increased numbers of persons needing education to help manage chronic conditions or information about new diagnostic and treatment services, and increased consumer interest in making health decisions.

## Coordination

To meet the various education needs of patients, relatives, or friends in the preadmitting, admitting, inpatient, outpatient, and discharge stages of care, patient education goals and activities should be planned and coordinated at three levels: the entire hospital; specific patient populations, such as those with hypertension or on low-sodium diets; and individual patients and families. The education planning process is applied to all three levels.

In order to implement planned, coordinated patient education services, the responsibility should be assigned to a hospital committee, department, or staff person. The responsible individual or group should possess education and management skills and should enable the hospital to implement staff policies and procedures on the roles and responsibilities of persons providing patient education, staff training programs, staff performance evaluations that include patient education activities, documentation of patient education services as part of patient care, and evaluations of patient education services and subsequent implementation of changes in program content.

The coordinating committee, department, or staff person should involve the medical staff and individuals in various hospital departments and hospital committees, as well as selected patients, in making decisions about the content of and methods for conducting patient education services. These decisions help to determine the staff skills, the time, and the space needed to implement patient education services.

## Human resources

The assignment of responsibility for planning and coordination should enable the hospital and its staff to use their time and skills more effectively and efficiently. Although the responsibility for planning and coordinating patient education services is assigned, direct care staff, including physicians, nurses, dieticians, pharmacists, and others, are involved in patient education as part of the delivery of high-quality patient care services. Other individuals in the hospital, such as librarians, patient representatives, and selected patients and family members, can assist in the development and provision of patient education services. Trained volunteers and auxilians [auxiliary personnel] also can be a valuable resource.

## Financial resources

In order to implement planned coordinated patient education services, hospitals should provide the necessary staff and financial resources. Expenses for providing patient education services directly related to patient care should be treated as financial requirements under third-party agreements.

## Community resources

Community agencies may be a source of funding, and they also may have patient education materials, staff expertise, and patient education services. To assist patients needing patient education after discharge, as well as to expand their patient education resources and those of their community, hospitals should work with these agencies to refer patients, to develop cooperative activities, and to share resources.

# APPENDIX 2.3

## American Society for Healthcare Education and Training Resolution on Health Promotion*

Whereas, Health promotion (including health information and education) is the process of fostering awareness, influencing attitudes and identifying alternatives so that individuals can make informed choices and modify their behavior in order to achieve an optimum level of their physical and mental health and improve their physical and social environment and

Whereas, Each individual, to the extent he or she is able, has the personal responsibility for protecting his or her own health and

Whereas, Hospitals and other health care institutions have a responsibility for improving the health status of the communities they serve as well as for treating illnesses and

Whereas, The Council on Wage and Price Stability stated, "Health education can reduce health care costs in several ways. Education as to proper nutrition and exercise can help reduce the incidence of illness, and counseling services on alcoholism and emotional problem areas can reduce the incidence of physiological and mental illness," making health promotion an appropriate activity for institutions concerned about rising costs of health care

THEREFORE, BE IT RESOLVED that the American Society for Healthcare Education and Training encourages hospitals and other health care facilities and organizations to work closely with all health professionals, voluntary health agencies, school systems, local government, business and industry as well as the mass media to provide health promotion programs for employees, students, patients, and the community at large.

*Reprinted with the permission of the American Hospital Association.

# APPENDIX 2.4

## American Medical Association Statement on Patient Education (AMA House of Delegates Meeting, June 1975)*

Resolutions 37 and 41 (C-74) dealing with patient education were referred to the Board of Trustees for study and report at the 1975 Annual Convention.

Both resolutions called for planned programs of patient education developed and supervised by patient education committees whose membership would include health professionals, educators, and consumers. Both would have required that such programs be prescribed by a physician and documented on the patient's charts, as a basis for third-party reimbursement.

The American Medical Association's Department of Health Education and Division of Medical Practice have been exploring the overall subject of planned patient education programs and have arrived at the following general findings and recommendations in response to Resolutions 37 and 41 (C-74).

### DEFINITION AND ROLE OF PLANNED PATIENT EDUCATION PROGRAMS

It is recognized that increasingly complex patterns of health care, along with the patient's environment, attitude, lifestyle, and cooperation, all play an important part in effective treatment. Informed, motivated, and supportive participation in treatment by patients and their families can aid the recovery of the patient and enhance the quality of his health. Patient education, as an integral part of high-quality health care, provides an avenue to such improved participation.

Education of the patient has always been part of the ongoing professional responsibility of physicians, nurses, dietitians, therapists, and all other members of the health team. Health professionals have traditionally provided patients with some information about their illness and

*Reprinted with the permission of the American Medical Association. Copyright © 1975 by the American Medical Association.

the prescribed course of treatment. Some health instruction has also been provided. In some situations, there is a need indicated for a structured educational effort beyond that which individual members of the team can provide. It is in these situations that planned patient education programs may be expected to serve.

The provision of patient education services, designed to assist the patient and his family in the effective management of individual health, is a shared and continuous responsibility of both the physician and the patient. Patient education directed toward the effective management of individual illness and maintenance of health commences with the patient's entry into the health services. A positive personal experience between the physician and the patient at first contact will greatly contribute to the success of an effective patient education program.

The following factors define planned patient education:

**1.** Programs are distinguished from general health education of the public in that they focus on individuals who present themselves for medical services in institutions and in physicians' offices.

**2.** Programs are directed at the patient's understanding of his specific disease entity or physical or mental disability.

**3.** Programs assist the patient (and/or sometimes family members) to cooperate in the treatment of the disease or disability.

**4.** Programs involve patients with diseases or disabilities in which there are substantial grounds for belief that the patient will be better able to participate in treatment and that the treatment will be more effective with such a planned program than without it.

It should be clear from these four factors that planned patient education programs are distinct from general health education programs for the public and from programs intended as education for prevention of disease or for health maintenance. The planned program is for patients under treatment.

As the relationship between the physician and the patient is established, the physician determines the patient's level of knowledge concerning his illness or health, and the patient's educational needs. In this relationship, it is incumbent upon the patient to provide the necessary health history and medical information, and to comply with the prescribed medical regimen. Adherence to a prescribed treatment program is dependent upon the patient's understanding and acceptance of his condition, recognition of the importance of his role in the daily management of his prescribed treatment, and satisfaction with health services provided. It is in these areas that a planned patient education program can enhance quality care.

## REIMBURSEMENT

Planned patient education is a legitimate reimbursable item of patient care, when prescribed by a physician appropriate to the patient's condition and substantiated by entries on the patient record. Planned patient education should be eligible for reimbursement under the various health insurance and other three-party payment programs.

## BENEFITS

Properly planned programs of this type will improve care and can reduce the overall cost of treatment. Enabling patients to play a greater part in their own treatment can reduce unnecessary utilization of trained health professionals and of health care facilities. However, potential benefits such as cost containment, shortened recovery time, and improved patient morale may not be immediately achievable. Any new interdisciplinary program takes time to develop and to become effective.

## CONTENT AND ORGANIZATION

Planned patient education programs should be based on identified objectives, should make use of sound educational methods, should have approved content that is scientifically accurate, and should be adaptable to the individual needs of patients.

Objectives need to be clarified at the outset, along with specific criteria for measuring their achievement. The success or failure of the program should be determined by how well the objectives are realized.

## RECOMMENDATIONS

The Board of Trustees believes the general findings and recommendations contained in this report respond to Resolutions 37 and 41, and recommends that the report be adopted and Association activities to improve effective patient education be continued.

# APPENDIX 2.5

## American Hospital Association Policy and Statement on the Hospital's Responsibility for Health Promotion*

### POLICY

Hospitals have a responsibility to take a leadership role in helping ensure the good health of their communities. In addition to the primary mission of providing health care and related education to the sick and injured, the hospital has a responsibility to work with others in the community to assess the health status of the community, identify target areas and population groups for hospital-based and cooperative health promotion programs, develop programs to help upgrade the health in those target areas, ensure that persons who are apparently healthy have access to information about how to stay well and prevent disease, provide appropriate health education programs to aid those persons who choose to alter their personal health behavior or develop a more healthful lifestyle, and establish the hospital as an institution in the community that is concerned about good health in addition to one concerned about treating illness.

### STATEMENT

Increasing numbers of people are seeking information about their health and making decisions without the direct consultation of physicians or other health professionals. The American Hospital Association has supported and encouraged this trend toward greater personal responsibility for health in its *Statement on Provision of Health Services under Universal Health Insurance*: "Each individual, to the extent he or she is able, has the

*Reprinted with the permission of the American Hospital Association, copyright 1979.

In 1978, the American Hospital Association identified the need for a policy to encourage and guide hospitals in expanding their role as the center for health, not just illness, in the community. In August 1979, the American Hospital Association's House of Delegates approved the *Policy and Statement on the Hospital's Responsibility for Health Promotion*. A companion document, published by the Association in 1975, is the *Statement on Health Education: Role and Responsibility of Health Care Institutions* (S010).

personal responsibility for protecting his or her own health . . ."[1] The statement also identifies an active role for health care providers in helping the consumer achieve this goal: "The system should be oriented to the maintenance of personal good health and to the prevention of illness, as well as to the treatment of acute illness" and the hospital should consider developing and participating in "community-wide health educational and informational activities to actively encourage responsible decisions about health, as well as responsible use of health services by its community." Indeed, hospitals traditionally have been involved in health promotion activities.

## The hospitals' image: center for health

In many communities, the hospital is identified by the public as the center for health and thus is looked to as the logical source for all types of information relating to health as well as sickness. It is to the hospital's advantage to encourage this positive image through management support and governing board policy. Further, people look to health professionals as exemplars or models. Thus, hospitals should take a leadership role in providing appropriate health information and education to their communities and to their employees.

## The hospital as a catalyst

Hospitals, physicians, and other health professionals should serve as catalysts to stimulate the interest of, encourage the participation of, and develop strong working relationships with voluntary health agencies, other health provider groups, educational institutions, local businesses and industries, and other groups within the community that influence and/or control the resources needed to carry out these health promotion and education responsibilities. The fulfillment of these responsibilities will help ensure that patients, hospital employees, and community members have the information needed to enable them to make informed choices about their personal health behavior, their lifestyles, and the environment in which they live, since the responsibility for these decisions ultimately rests with the individual.

## Health promotion: informed choice

Health promotion (including health information and health education) is the process of fostering awareness, influencing attitudes, and identi-

---

[1] American Hospital Association, *Statement on Provision of Health Services under Universal Health Insurance* (Chicago: American Hospital Association, 1977).

fying alternatives so that individuals can make informed choices and change their behavior in order to achieve an optimum level of physical and mental health and improve their physical and social environment. Health promotion programs offered by hospitals should facilitate this informed choice, but should not have as their goal forcing specific habits or lifestyle choices (unless it can be demonstrated that an individual's health practices adversely and seriously affect the health of others).

## Protecting individuals' rights

In those areas where it can be demonstrated that the actions of one individual adversely and seriously affect the health of others, such as through alcohol or drug abuse or sidestream smoke, the hospital has a responsibility to take appropriate steps to protect the rights of the affected individuals within the institution. For example, hospitals have a responsibility to protect the rights of nonsmoking patients, employees, and visitors within their institutions. To the extent feasible, they also have a responsibility to work with others in the community—such as physicians, voluntary health agencies, health provider groups, educational institutions, local businesses and industries, and other interested groups—to make information available on the hazards to others of reckless driving, alcohol and drug abuse, smoking, and other harmful practices, as well as to make appropriate behavior change programs available. As with all hospital services, steps should be taken to assure confidentiality.

## Lifestyle

Hospitals have long supported the concept of educating patients about managing disease and illness. The phrases "responsible decisions about health" and "maintenance of personal good health," as contained in the *Statement on Provision of Health Services under Universal Health Insurance,* however, imply a role that goes beyond disease-related information and takes hospitals into the area of lifestyle and personal behavior. (Lifestyle includes such personal choice factors as the use or abuse of alcohol, drugs, tobacco, and the automobile, as well as exercise, nutrition, and sleep habits.)

## Cooperative efforts

In order to ensure the most effective use of community resources, including funding, and to achieve the broadest possible benefits from health promotion programs, it is appropriate and necessary for hospitals to work with others in the community to provide information and education about the value of and techniques for achieving a healthful lifestyle, the potential dangers to the individual and to others from certain personal health habits, methods to prevent disease, and opportunities for early disease detection and treatment. This may include stimulating, encouraging, and working closely with physicians and other health professionals, hospital auxiliaries and volunteers, voluntary health agencies, health provider groups, third-party payers, public health departments, and other interested groups, as well as developing new and stronger health promotion channels through cooperation with school systems, religious organizations, local government, local businesses and industries, and the news media.

## Health promotion and costs

Many personal health and lifestyle factors are related to expensive and preventable illnesses and accidents. The Council on Wage and Price Stability stated, "Health education can reduce health care costs in several ways. Education as to proper nutrition and exercise can help reduce the incidence of illness. So, too, can counseling services on alcoholism and emotional problem areas reduce the incidence of physiological and mental illness."[2] Thus, health information and education programs relating to lifestyle and personal health behavior are appropriate activities for institutions concerned about rising costs of health care.

However, the financing of health promotion activities often poses problems for hospitals, especially in an environment of conscientious cost containment. Experience shows that hospitals are utilizing a wide range of appropriate financing mechanisms to balance the commitment to helping ensure good health and the commitment to containing costs. These financing mechanisms include third-party reimbursement, fee-for-service, donations from consumers, contributions and gifts, grants and contracts, and the extensive use of volunteers.

[2]*The Complex Puzzle of Rising Health Care Costs: Can the Private Sector Fit It Together?* (Washington, D.C.: Council on Wage and Price Stability, 1976), p. 169.

# APPENDIX 2.6

## Excerpts from American Hospital Association Professional, Accreditation, and Legal Statements Supporting Patient Education*

Because education of patients is an integral part of the care of patients, it is important that patient education activities in hospitals be based on defined outcomes, documented on patient charts, and evaluated for efficiency and effectiveness. The following is a review of relevant documents on accreditation, informed consent, and patients' rights as well as statements of professional health care organizations.

## PATIENT EDUCATION AND ACCREDITATION

The 1976 edition of the *Accreditation Manual for Hospitals*, published by the Joint Commission on Accreditation of Hospitals (JCAH), includes specific statements regarding the scope of patient education programs. These statements relate to quality of professional services, patients' rights, emergency services, hospital-based home care, medical record services, nursing services, and outpatient services.

### Quality of professional services

The most comprehensive of the JCAH statements relates to quality of professional services: "Evidence of the quality of patient care provided in the hospital shall be demonstrated by measurement of actual care against specific criteria. . . . Criteria must be explicit and measurable, and must reflect the optimal level of care that can be achieved through current medical and related health-science knowledge. . . . Criteria shall include . . . *demonstrated knowledge* (emphasis added) of the patient concerning his health status, level of functioning, and self-care after discharge" (page 27 of *Accreditation Manual*).

*Reprinted from American Hospital Association, *Professional, Accreditation, and Legal Statements Supporting Patient Education*, AHA catalog No. P014 (Chicago: American Hospital Association, 1977), and American Hospital Association, *Implementing Patient Education in Hospitals Manual*, 1978, by permission of the American Hospital Association.

## Patients' rights

According to the JCAH manual ([1978] page 24), "The patient has the right to be informed as to the nature and purpose of any technical procedures that are to be performed upon him, as well as to know by whom such procedures are to be carried out . . . and to receive from [persons responsible for his care] adequate information concerning the nature and extent of his medical problem, the planned course of treatment, and the prognosis. In addition, he has a right to expect adequate instruction in self-care in the interim between visits to the hospital or to the physician."

## Emergency services

Policies and procedures for the medical staff providing emergency services should include "instructions to be given to the patient and/or family in regard to follow-up care" (page 73).

## Hospital-based home care

The written plan of care for each patient in the hospital-based home care program should refer to the "patient and family teaching program, if applicable" (page 89). The medical record shall include a "statement completed at the time of discharge from home care program, showing that the patient or his representative has received written instructions for his future care" (page 91).

## Medical record services

"Evidence of appropriate informed consent" should be included in the medical record (page 95). The final progress note should include "the specific instructions given to the patient and/or family, particularly in relation to physical activity, medication, diet, and follow-up care" (page 97).

## Nursing services

A brief and pertinent written nursing care plan should be developed for each patient. The plan should indicate what nursing care is needed, how it can best be accomplished, what methods and approaches are believed to be most successful, and what modifications are necessary to ensure the best results. The written nursing care plan may include "patient and family teaching programs" (page 124).

## Outpatient services

With regard to the development of policies and procedures for outpatient services, the JCAH manual states that "If outpatient surgery is performed, the written procedures shall include provisions covering . . . written preoperative instructions to patients" (page 128). In addition, "Written instructions for follow-up care shall be given to the patient. All patients shall be advised about contacting the appropriate physician for help in the event of postoperative complications" (page 129).

"Special procedures should be developed to ensure that patients are adequately informed of other sources of services and of any steps that must be taken to arrange for such services" (page 129).

"The patient shall be informed of the identity of the physician(s) primarily responsible for his care. If trainees participate in patient care, reflecting the concept of team care, the patient shall be so informed and his consent obtained. To the extent possible, the patient shall be informed by a physician as to the general nature of his medical problem, the general prognosis, if feasible, and the nature and purpose of the treatment and procedures that are contemplated. Appropriate instruction in self-care shall be given to the patient" (page 129).

## PATIENT EDUCATION AND INFORMED CONSENT

*Nursing and the Law*, published in 1975 by the Health Law Center, Aspen Systems Corporation, describes two tests, both directed to the education activity of the physician in answering legal questions concerning the performance of procedures on patients:

**1.** The "objective" test: Did the physician give the patient as much instruction concerning the nature of a given procedure as other physicians in the community would have given?

**2.** The "subjective" test: Was there sufficient assurance that the patient was adequately informed, especially concerning risks and probable consequences, regarding the procedure to the extent that his understanding was beyond reasonable doubt?

An additional crucial issue is to determine what documentation will be used as evidence to show that *informed* consent actually was obtained.

The question has two aspects:

**1.** What format will serve best? (This is especially pertinent to the design of consent forms.)

**2.** What supportive documentation reflective of care-provider intervention will best enhance and illustrate the processes by which patient education was undertaken and accomplished?

## PATIENT EDUCATION AND PATIENTS' RIGHTS

A *Patient's Bill of Rights* was approved by the American Hospital Association's House of Delegates in 1973. One of its purposes was to show that hospitals recognize certain rights of persons who come to hospitals for treatment. Six of the twelve sections refer to the patient's right to obtain specific information from the physician or the hospital as indicated below:

*Section 2.* Diagnosis, treatment, and prognosis (physician).

*Section 3.* Procedures determined necessary for the patient's care (physician).

*Section 7.* Needs for and alternatives to transfer to other facilities (hospital).

*Section 8.* The relationship between the hospital and other health care and educational facilities (hospital), and relationships among those treating the patient (physician).

*Section 9.* The existence of research projects that may affect the patient (hospital and physician, see [Section] 2 above).

*Section 10.* The patient's requirements for continuing health care following discharge (physician).

Some hospitals have developed statements on both patients' rights and patients' responsibilities concerning health care. Such statements serve to clarify the relationship between the consumer and the provider.

## PATIENT EDUCATION AND PROFESSIONAL PRACTICE
## ACTS AND STATEMENTS OF PROFESSIONAL ASSOCIATIONS

Patient education is integral to the clinical practice of several health professions. In this document four professional groups—medicine, nursing, dietetics, and pharmacy—are used as examples.

Although legislation in various states defines practice in several fields, the language of practice acts varies from state to state. Regardless, legal definitions of practice must be thoroughly understood both by the practitioner and the hospital in which the practitioner works, for two important reasons: (1) the individual can be held liable for practice that does not conform to the legislated definition and (2) the hospital in which the practitioner works can be held liable for failure of the practitioner to conform to the definition. Health professions' statements on patient education may be admissible as evidence in legal proceedings related to the role of health professionals and their employers.

## Medicine

In 1975, the American Medical Association's House of Delegates adopted its *Statement on Patient Education*. It states, "The provision of patient education services designed to assist the patient and his family in the effective management of individual health is a shared and continuous responsibility of both the physician and the patient."

In January 1977, the Association for Hospital Medical Education adopted its *Policy Statement re Health Education Programs*. This statement supports health education activities and encourages the involvement of the hospital medical education officer in both the definition and delivery of such programs. Although the statement does not prescribe educational program content, it makes specific reference to "community education programs" that focus on the needs of patients with chronic disease and programs whose purpose is to teach general preventive health measures.

The Michigan Medical Practice Act of 1976 defines the phrase *to practice medicine* as "to diagnose, treat, prevent, cure, or relieve a human disease, ailment, defect, complaint, or other condition, whether physical or mental, by attendance or *advice*, or by a device, diagnostic test, or *other means*, or to offer to undertake, attempt to do, or hold oneself out as able to do, any of these acts" (emphasis added). In Michigan, at least, the education of patients falls within the purview of medical practice.

## Nursing

The specific language of nurse practice acts varies in different states, and reference to patient education may be either implicit or explicit. For example, the 1975 Illinois Nursing Act defines professional nursing as "the performance for compensation of any nursing act . . . in the observation, care, and *counsel* of the ill, injured, or infirm" (emphasis added). The Illinois act adheres closely to the definition of professional nursing developed by the American Nurses' Association. Neither the Illinois nor the ANA document defines *counsel*. However, the *American College Dictionary* published in 1964 by Random House defines *counsel* as "advice, opinion, or instruction given in directing the judgment or conduct of another." On the basis of this definition, it appears that teaching patients is considered to be a function of professional nurses, at least in those states that have adopted the ANA-recommended language in defining nursing and nursing practice.

Further evidence of the importance of teaching patients is found in official professional nursing association statements on the role of nursing and patient education. A 1975 ANA publication entitled *The Professional Nurse and Health Education* provides "guidelines for the professional nurse's participation in health education activities." It states, "As a health care provider, every professional nurse is responsible and accountable to the patient and family for the quality of nursing care the patient receives. This responsibility includes teaching the patient and family relevant facts about specific health care needs and supporting appropriate modification of behavior." Supporting this premise, the document goes on to state that the responsibilities of nurses in hospital settings are identified as "assessing the patient's knowledge about his illness, rehabilitation, and health maintenance." According to the guidelines, these activities should include "diagnostic preparation and procedures, preoperative and postoperative care, treatment and drugs, and discharge planning and follow-up."

Another ANA publication, *Standards of Nursing Practice*, published in 1973, specifies how these activities are to be accomplished. Standards IV, V, and VI address nursing's responsibility for planning care, providing client/patient participation in health-related activities, and maximizing client/patient health capabilities. These standards specify the need for behavioral objectives concerning the patient education program and content. In support, *The Professional Nurse and Health Education* [1975] emphasizes that such efforts are "not new to nursing; [they are] an integral part of nursing practice."

## Dietetics

Registration of dietitians is accomplished through an examination conducted under the auspices of the American Dietetic Association. The ADA supports nutrition teaching as a function of registered dietitians.

In its 1975 position paper *Guidelines for Diet Counseling*, the ADA recommends that dietitians counsel individuals and families in nutritional principles, dietary plans, and food selection; communicate appropriate dietary history and nutritional care data in the medical records; and compile and develop nutrition education materials.

Guidelines for diet counseling by registered dietitians were developed in 1976 by a special committee of the ADA in its *Position Paper on Recommended Salaries and Employment Practices for Members of the American Dietetic Association*. In the paper, *diet counseling* is defined as a three-part program of patient interview, patient counseling, and patient consulting for the purposes of therapeutic treatment, general nutritional assessment, nutrition, and other related purposes. The guidelines, which rest on the premise that dietitians should become proficient in counseling, state, "Proficiency in diet counseling is, or should be, a basic skill of the dietitian concerned with patient care."

Guidelines entitled *Recording Nutritional Information in Medical Records* were prepared by a joint committee of the American Hospital Association and the American Dietetic Association in 1976. The guidelines emphasize the need for including information on nutrition education in the patient's medical record.

Other ADA position papers and statements noting the importance of nutrition education include *Promoting Optimal Nutritional Health of the Population of the United States* (1969), *The Role of the Dietitian in Consultative Services to Group Care Facilities* (1975), *Nutrition and the Aging* (1972), *Child Nutrition Programs* (1974), and *Nutrition Services in Health Maintenance Organizations* (1972).

## Pharmacy

The Illinois Pharmacy Act of 1955 includes the following in its definition of the practice of pharmacy: "recommending or advising concerning contents and therapeutic values" of various medicinal agents. It makes no other direct mention of specific patient education functions.

In 1975, [the] *Statement on Pharmacist-Conducted Patient Counseling* was approved by the board of the American Society of Hospital Pharmacists (ASHP). This document states, in part, that the pharmacist should "inform, educate, and counsel patients about [specific issues concerning] each medication in the patient drug regimen," including

- Name (trademark, generic, common synonym, or other descriptive name[s])
- Intended use and expected action
- Route, dosage form, dosage, and administration schedule
- Special directions for preparation
- Special directions for administration
- Precautions to be observed during administration
- Common side effects that may be encountered, including their avoidance and action required if they occur
- Techniques for self-monitoring of drug therapy
- Proper storage
- Potential drug-drug or drug-food interactions or other therapeutic contraindications
- Prescription refill information
- Action to be taken in the event of a missed dose
- Any other information peculiar to the specific patient or drug

# APPENDIX 2.7

## The Concept of Planned Hospital-Based Patient Education Programs*

The ultimate goal of planned in-hospital patient education programs is to help individuals acquire new knowledge, attitudes, and behavior that will promote their ability to care for themselves more adequately. It requires accepting the premise that most patients have an inalienable "right to know" the status of their health, the nature of an existing health problem, what community health resources are available to them and their family, and what they can do to achieve and maintain an optimum state of health and to prevent future recurrences of illness.

With an increasing focus on preventive health measures and new ways of providing health care, many health professionals concur it is essential that planned in-hospital education programs become an integral component of health care services to augment patient compliance with prescribed medical regimes.

Mounting evidence indicates that when a selected population of patients with similar medical problems are provided with planned educational experiences and take an active participatory role in their own care, they are able to cope with and follow prescribed medical programs more adequately than those individuals who are not offered comparable experiences. Compared with control groups, their hospital readmissions and total readmission days are significantly reduced. Families have also been found to be more responsive and cooperative when they are included in the educational process during the hospitalization, preparation for discharge, and follow-up care of a family member.

Patient education programs, however, cannot be realized without the support of health professionals, including hospital administrators; nor will they be operational without carefully designed programs to assist physicians, nurses, and other allied health workers in the art of patient education as a team endeavor.

In addition, evaluation of the educational component in patient care becomes important not only in identifying successful approaches to patient teaching but in learning what practices are not conducive to patient improvement.

---

*Editor's Note: This is a synopsis of a position paper by the same title, submitted by the Task Force on Patient Education on February 28, 1972, for consideration by the President's Committee on Health Education, *Health Education Monographs*, 2(1), Spring 1974.

# EXERCISES

1.    Think of an educational experience that you had that was positive, that helped you make an important decision, or that helped you make a significant change in your life, helped you take care of important business, or made you feel more powerful. On a separate sheet of paper, list all the characteristics of the leader, the participants, the educational methods, the pervading values, the environment, the impact on you and others in the group, and so on, that made this experience so special to you. As a result of this recall, design a statement of educational philosophy to guide your professional and personal decisions about health education over the next several months. In writing, describe three such decisions coming up soon and say how your statement of philosophy would affect them.

2.    In writing, prepare a rationale for a community outreach program that, if funded as proposed, will be initiated by a 200-bed community hospital in a suburban community in your state. Describe how professional, accreditation, or legal statements, organizational policies and goals, and your own philosophy and beliefs influenced the statement of rationale.

3.    You are approached by Dr. Jenkins to develop some materials for her diabetic patients. You are glad that she has come to you because you have wanted to involve her in health education planning for years. She is a popular physician among her peers and usually is quite skeptical about health education. As an endocrinologist, Dr. Jenkins sees many adult diabetics. A large percentage of her patients are obese. She has followed many of these patients for years and feels that they would be better off if they lost weight. She has tried everything that she knows—counseling, admonitions, bullying— but none of these techniques has worked. Out of desperation she has come to you. She wants you to write a pamphlet to "make" her patients lose weight. Write a position statement that you could use to respond to Dr. Jenkins's request. Your task is to create a situation where you both can win.

# RESOURCES

*Health Education: Role and Responsibility of Health Care Institutions*, 1975. APHA Catalog No. S010. Available from American Hospital Association, 840 N. Lake Shore Drive, Chicago, IL 60611.

*A Patient's Bill of Rights*, 1975. AHA Catalog No. S009. Available from American Hospital Association, 840 N. Lake Shore Drive, Chicago, IL 60611.

*White Paper: Patient Health Education*, 1974. Available from Health Care Services, Blue Cross Association, 840 N. Lake Shore Drive, Chicago, IL 60611.

American Nurses' Association, *The Professional Nurse and Health Education*. Available from the American Nurses' Association, 2420 Pershing Road, Kansas City, MO 64108.

American Society of Hospital Pharmacists, *Statement on Pharmacist-Conducted Patient Counseling*. Available from the American Society of Hospital Pharmacists, 4630 Montgomery Avenue, Washington, D.C. 20014.

American Medical Association, *Statement on Patient Education*, 1975. Available from the AMA's Department of Health Education, 535 N. Dearborn Street, Chicago, IL 60610.

"Guidelines for Diet Counseling." *Journal of the American Dietetic Association.* 66 (June 1975): 571–573.

# 3

## The health educator's roles in medical care

MEDICAL CARE ORGANIZATIONS, including hospitals and clinics, have recently become major employers of health educators. In this chapter we explore the role of the health educator. We present case examples of health educators in various medical settings, and then analyze the roles of the health educator: manager, coordinator, instructor, trainer, and consultant. Finally, we examine role ambiguity and role conflict as they influence the effectiveness of the health educator, as well as possible ways to resolve such dilemmas.

This chapter concludes the part of this book that lays the foundation for health education practice in medical care. With this foundation comfortably laid, the reader is then ready to work with the next section, which deals with planning and implementing patient education and health promotion services.

### VARIED ROLES, CONFLICTING EXPECTATIONS

One of the greatest challenges facing health educators is to clearly define our roles and responsibilities. In the course of a typical day, we perform a wide array of tasks. Figure 3.1 shows a sample page from a health educator's calendar. The educator may conduct an educational program, attend a budget meeting, train physicians in educational principles, coach an employee, chair a program-planning committee, and counsel a patient

| Wednesday, April 18 | | |
|---|---|---|
| **8** Department manager's meeting | Lunch | 1 |
| **9** Conduct employee performance evaluation | Evaluation training for health education instructors | 2 |
| **10** New staff orientation | Meet rep of American Cancer Society to discuss | 3 |
| **11** Teach hypertension class | cosponsoring new program | 4 |
| **12** Diabetes education committee meeting | Drop off promotional flyers to printer | 5 |
| | Evening | |

**Figure 3.1   Health educator's calendar**

who has recently been diagnosed with a chronic disease. Moreover, we come from varied backgrounds. We may be professionally trained health education specialists, registered nurses, or other health professionals with hands-on clinical experience. As a result, our colleagues may have differing and conflicting expectations of us and may not know how to best use our skills. Because our profession is so diverse, we are often challenged with defining our own roles and responsibilities and communicating that knowledge to the health care community.

The following examples describe the roles of three health educators working in medical care. In the first example, the responsibilities of the health educator are institution-wide, encompassing the entire medical center as well as the community it serves. Here, the health educator's role as a manager is clearly established. In the second example, the health educator has responsibilities at a programmatic level, aimed at specific groups of patients sharing common health problems. His degree in nursing allows him to develop patient education programs for nurses for use in patient teaching. In the third example, the health educator's responsibilities are directed primarily at an individual or client level. Instructing and counseling patients individually as well as in small groups are major responsibilities of her position.

As you read through each of these examples, notice varying leadership, coordinator, and provider functions. How does each position differ with regard to job title, reporting relationships, and required skills?

## In a large medical center

In this first example, the health educator (let us call her Marge Benz) is the full-time director of health education in a 400-bed medical center located in a large urban area, such as St. Louis, Missouri. The medical center employs 1,800 people and provides comprehensive outpatient and inpatient services. The health education services have operated for twelve years, although the services were not given through a formal health education department until four years ago. A patient education advisory committee, composed of medical and managerial personnel, advises the health education department on program development and helps set long-range and short-term patient education goals.

The director has primary responsibilities in the areas of management and supervision. Benz developed a policy statement, shown here, that defined the role and function of an integrated health education department:

**1.** *Purpose:* To identify and articulate the role and responsibilities of Community Hospital staff in the development and provision of new health education services.

**2.** *General:* The provision of health education services is the responsibility of the departments providing the related patient care. Medical Center-wide coordination and consultation, and some program implementation, are provided by the Department of Health Education.

**3.** *Policy:* It is the policy of Community Hospital to offer coordinated health education services to patients to complement medical care and/or prevent disease. All health education services receive initial approval of the appropriate department head and administrative designee, are reviewed by the Health Education Coordinator, and finally, must receive approval of the Medical Center Administrator and Physician-in-Chief. Budgetary responsibility for services belongs to the department providing patient care which the educational program complements. When programs emanate directly from the Department of Health Education or are aimed at the community, budgetary responsibility belongs to the Department of Health Education.

   **4.** *Responsibilities*
      4.1. *Chief of Patient Education:* Responsible for the general direction of health education program and staff.
      4.2. *Health Education Coordinator:* Responsible for continuity of health education services, effective use of resources and

avoidance of duplication in health/patient education services in the Medical Center.

   a. Coordinates services/programs that involve more than one department.

   b. Documents patient education/health promotion activities offered at the Medical Center.

   c. Acts as consultant and resource person to entire Medical Center for the development, administration, and evaluation of health and patient education programs at the facility.

   d. Supervises health education staff.

4.3. *Patient Education Committee:* Responsible to assess health and patient education needs in the Medical Center and make recommendations regarding the meeting of these needs to the administrative team and medical staff.

4.4. *Department Managers and Chiefs of Services:* Responsible to approve allocation of departmental resources for use in health education services and to obtain approval of administrative designee and/or Physician-in-Chief, as required by their departmental procedures.

4.5. *Medical Center Administrator and Physician in Chief:* Responsible for final approval of all health education services to be implemented in the Medical Center.

4.6. *Instructors:* Responsible for:

   a. Designing and conducting education programs (one-to-one or group).

   b. Working with Health Education Coordinator as needed for assistance in program development and coordination with other departments.

   c. Providing Health Education Coordinator with data sheet (updated annually), written objectives, content outline, teaching materials, and evaluation tool for documentation purposes.

   d. Ensuring that registration and attendance records are maintained (either by themselves or by the appropriate clerk) and submitting attendance figures to Health Education Coordinator at specified intervals.

Benz also developed a proposal for administration that outlined departmental budget and staff needs (Brekon, 1982). In addition, she implemented programs that the administrative team of the medical center had identified as priorities and that had strong physician and nursing input, visibility, and available resources. These projects included designing and coordinating a closed-circuit television system, and organizing and subsequently coordinating educational services for cancer patients. Because these projects involved interdepartmental, interdisciplinary working groups, Benz's department affected the entire organization.

Currently the director supervises nine employees and administers a budget of $210,000. Forty programs (inpatient and outpatient) are coordinated through the department year-round. Benz has a master's degree in public health education and five years' experience working in medical care. These minimum requirements for her position are set by her organization. She needs experience in supervising professional staff because master's-level librarians, health educators, and psychologists report directly to her. The director reports to the hospital administrator. She also reports to a physician who has been designated chief of patient education for professional guidance and direction in areas related to patient care and physician support and liaison. This chief serves as the chairperson of the hospital's patient education committee and as a link between the health education staff and physicians. The organization chart is shown in Figure 3.2.

The scope of the director's work is defined within the general goals of the health education program. Annually, departmental objectives are

**Figure 3.2  Medical center-wide organization chart for health education**

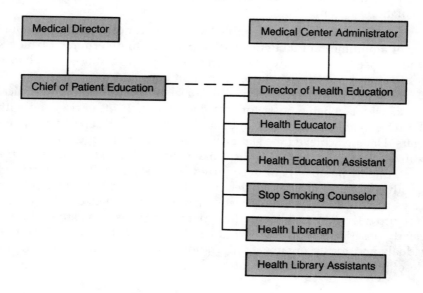

established based on the four goal areas. The general goals, along with a partial sample of one year's objectives, follow:

## General Goals

**1.** To improve the quality and effectiveness of current health education services throughout the medical center

**2.** To integrate educational activities in total patient care by bridging the gap between hospital, clinic, and home

**3.** To develop new health education approaches that are responsive to perceived needs of consumers and providers

**4.** To evaluate the effect of educational intervention in patient care

## Annual Objectives

**1.** By October, nurse practitioner- and physician-referred patients to health education programs will reach 25 percent.

**2.** By September, 75 percent of health education programs will be documented in the patients' medical record so that health providers are aware of their patients' participation in educational programs.

**3.** By November, 80 percent of health education instructors will participate in one of three eight-hour training programs on health education teaching and methodology that will include a follow-up individual evaluation session.

**4.** By September, the health educator will conduct a telephone survey of a minimum of 90 hypertensive patients, to determine if patients who choose to attend a hypertension class differ from those who choose not to attend with respect to select patient behaviors.

These goal areas define the director's position as one that is medical center-wide, so Benz must work closely with chiefs of service, and with the nursing, hospital, and clinic administrators and department managers. Having achieved the status of a department manager, the director is in a better position to establish, maintain, and direct the goals of the department. Because Benz recognized the need to sell the concept of health education, not only to decision makers but also to providers, she gives presentations before department managers, chiefs of service, and care providers. An essential requirement of her position is the ability to clearly describe the outcomes and benefits of health education to individuals and to the organization. The director of health education's job description is presented in Figure 3.3.

## Figure 3.3   Job description: director of health education

1.  Identifies overall opportunities for health education within the medical center and helps medical center administrative, managerial, and medical staff to identify, analyze, plan, and evaluate the health education component of programs and services, and to set program priorities.

2.  Coordinates the development and implementation of organized inter-disciplinary health education programs by determining the factors that contribute to the behavioral aspects of health problems, such as (a) the patient's knowledge, attitudes, values, and perceptions; (b) availability of organizational resources, accessibility of services, referrals, and patient skills; and (c) the attitudes and behavior of health care professionals, peers, patients, and employers.

3.  Supervises the health educator, smoking cessation counselor, education assistant, health librarian and library staff, and M.P.H. field-training health education students.

4.  Plans and manages yearly budget for health education.

5.  Designs a system to objectively evaluate expected outcomes of educational programs and individual participation.

6.  Recommends and/or plans staff development courses for health providers and other members of the health team on aspects of health education diagnosis, planning, or evaluation.

7.  Prepares health education protocols, using the systematic application of health education theory and health behavior change theory, or delegates this to appropriate staff.

8.  Designs methods to document health education activities in patient records to assure their integration into the total care process.

9.  Prepares reports for publication or for administration as required.

## In a small rural hospital

In the second example, the health educator (let us call him Tom Waite) was hired for the position of patient education coordinator. He works in the 99-bed Canton County Community Hospital in a semirural area, Paradise, California. The hospital employs approximately 450 people and provides inpatient services in medical and surgical care, obstetrics and gynecology, pediatrics, and emergency room care. The position was originally held by the discharge planner, who relinquished her responsibilities as patient education coordinator because she was unable to perform both jobs.

Waite has been in his position for six months. Prior to this he worked as a staff nurse and nursing educator at the hospital. A background in nursing, program planning, and supervision was required for the patient education coordinator position. At this time Waite has an annual budget of $2,000. He reports to a nursing education coordinator, with whom he shares a secretary. The organization chart is shown in Figure 3.4.

Waite's relationship to his supervisor is shaped by the overall coordination of the educational program. He schedules most of his own work activities, which are defined by the identified need to formalize and revitalize previously neglected educational programs. Although formal needs assessments have not been conducted within the medical center, the hospital managers along with physician chiefs of service have identified several program priorities for the patient education coordinator. The cardiac rehabilitation program, the pediatrics and adult preoperative education programs, and the diabetes program are the four projects that demand immediate attention.

Waite's prior nursing experience at the hospital and his reputation as an effective nursing educator made him a good candidate for patient education coordinator. At the time he was hired, this position initially demanded skills in planning and coordination. More recently he has acquired the additional responsibility of training the nursing staff to develop their skills in teaching patients. His job description is presented in Figure 3.5. Although all patient teaching is done on a one-to-one basis by hospital nurses, the patient education coordinator must work closely with physicians and nurses to earn their support and their subsequent referrals to patient education programs.

The patient education coordinator is required to explicitly outline the steps of patient education, whether for diabetic, preoperative, or cardiac rehabilitation education. Flow charts, checklists, and audiovisual aids are used by the nurses when they are teaching patients. Sources for such aids are listed in the Resources section at the end of this chapter.

**Figure 3.4  Department of nursing organization chart for patient education**

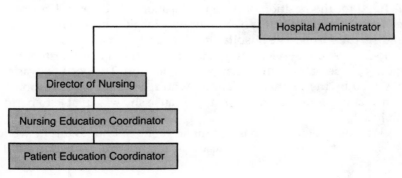

**Figure 3.5   Job description: patient education coordinator**

1. Participate in formulating patient education goals and policies by helping to identify and analyze the educational components of these goals.

2. Assess the needs of "patient communities" in relation to patient education goals.

3. Plan a course of action appropriate to these needs and goals.

4. Determine the health behaviors and actions contributing to the specific health problems presented by the patients that are served.

5. Identify the health problems that are amenable to education intervention. Design educational protocols for use by health providers.

6. Serve as consultant to members of the medical center staff in analyzing educational problems and in defining target groups, identifying desired behavioral change, and selecting communication methods.

7. Coordinate the implementation of organized interdisciplinary patient education programs.

8. Evaluate the education interventions to see if they made a difference in patients' health status, as well as in meeting the organization's goals.

9. Design methods to document health education activities in patients' records to assure their integration into the total care process.

10. Plan staff development programs for health providers and other members of the health team on how to teach learning strategies and methods.

11. Help select, prepare, and distribute educational materials to be used in patient education programs.

Waite's primary responsibilities are (1) to develop these teaching plans, with assistance from physicians and nurses and (2) to train the nursing staff to teach cardiac patients.

Waite will decide on future program development once he completes a needs assessment. This assessment will be based primarily on inpatient needs, hospital statistics, demographics, and interest level of the physicians and nursing staff. Once he completes the needs assessment, he will begin to organize the patient education programs offered at the hospital. Initially, this will involve completing an inventory of all classes taught at the medical center. A sample of an inventory data sheet is shown in Figure 3.6.

### In a primary care clinic

In the third and last example, the health educator (let us call her Joan Kimura) has worked in a primary care clinic since its inception two years

**Figure 3.6 Patient education inventory data sheet**

## Patient Education Inventory Data Sheet

1. Name of program: _____

2. Department offering program: _____

3. Instructor (Names): _____ Extension: _____

4. Description of program (Please attach teaching plan and samples
   of handouts) _____

   _____

5. Objective(s): _____

   _____

6. Group teaching: ____ One-to-one teaching: ____
   Audiovisual only: ____

7. Methods of evaluation: _____

8. When and where offered: _____

9. Target population: _____

10. Criteria for entry into program: _____

11. Are fees charged?   Yes ____ No ____ Amount $_____

12. Estimated annual cost:

    Personnel: _____   $ _____

    _____   $ _____

    Supplies: _____   $ _____

    _____   $ _____

13. Other information: _____

    _____

    _____

    _____

    _____

ago. In addition to Kimura, the clinic staff consists of a clinic director, two physicians, six nurse practitioners, a mental health coordinator, and support staff. Together, they provide primary care services for approximately 12,000 individuals. The stated goals of the clinic are

**1.** To provide primary care services

**2.** To match sick and well care needs with the most appropriate resources (physician, nurse practitioner, health educator, mental health professional, and/or audiovisual materials)

**3.** To increase adherence to treatment through intensified follow-up

**4.** To encourage new clients to develop a personalized health improvement program with the collaboration of the clinic team

From the onset of clinic operation, the structure and overall goals and policies of the clinic clearly identified a meaningful role for the health educator. The clinic director had allocated a budget, space, and other resources for health education services. A health education assistant and part-time secretary were hired as support staff. The organization chart is shown in Figure 3.7.

The health educator functions primarily as a provider of direct educational services. Kimura sees patients individually and consults with other providers about the progress of particular patients. For example, a physician might direct to her a hypertensive patient who wants to start an exercise program. The health educator's flexible schedule and formal health education background allow her to conduct a deeper and more thorough needs assessment, and to give the client a better perspective of what is involved in establishing an exercise program that could be sustained over time. In order to perform effectively in this role, Kimura obtained additional training beyond the required degree (master's of public health education) by taking coursework in counseling, clinical skills, nutrition, exercise, and stress management. Her job description appears in Figure 3.8.

**Figure 3.7   Primary care clinic organization chart**

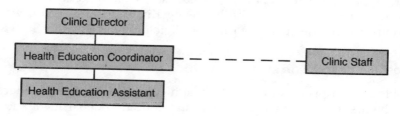

**Figure 3.8   Job description: health educator**

1. Provide direct patient care, conduct health education interventions for individual clients and groups, and provide consultation for patients referred by the clinic staff

2. Assemble data concerning the health status of clients entering the primary-care clinic, select those behaviors requiring modification that are most amenable to change, and plan health education interventions to implement these changes

3. Help design patient education progress forms to be included in the client medical record, and document health education activities in patient medical records

4. Administer a fitness test and health hazard appraisal program, and help patient interpret results

5. Select and/or develop cost-effective, creative, and relevant educational methods for influencing health behaviors and actions

6. Make recommendations to the clinic director and assist in the formulation of short- and long-term health education goals

In her role as direct provider, Kimura initially designed a health improvement self-assessment questionnaire that became part of the medical chart. The questionnaire (which is shown in Chapter 9) goes beyond clinical measurements and observations to include educational diagnosis.

Since one of the clinic's goals is to include health education as part of primary care, the health educator is also involved in redirecting staff orientation from an emphasis on sick care to both sick and well care. Kimura designed and conducted part of an intensive training program on how to effectively incorporate educational principles into the therapeutic encounter. Currently, she regularly reviews charts with clinic staff to ensure that they effectively document educational intervention and follow-up. Kimura also documents all her visits with clients. A sample of her patient education documentation is shown in Figure 3.9.

Because the staff refer clients regularly to the health educator and because clients themselves experience health education as an important part of their medical care, the health educator's role is closely linked with the rest of the clinic staff. Withdrawing Kimura's contribution would seriously affect the quality of care the clinic provides.

## Position description summary

Table 3.1 is a profile of the three health educators. The health educator in the first example manages the health education department and has

## Figure 3.9  Example of chart documentation

*Key*

| | | | |
|---|---|---|---|
| BP | blood pressure | CV | cardiovascular disease |
| ↗ | elevated, or increased | DM | diabetes mellitus |
| FBS | fasting blood sugar | 35 y.o. | 35 years old |
| Chol | cholesterol | RTC | return to clinic |
| Fam hx | family history | prn | when needed |

Symptom: Pt. referred by Smith M.D. for lifestyle change. Reports health conditions of ↗ BP, ↗ FBS, ↗ Chol, Fam hx CV and DM, poor results of physical fitness test. 35 y.o. white male Franciscan brother lives in Franciscan home. Meals cooked for him, often hi fat, lg. desserts, much soda, 0 reg. eating or exercise pattern. High stress due to class work overload. Has 2 brothers at house to talk with re personal concerns and with mutual behavior change interest. Feels good about living situation and work. Fearful of impaired health status and feels ready to make lifestyle change.

Objective: BP: 146/94. FBS: 129. Chol: 324.
Pt. stated link between lifestyle and health conditions. Able to identify alternatives and avenues for ↗ support.

Assessment: High-Risk Status--Cardiovascular problems. Good support system. Temporary stress situation due to school pressures. Very fearful of CV and DM complications he has seen in family members.

Plan:
1. Discuss alternative menu plan with cook.
2. Keep 7-day food and exercise records to observe patterns.
3. Discuss support possibilities for behavior change with other brothers in house.
4. Reinforced concern/interest and motivation at this time.
5. RTC 2 weeks. Call prn.

institution-wide responsibilities. The health educator in the second example develops patient education programs operating at a programmatic level. The health educator in the third example provides direct patient services and therefore functions at the individual level. Notice from the chart that the reporting relationships, size of staff, and budget allocation will depend on the position's requirements and on departmental history.

**Table 3.1   Position descriptions: summary**

| Primary level | Institutional example | Programmatic example | Individual example |
| --- | --- | --- | --- |
| Title | Director, health education | Patient education coordinator | Health educator |
| Major role | Manager | Coordinator | Provider |
| Professional training (degree) | Master's in Public Health Education | R.N., B.S. in Nursing | Master's in Public Health Education |
| Supervisor's title | Hospital administrator/ chief, patient education | Nursing education coordinator | Clinic director |
| Number of employees | 9 (health educator, counselor, librarian, and library assistants) | None | 1 (health education assistant) |
| Budget (includes salary and benefits) | $210,000/year | $26,000/year | $50,000/year |
| Salary/month (range) | $2300–$2800 | $2100–$2500 | $1900–$2300 |
| History of health education department | Yes, 13 years | No | No |
| Type of hospital | Fee-for-service medical center | Community hospital | Primary care clinic |
| Size of hospital staff | 1,800 | 450 | 20 |

## ROLES OF THE HEALTH EDUCATOR

The three examples just given show health educators functioning in five primary roles: manager, coordinator, provider, trainer, and consultant. In the following section, we examine the major responsibilities associated with each of these roles.

## Health educator as manager

Health educators often become managers without much formal management training. As managers, our primary responsibility is to supervise the health education staff and direct the activities of the health education department. We must forecast and operate within budgets, which may include generating revenue for our departments. We must hire, train, and evaluate health education staff. We must direct the educational efforts of the medical care setting. And we must oversee the planning, development, coordination, and evaluation of educational programs for clients and staff.

**Leadership qualities of the manager.**  As managers, the ability to lead and define our purposes is critical. In Example 1, the director of health education could never have developed a staff of nine people and implemented forty educational programs without a vision of the potential for organization-wide health education services. In a health care setting that has already been established, has firm ground rules, and that may not be entirely pliant to the visions of a beginning health educator, such an educator must have strong leadership qualities. And in fact, Benz had both a purpose and the ability to encourage, excite, influence, and direct those around her to realize that purpose.

As health educators, we must be able to use formal and informal channels of communication and to articulate the needs of our department. And our ability to lead must reflect an understanding for the people we are working with—whether they be colleagues, clients, administrators, or supervisors. Certain abilities are critical: to demonstrate the success of past efforts, to document the effective use of resources, and to clearly demonstrate the interrelationships between the goals, philosophies, and practices of the organization and those of the health education department. We may need all the foregoing skills, for example, in discussing the integration of an educational service into the treatment of a certain category of patients with a chief of service over lunch, or in giving a presentation at a department managers' meeting.

**Personnel management.**  Personnel management and development, a skill acquired through experience, is of particular importance to the health education manager. As managers, we must be able to develop job descriptions; hire, train, and dismiss staff; establish performance standards; and conduct performance appraisals (Chapman, 1975). Although many organizations provide training workshops in management development, applying general supervisory principles and policies to specific situations can be difficult—as in firing an employee, for example. The general policy provides information regarding the process. If the employee's performance does not improve, the manager then completes progressive disciplinary action, which includes counseling memos, letters of warning, suspension, and termination. The policy, however, does not tell how to discuss the problem with the employee, nor how to conduct an exit interview. Similarly, a policy statement on hiring new employees may state the steps to follow in the hiring process, but does not aid in interpreting résumés or provide skills for conducting a good interview. The following list gives several points for conducting good interviews that do not appear in departmental hiring policy (Dickelman and Broadwell, 1977):

**1.** Prior to the interview, review the job description and the applicant's résumé. Take note of unexplained lapses in employment, number of jobs held within a given year, the relationship between prior work experience/education and the position.

**2.** Set a comfortable climate for the interview. Face the applicant directly, avoid sitting behind a desk, offer a beverage, and begin the interview with a reference to an item in the résumé that impressed you.

**3.** Ask open-ended questions: "Please describe your present job and responsibilities." "Discuss some of the problems you encountered on your job." "What in your background particularly qualified you to do the job?" "What position would you like to have in five years? Ten years?"

**4.** Avoid sensitive questions regarding age, child care, arrest records, religious practices, disabilities, marital status, ethnicity, or whether the applicant is a U.S. citizen. (In many states such questions are illegal.)

**5.** Once you have been given information about the applicant's qualifications, provide the applicant with information about the position: its duties and responsibilities, promotion potential, the challenges and rewards the job offers. Close the interview by telling the applicant the steps that will follow.

**6.** Evaluate the applicant. Immediately record your impressions, consider strong and weak qualities, and compare to other applicants.

**Personal qualities of a manager.**   The health education manager, like any other manager, must possess certain personal qualities that demonstrate an ability and interest in working with people on the staff. The supervisor must be impartial, open-minded, and able to express concerns and draw on the qualities of the staff. Arbitrary decisions, threats, and ambiguous directions detract from employee trust and respect. The manager who is able to communicate effectively, who leads rather than controls, who is straightforward and honest, and who can delegate with encouragement will attract and promote skilled, competent, and motivated employees (Eddy and Warner, 1980).

## Health educator as coordinator

As coordinators, we are responsible for organization-wide development and coordination of comprehensive, consistent, and well-integrated health education services. Health education services are comprehensive when they provide a balance of educational services for both sick and well clients, consistent when the program adheres to prescribed medical policies, and integrated when they are a meaningful aspect of all inpatient, outpatient, home health, and rehabilitation patient care services.

How do we provide programs that are comprehensive, consistent, and well integrated? One way is to help the hospital or clinic confront and solve problems related to health education services. For example, if the nutrition and medical departments offer their own hypertension education programs, we are responsible for ensuring that they reinforce and complement each other rather than duplicate or contradict each other. Consumers would be understandably angry if they attended two programs covering the same information. Similarly, we ensure that the information given to an expectant mother in a prenatal class coincides with what will actually happen to her in the prenatal clinic. The following situations also pose problems, yet are typical of the kinds of issues coordinators face and are expected to resolve:

- An instructor has an alcoholic in his or her stop smoking group.
- A physician has filed a complaint against a program or instructor.
- Two powerful members of the staff have opposing views about how to approach an identified need.
- A class has a high attrition rate or low enrollment.
- Two instructors want to co-teach a program that has been budgeted for one instructor.

It is the task of the health educator to work with the individuals, departments, administration, and clients involved to resolve these problems before they create barriers to providing quality health education services.

We also need to be able to work effectively in committees. Health educators often establish planning committees in order to involve the staff as much as possible in program development. The committee may be an interdisciplinary committee composed of key representatives from various hospital departments or an ad hoc committee representing people with expertise on the identified topic. Whenever possible we need to choose committee members who can best contribute in terms of advice, interest, support, influence, and technical expertise. Sometimes, however, we may want to involve a key individual who is unsupportive but whose support, if enlisted, could positively affect the acceptance and outcome of the program. At other times, we may not have the authority to choose committee members.

As members of the planning group, health educators are responsible for facilitating a team effort. We act as mediators, to help individuals with different viewpoints understand and agree on the issues; as facilitators, to encourage others to contribute and give feedback; and as liaison between relevant parties, to improve communication and build trust. For example, in planning a preoperative education program, we may need to involve representatives of nursing, volunteers, surgery, anesthesiology, admitting, laboratory, and administration. All these players have valuable contributions to the program's success. Our role is to gather and synthesize pertinent information, get agreement on the plan, write the

**Figure 3.10    Time line for preoperative education program**

| Activity | J | F | M | A | M | J | J | A | S | O | N | D |
|---|---|---|---|---|---|---|---|---|---|---|---|---|
| • Administration/patient education committee approves concept of preoperative program. | — | | | | | | | | | | | |
| • Form preoperative task force. | — | | | | | | | | | | | |
| • Develop and get approval of preoperative program proposal. | | — | — | — | | | | | | | | |
| • Recruit staff. | | | | — | | | | | | | | |
| • Provide staff training and development. | | | | | — | | | | | | | |
| • Develop preoperative patient checklist: list of steps to complete prior to surgery. | | | | — | — | | | | | | | |
| • Obtain relaxation tape, pamphlets, and visual aids for program. | | | | — | — | — | | | | | | |
| • Develop program publicity (flyers, newsletters, preview of preoperative film); present at physician meetings. | | | | | — | — | | | | | | |
| • Implement pilot program. | | | | | | | | | — | — | | |
| • Preliminary evaluation; make necessary changes. Implement revised program. | | | | | | | | | | | — | — |

proposal (including objectives, lesson plans, criteria for evaluation, program budget), and distribute the proposal for further input. During this process, we continuously balance the need to gather sufficient information with the desire to move the project along to completion. The timeline shown in Figure 3.10 illustrates one program-planning tool balancing the sequence and timing of activities to implement a preoperative education program.

## Health educator as provider

In some health care settings, health educators are required to provide direct health education service to clients. For example, the health educator employed in a primary care clinic discussed earlier sees clients individually about identifying specific health risks and embarking on a personal plan to minimize those risks. More commonly, however, we provide services to clients in groups. For example, we might lead a stop smoking group or conduct a hypertension class. Ideas about how people learn have changed dramatically over the years, and this change has greatly influenced the health educator's role as instructor (Knowles, 1978). The focus has shifted from the teacher to the learner, from the content to the process. A few of the major changes are shown in Table 3.2.

**Table 3.2   Factors that inhibit or facilitate learning**

| Inhibits learning | Facilitates learning |
| --- | --- |
| • Instructor is authority figure—behavior is stiff and professional. | • Instructor is facilitator—behavior is friendly and informal. |
| • Instructor maintains teacher/student relationship. | • Instructor treats participants as equals and as self-directors. |
| • Instructor transmits content. | • Instructor involves participant—participants teach each other. |
| • Instructor is unapproachable. | • Instructor encourages sharing of feelings, including his or her own. |
| • Instructor cuts off participants. | • Instructor responds to participants. |
| • Instructor determines needs and sets objectives. | • Instructor and participants mutually negotiate objectives. |
| • Instructor assumes participant experience is of little worth. | • Instructor taps rich resources of the group. |
| • Instructor evaluates participants. | • Instructor and participants mutually measure progress. |

**Assessing group needs.**   As instructors, health educators need to be able to assess a group's needs and tailor the lesson plan accordingly (Freedman, 1978). Although lesson plans are important because they help us organize content, they become meaningless if the information is not relevant to the group. Before beginning the program, we can benefit from assessing what the group members want to know about the topic and what they already know. During the program, we need to continue monitoring and responding to class participants. If, for example, a group of cancer patients of varying ages and educational levels may need learning exercises that will bring them together as a group regardless of their individual differences. In this case, prior information about the group composition helps prepare for the program.

**Selecting teaching methods.**   Another function of an instructor is to select and use a variety of educational approaches (Davis, 1976; Pfeiffer and Jones, 1975). Many of us choose teaching methods because we feel comfortable using them even though they may not always be appropriate. A better approach would be to review the numerous educational methods—which include such activities as role playing, group discussion, and brainstorming—and to carefully weigh the advantages and disadvantages of each. A few criteria we can use when selecting teaching methods are size of group, learning objectives, course content, competence and comfort level of instructor, time available, potential for increasing participant involvement, and the audience's experience and background. Chapters 5 and 6 describe further how instructors can better assess and respond to class participants as well as choose and apply appropriate educational methods. Chapters 7, 8, and 9 cover individual patient assessment and counseling.

## Health educator as trainer

As trainers, health educators are responsible for employee training, specifically as it applies to health education. Our role is to help staff develop and improve their skills in patient teaching, in educational assessment, in educational intervention, and in referral. Typically, we design and teach courses on educational theory and practice for those staff members who are instructors of patient education programs. Training other health professionals requires the necessary content expertise as well as skills in communication, group process, and teaching (Ingals, 1973). And we need to accomplish all this in a nonthreatening and supportive manner. Throughout the training process, we must be keenly aware of the potential for territorial conflict and must support in theory and in practice the concept of team effort.

As health educators, we are in a unique position to stimulate and encourage instructors to share their experience and expertise. By holding formal meetings of all instructors, we can provide a forum for the exchange of information and skills. The following example shows the objectives for a training workshop given to a group of health education instructors in a teaching hospital in Minnesota: by the end of the workshop, each participating instructor should be able to

**1.** Analyze an audience and adapt class plans and teaching methods to meet the needs of each group

**2.** Increase student participation by practicing different teaching methods

**3.** Effectively use instructional media/materials

**4.** Understand the overall role of the health education department and identify ways that the department can better support educational classes

**5.** Identify and discuss methods to evaluate his or her ongoing class as a means to assess the effectiveness of his or her presentation

**6.** Develop an action plan that will specifically outline future changes in his or her class

As you review the workshop objectives, note those objectives that go beyond instructor skill development to promote the concept of instructor team development. An offshoot of the training was the establishment of noon-time health education workshops (continuing education training). These miniworkshops, or brown-bag lunch meetings, bring together all health education instructors.

The impact of the training and support group benefits both the instructors and the health education department. Instructors use the support group as a place to share ideas and skills and to consult with one another on specific class problems or innovative teaching methods. The training helped foster a feeling of identification with the health education department. The workshop helped instructors recognize that their classes were linked to one another. For example, the hypertension class instructor now refers a hypertensive patient who may need additional help in losing weight or stopping smoking directly into the weight control or stop smoking clinic. Also, as a result of the workshop several instructors worked with the health educator to develop a health education patient referral form for use by instructors and hospital staff.

**Health educator as consultant**

As internal consultants, we assist departments in identifying and pursuing their health education goals. For example, we may be asked to consult with a department on methods for (1) setting priorities for the educational needs of the department, (2) developing a systematic method for referring clients to educational programs, (3) reviewing and revamping existing educational programs, (4) designing a means of chart documentation for patients attending educational programs, or (5) helping staff members assess their skills in patient teaching.

As consultants, we help solve the health education problems of other departments and make recommendations. In the examples just mentioned, we must be aware of constraints, such as staff shortages, financial constraints, and other more pressing departmental priorities that may block our recommendations (Mullen and Zapka, 1982).

Up to now we have outlined a number of roles that health educators fill in medical care settings. These descriptions were fleshed out of our own experiences and the experiences of hundreds of colleagues in the field. However, in any one institution, key individuals may not understand the range of competencies and services that health educators offer.

## THE AMBIGUOUS ROLE OF THE HEALTH EDUCATOR

The health educator's role in the medical care delivery system is often poorly defined. In fact, most health education positions require the ability to function in all the roles we have just described. Although a policy statement approved by top-level decision makers can help provide legitimacy and organizational commitment to health education services, ambiguity may still exist. You will find a different set of expectations for the role of health educator depending on whom you talk to—an administrator, nursing supervisor, chief of service, or consumer. We also have our own professional standards, which dictate our role expectations. This lack of agreement about the role of a health educator has both benefits and drawbacks, as discussed in the next sections.

### Benefits of ambiguity

Discretionary power is the most important benefit of our fluid, dynamic role definition. We are often free to clarify and pursue our own priorities for health education based on our professional knowledge and experience. We can define, within broad guidelines, what we expect to accomplish and how we expect to accomplish it. If we, for example, determine that documentation of program attendance and patient progress in the medical chart is a priority, we can rally support from physicians and/or administrators and pursue this objective.

In fact, we are sometimes referred to as "jacks-of-all-trades" because we are not limited by a narrow perspective of our role. Since a health educator's tasks are predominantly self-scheduled, we have the flexibility to adapt to changing priorities as the need arises. We are not limited by policies and procedures that dictate every action or decision. A flexible job allows us to accomplish the most pressing tasks first. Ultimately, this flexibility allows the most creative contributions to emerge.

## Drawbacks of ambiguity

Sometimes, however, a lack of consensus concerning job expectations can have unhappy consequences. When the role expectations of various client groups conflict or are unclear, it is impossible to meet them all. At the same time, it is difficult to judge our own job performance. Differing role expectations, both overt and covert, continuously vie for position. One minute we are champions for consumer rights and the next bureaucrats appeasing angry clients who must wait three months for a stop smoking group.

Caught in the middle between client demand and organizational constraints, we must respond to a wide array of conflicting demands. For instance, the administrator may want proof of the financial benefits of specific programs before allocating resources to health education. Potential benefits may include decreased costs and measurable health outcomes of financially self-supporting programs. Based on these criteria, for example, the administrator may be unwilling to pay for a weight control class. Yet physicians, weight control instructors, and clients may demand services regardless of cost or proven effectiveness.

Our own expectations for health education, based on our own professional training and personal interests, may also conflict with the expectations of other professionals. For example, co-workers may expect us to develop and distribute informational pamphlets for their departments. However, our approach is to examine various educational methods and then decide on the method that best fits the intended purpose. Sometimes pamphlets do not fill the need.

With limited resources, we cannot possibly meet all these expectations. Unfortunately, health education often spreads its resources too thin; it ends up devoting only little effort to any one expectation and thus fails to achieve anything significant. And sometimes health education focuses its resources but leaves too many expectations unmet—

which again results in a serious lack of credibility. For example, providing educational services for stroke patients and their families may be a priority that is identified at the institution in which you work. You may only have the resources to provide one two-hour seminar and discussion group, four times a year. Will this type of educational service have the medical and social outcomes that you, your clients, and the providers expect?

Table 3.3 summarizes some of the benefits and drawbacks of fluid role definitions. Can you think of others?

## Role conflicts

Many jobs in hospitals or clinics involve challenge. That challenge stems from the pivotal role that we are often asked to play among various health professionals. Three potential areas of conflict that can arise are (1) promoting interdepartmental cooperation in developing health education

**Table 3.3    Benefits and drawbacks of an ambiguous role**

| Benefits | Drawbacks |
|---|---|
| • Latitude in program development | • Conflicting role expectations |
| • Freedom to set own priorities | • Difficulty in measuring performance |
| • Ability to define own standards of success | • Lack of credibility |
| • More creativity | • Increased territorial conflicts |
| • More discretionary power | • Less recognition |
| • More control over job (able to increase job scope | • Lack of relevance to the organization |
| | • Feelings of low self-esteem or job burnout |
| • Less "red tape" (don't have to go through oppressive approval process) | • Low visibility |
| • Freedom to choose whom you want to work with | • Poor interdepartmental cooperation |
| • Increased job flexibility | • Too many organizational expectations for limited resources |
| • Ability to accomplish more | |

programs, (2) supervising staff with different professional affiliations who conduct these programs, and (3) being accountable for high-quality programs but not always having the power to achieve and/or maintain that quality. These three conflict areas are discussed next, followed by a few suggestions for overcoming these and other conflicts characteristic of our role.

**Promoting interdepartmental cooperation.** In order to ensure a health education program's eventual success, we often bring together the skills and expertise of many health professionals. For example, we may form an advisory committee composed of representatives from various departments to develop a preoperative education program. Among other reasons, we want to ensure that the information in the program is accurate and relevant, as well as to promote joint ownership and eventual patient referral to the program.

However, enlisting cooperation from a vast array of people with different professional and management functions creates many challenges. Depending on their professional training and socialization, these individuals may operate quite differently. For instance, health educators are trained as compromisers who attempt to balance the demands and perspectives of others. Physicians and administrators may find this balancing act, with its preoccupation on involvement of others, and a focus on process rather than on problems, both tedious and a waste of time.

**Conflicts over supervision.** The role of the health educator as a supervisor of other health professionals is often a cause of role conflict. Because professionals have an identity or affiliation with their own professional group, they may challenge our right to supervise them. Whether a psychologist, social worker, nutritionist, or librarian, their affiliation to their own professional group is understandably greater than their commitment to health education. If they don't share our values and approaches regarding educational methodology and practice, the situation may lead to conflict. As trained health educators, we may see the diet prescription as just one component of a diabetes class, whereas the instructor may believe that the diet prescription is the purpose of the class. Similarly, in a weight control class, the psychologist may focus solely on the psychological issues of being overweight, neglecting diet and exercise components—which we believe are equally important. However, as health educators we are able to combine the instructor's content expertise with our own understanding of the behavior change process. As experts in health behavior change—the overall purpose of education programs—we are eminently qualified to supervise health education instructors.

**Responsibility without power.**   A major role conflict occurs when we struggle to carry out our assigned responsibilities but feel frustrated because we haven't been given sufficient power to do what needs to be done. Technically, we often act as consultants when assisting various departments in matters pertaining to health education services. In these cases, we have no real authority to make the decisions that affect these services, yet we are held responsible for the services.

For instance, we may determine that the format, curriculum, and teaching methods used in a hypertension class are outdated and ineffective. We may advocate that a series of classes, as opposed to a single class session, will improve patient compliance. Even though the literature, the instructor, and the supervisor support the proposed program changes, the chief of medicine, who controls the budget, may be unsympathetic toward health education or may feel a more pressing use for valuable staff time. In this example, we have no direct power to make the necessary improvements. Nevertheless, we are responsible for the success and quality of the program.

In another example, the health education department may want to work jointly with the dietary department to offer a comprehensive diabetes teaching program that includes medical and nutritional components. The dietary department may instead choose to work independently, arguing that the nutritionist's schedule cannot be adjusted to accommodate classroom teaching and that the department's major responsibility is to prescribe diets. In this situation, the patient receives fragmented information as a result of having to attend both a general diabetes education program and a separate program on diet instruction. Even though cooperation between health education and the dietary department could prove to be mutually beneficial in terms of ensuring continuity of care and improving patient services, the health educator in this case does not have the authority to make these changes.

## Conflict resolution

Since conflict is an inherent characteristic of the role, our ability to recognize and effectively manage conflict is critical. By training or disposition we may tend to avoid conflict; our liking for compromise and/or a fear of negative repercussions can block our ability to recognize its positive aspects and its power for change. Several strategies for resolving conflict are as follows:

Strategy 1. *Get support.* Build relationships with powerful figures in the organization, among peers, and with clients who use health education services. All these resource people can give health education needed backing and support as well as provide important channels of communication. In the aforementioned example, you might enlist the support of a physician with administrative authority to seek a solution to fragmented diabetic education services.

Strategy 2. *Be part of the solution.* In order to increase relevance to and visibility within the organization, you must have a firm handle on larger organizational problems, goals, needs, and systems. How can the health education department help solve these problems? Do the goals of the health education department reflect the goals of the organization? What added responsibilities can you assume that have organization-wide significance?

Strategy 3. *Seek help.* In some situations, it may be appropriate to ask for assistance from an outside arbitrator. Internal consultants, often called "organizational development specialists," specialize in conflict negotiation and resolution. They may work with groups of employees or with employees and their supervisors via role clarification, problem solving, constructive confrontation techniques, and team-building methods to improve their interdependent efforts (Ross and Mico, 1980).

Strategy 4. *Weigh the options.* Another option is to recognize when it is to your advantage to fight for what you want and when it is better to pursue other goals that you can better achieve. Sometimes you must be satisfied with planting seeds and waiting for their fruition. You need to possess special qualities of optimism, patience, and especially perseverance (Squyres, 1982).

Strategy 5. *Identify and sharpen your skills.* Health education students need the benefit of a field placement experience to help them develop their skills and interests. The placement should be long enough in duration and complex enough in scope to provide an introductory experience of health education practice to the student approaching graduation.

We must not be led to believe that, because we are generalists, we can successfully meet the responsibilities of all roles. Our professional training is often weak in preparing us for certain managerial tasks such as personnel management and financial analysis. Likewise, depending on the requirements of the position, we may be weak in certain clinical skills such as psychosocial assessment of individual patients or interpreting medical charts.

As practicing health educators, we need to enroll in continuing education courses to develop those skills required for a position in medical care. Community and state colleges, universities, and community agencies such as the American Cancer Society or the American Heart Association offer many courses in health education and related topics. Employers may also sponsor employee development and training workshops. In addition, we can join professional associations, including the Society for Public Health Education (SOPHE), the American Public Health Association (APHA), or the American Society for Training and Development (ASTD). These organizations encourage information sharing, skill development and professional support.

Strategy 6. *Clarify your role.* Finally, as health educators become more prevalent in medical care, it is increasingly important that we sharpen the definition of our role. We need to develop job standards that clarify our role, work with administrative teams to set goals for health education, and develop policy statements that define our departments and the services we provide. We must accept the challenge to critically evaluate our role in medical care and help shape our future.

These six strategies serve to reduce role conflict. They also serve to clear the decks for making decisions about how to set up a program, as is discussed in the chapters of Part Two, especially in Chapter 4.

# EXERCISES

1.  *Role ambiguity:* A variety of expectations often accompanies the role of health educator in medical care. The chart on page 87 lists some of these expectations (or performance indicators) down the left side and health education client groups across the top.
    a.  Complete the grid on the chart. For example, ask yourself if reducing costs—the first item listed under "expectations/performance indicators"—might be an expectation that the hospital administrator has of the health educator. If so, check the square as shown. Continue to ask yourself this same question as you move across the top "client groups" grid to physicians, nursing department, and so on. Feel free to add any additional expectations or client groups to the chart.
    b.  As you completed the grid, what criteria did you use to match the expectations in the lefthand column with each client group? On a separate sheet of paper, list the criteria, with a rationale for each. If possible, interview representative(s) from each client group and test the accuracy of your predictions.

| Expectations/Performance Indicators | Client Groups | | | | | | | |
|---|---|---|---|---|---|---|---|---|
| | Hospital Administration | Medical Doctor/ Nurse Practitioner | Instructor | Advisory Group | Clients | Staff | | |
| *Example:* Reduce costs | ✔ | | | | | | | |
| 1. Improve community relations | | | | | | | | |
| 2. Improve client health status | | | | | | | | |
| 3. Meet needs of client | | | | | | | | |
| 4. Enhance client satisfaction | | | | | | | | |
| 5. Provide consumer advocacy | | | | | | | | |
| 6. Provide community services | | | | | | | | |
| 7. Increase health promotion | | | | | | | | |
| 8. Increase patient education | | | | | | | | |
| 9. Increase use of educational service | | | | | | | | |
| 10. Increase physician satisfaction | | | | | | | | |
| 11. Increase physician involvement | | | | | | | | |
| 12. Improve departmental relations | | | | | | | | |
| 13. Provide employee health programs | | | | | | | | |
| 14. Increase department accountability | | | | | | | | |
| 15. Maintain low profile | | | | | | | | |
| 16. Maintain high visibility | | | | | | | | |
| 17. Provide loyalty/support | | | | | | | | |
| 18. Increase department credibility | | | | | | | | |
| 19. Enhance personal leadership/recognition | | | | | | | | |
| 20. Broaden staff acceptance of health education | | | | | | | | |

2.  *Skills inventory:* Whether you are a student beginning a new career or considering a job change, identifying your own special likes/dislikes, strengths/weaknesses can help you obtain a satisfying position in health education. The chart on pages 89–90 lists a number of common skills required for a health education position.

    a.  Complete the "role(s)" column on the chart by determining the role or roles that pertain to each of the skills listed. Use the following code for the roles: M = Manager, C = Coordinator, T = Trainer, P = Provider, and CN = Consultant.

    b.  Assess whether and at what level you possess each skill. Rate your proficiency level in Column B and interest level in Column C on a scale from 1 (lowest level) to 5 (highest level). Think about your past work and volunteer experiences, courses you have taken, and tasks that you have found easy or difficult to perform.

    c.  After you have completed the chart, summarize your strengths and weaknesses. Star (*) the skills you both enjoy using and are good at. Note which roles and/or skills appeared repeatedly. Check (✔) the skills that you are interested in developing but do not have proficiency in. Then write an action plan on a separate sheet of paper. Your action plan should be specific, goal directed, reasonably achievable, and something you can begin to work on now. For example, if you choose to develop computer skills, your action plan may include taking an introductory computer course at the local community college beginning in three weeks.

| Strengths (*) | Weaknesses (✔) | Action Plan |
|---|---|---|
| 1. _____ | _____ | _____ |
|  |  | _____ |
| 2. _____ | _____ | _____ |
|  |  | _____ |
| 3. _____ | _____ | _____ |
|  |  | _____ |

3.  *The Job Interview:* Finding a good fit between the health educator role set out in a job description and your special talents and interests is not an easy task. But remember, an interview is a two-way communication process. Interviewing the interviewer is an important

| Skill area<br>Ability to . . . | A. Role(s) | B. Proficiency<br>Level (1–5) | C. Interest<br>Level (1–5) |
|---|---|---|---|
| • Lead and manage<br>people | M | | |
| • Analyze and solve<br>problems | | | |
| • Work in unstructured<br>situations using<br>creativity | | | |
| • Organize information<br>or systems | | | |
| • Carry out and follow<br>through on projects<br>and instructions | | | |
| • Work with people to<br>inform, train,<br>develop, help | | | |
| • Build power and<br>enlist support to<br>accomplish goals | | | |
| • Persuade and<br>influence others | | | |
| • Manage money,<br>develop budgets,<br>allocate resources | | | |
| • Handle many tasks<br>and responsibilities<br>simultaneously | | | |
| • Mediate and<br>negotiate conflict | | | |
| • Address large or<br>small groups | | | |
| • Bring about change | | | |
| • Make difficult<br>decisions | | | |
| • Take risks | | | |
| • Facilitate meetings | | | |

*(Continued)*

| Skill area<br>Ability to . . . | A. Role(s) | B. Proficiency<br>Level (1–5) | C. Interest<br>Level (1–5) |
|---|---|---|---|
| • Plan, implement, and monitor educational programs | | | |
| • Get diverse groups to work together | | | |
| • Apply special understanding of health related topic(s) | | | |
| • Evaluate staff performance | | | |
| • Identify health education needs | | | |
| • Set priorities | | | |
| • Create, acquire, review, use teaching materials | | | |
| • Provide educational consultation | | | |
| • Represent others | | | |
| • Predict behavior outcomes of health education strategies | | | |
| • Apply educational principles | | | |
| • Communicate orally and in writing | | | |
| • Employ group process techniques | | | |

skill that you can develop. Be sure about your assessment of the job and whether it interests you before you accept a new position.

Choose one of the three job descriptions used in the case studies. See Figures 3.3, 3.5, and 3.8. Imagine you are applying for this job. List ten questions you might want to ask a prospective employer (such as "How are priorities for this department set?" and "Who is my immediate supervisor?").

# RESOURCES

Bolles, R. *What Color Is Your Parachute?* Berkeley, Calif.: Ten Speed Press, 1983.

An overview of career and life planning and principles of successful job hunting, updated annually. Includes helpful exercises to help you identify the job you would love to do and a step-by-step process for getting it. Specific information includes how to determine your functional and transferable skills, negotiate a salary, carry on a successful interview, write a résumé, and cope with rejection shock. The book also includes an appendix of additional job-hunting tools and resources.

Doyle, M., and Straus, D. *How to Make Meetings Work.* New York: Playboy Paperbacks, 1977.

Describes the interactive method of running meetings, which rests on four well-defined roles and responsibilities—group facilitator, recorder, member, and chairperson. Includes practical tools and techniques that can improve the quality of your meetings and make you more effective, whether as a leader of a group or a participant.

Josefitz, N. *Paths to Power.* Reading, Mass.: Addison-Wesley, 1980.

This book is addressed to people, especially women, who want to become more knowledgeable, more effective, and better prepared to face roadblocks to power. After discussing power, the author considers the various phases of work life: looking for a job, the first days at work, the early years, supervision, middle management, top executive level, and retirement.

Kradjian, C. (ed.). *The 1983 Guide to Health Information Resources in Print.* Daly City, Calif.: PAS Publishing, 1983.

This guide provides a comprehensive list of health information resources for educators. It is divided into three sections: "Materials for Professionals," which lists materials for staff training and development; "Materials for Patients," which provides sources for specific teaching aids in 150 categories of health and disease; and "Supplier" listings. The book includes over 3,000 low-cost resources.

Michelozzi, Betty Neville. *Coming Alive from Nine to Five*, 2nd ed. Palo Alto, Calif.: Mayfield, 1984.

This is a warm, witty, and practical guide to the entire process of career planning. Through self-assessment tests and exercises the reader gains awareness, confidence, and a realistic sense of available options. The book contains exercises on skills assessment and decision making and information on work places and work styles as they relate to the whole of one's life.

Plunkett, W. *Supervision: The Direction of People at Work.* Dubuque, Iowa: Brown, 1975.

> Plunkett discusses organizational structure, the managerial function, and the role of the supervisor. General topics include the role of the supervisor, human relations, leadership and management styles, personnel selection, review, discipline, and developing relationships with your boss. Tools of supervision are explained in detail.

Ross, H. S. Health Education Credentialing: The Role Delineation Project. *Focal Points.* Atlanta: Centers for Disease Control, July 1981.

> Ross outlines the skills and knowledge essential to competent performance of the entry-level health educator's role. The role includes seven areas of responsibility, each composed of a number of functions. Performing each function requires certain skills and knowledge. The information in this report was obtained from health educators in school, community, and medical-care settings, and from job descriptions for health educators and the literature on professional preparation.

# PART TWO

## STEPS IN PLANNING AND IMPLEMENTING EDUCATION SERVICES

# 4

# Setting up a program

THIS CHAPTER PAYS special attention to management skills that are pivotal during the planning and early implementation stages of a program. The chapter offers specific and practical guidelines for health educators who are setting up direct educational services for clients, working with other health professionals to plan educational services, or formalizing a health education program in a medical care organization. The message of this chapter is that health educators need not be content to make the best of given situations. Very often, we can make decisions and take actions that ensure that both our services to clients and our programs are successful and our status in the organization is enhanced.

## TIMING

Timing is probably one of the most important skills a health educator can master. It can make or break an individual counseling encounter, a whole program, and an organization-wide health education effort. Setting up a successful health education program requires a superior sense of timing as well as a mature capability for making sound judgments and politically sensitive decisions.

### The timing of direct service

How do you know that the time is right to work with a client on weight loss? When is the best time to suggest that a client join a support group?

When do you involve your client's spouse or parent? One key to those dilemmas is to have a handle on timing. One way to know if now is the time to enter an educational encounter with a client is to assess the situation. There are many questions you can ask yourself before you get started. Table 4.1 is a sample of just a few questions that you may want to begin with. After you read the list in Table 4.1, use a separate sheet of paper to jot down others that come to your mind.

Sometimes health educators can't spend much time assessing the situation before providing direct service to their clients. Clients may ask for guidance in setting up a stop smoking program for themselves. Patients

**Table 4.1   Questions to ask before beginning direct educational service to a client or a group of clients**

1. Do I have an existing relationship with these clients? Can the education be part of our regular, ongoing business (e.g., the provider/patient visit)? Have the clients registered for or referred themselves for an educational service (e.g., breast self-exam class, insulin injection instruction)?

2. Am I ready to begin or to stimulate an educational experience?

3. Am I prepared in both the educational content and in the educational process?

4. Am I prepared to follow through with these clients, even though the educational path may be bumpy or complicated?

5. Can I offer these clients a number of options to choose from that will lead to the educational goal?

6. Have the clients indicated an interest in taking action toward the educational goal?

7. How much do the clients want to add something or change something in their lives that will help them be healthier and happier?

8. Can the clients express their expectations of what they want this educational experience to yield for them? Can they express these expectations in their own words?

9. Have the clients asked for assistance, skills, resources, or referrals?

10. Are the clients ready to start working together with you right now?

11. Do you have the time, the space, and the resources to provide the kind of educational experience that both you and your clients desire?

12. Are there other people—either (1) other providers, educators, or administrators or (2) spouses, family members, or friends of the clients—who should be included during this assessment phase?

receiving medical care for diabetes may express disappointment in not having lost weight. During a visit for an immunization, a child's parent may let you know that the responsibilities of parenting are sometimes overwhelming. In these cases, a few preliminary, probing questions can demonstrate your interest in their problems and can allow you to gather more information. Within a short period of time, you may be able to decide if you are willing and prepared to begin the educational experience, if the client is truly ready for education, or if you had better refer the client to another educator or educational program.

It can be rewarding for you to follow an educational experience from beginning to end with one client. You can make return appointments with the client, document educational progress in health records or medical charts, and support the client through various steps to achieve the goal. Sometimes, however, you will not have the luxury of this kind of long-term relationship. You may only have an opportunity to start the educational process. Once you have paved the way, you may refer the client to a longer-term program in the community, to a structured self-instructional guidebook, or to another educator who can continue the work with the client.

## Timing the start of new programs

How do you know if the time is right to introduce an educational program for a specific target group? Is any time all right as long as there is client interest and demand? Is it the right time if you have an energetic, highly motivated clinician who will be the educator for a program? Is it the right time because the administrator has special interest in a particular topic? Table 4.2 shows the type of questions you may want to ask yourself. The answers to these questions can guide your sense of timing for the introduction of new programs. Once you have read these questions, write down on a separate sheet of paper two or three more that come to mind.

The case study that follows gives you an opportunity to think about the forces in the organization that affect your decisions on timing the start of new programs. Key questions to answer and a useful technique for setting priorities are given as tools you can use to marshal these forces when planning new programs.

A community hospital in one Midwestern town had a health education committee that worked closely with the health education coordinator to set priorities for developing new programs for the year. The committee decided several years ago that the hospital should provide health promotion classes as a service to the community. The hospital administrator gave the health educator coordinator a budget for these programs. The time came for the committee to advise the health edu-

**Table 4.2    Questions to ask before beginning new health education programs**

1. Does the educational program fit the objectives and mandate of the health education department within the organization?
2. Is the proposed program consistent with the priorities that have been set for the year?
3. Is simultaneous interest in this program being expressed by clients, providers, educators, managers, and administrators?
4. Does existing evidence support the proposed benefits of the program?
5. Are there sufficient space, resources, and expertise in the organization to support such a program?
6. Do you have the support and cooperation of the departments who should be, or will be, involved?

cation coordinator on two new programs for the coming year. Before they listed all the potential programs they could recommend, they restated their definition of a health promotion program as "an educational service that focuses on providing information, skills, and support, both physical and psychosocial, to well people who want to stay well, or to people who wish to contain or modify unhealthy activities."

The committee spent twenty minutes simply listing recommended potential health promotion programs for the coming year. The list included programs on

1. Immunizations
2. Health hazard appraisal
3. Weight management for adults
4. Weight management for teens
5. Self-care
6. Nutrition
7. Health behavior change
8. Drug abuse education
9. Family planning
10. Cardiopulmonary resuscitation
11. Accident prevention
12. Alcohol information

**13.** Smoking prevention

**14.** First aid

**15.** How to use the health care system

**16.** Stress management

**17.** Home blood pressure monitoring

**18.** Body image and self-concept

Once the list was developed, the health education coordinator asked the committee members to consider each proposed program on the list and to rate each program on (1) the magnitude of effort that it would take to plan, implement, and evaluate each program and (2) whether the program is a high priority or a low priority given the hospital's objectives for the year. Then the ten-member committee split into three smaller discussion groups. These small groups discussed, and then rated, each proposed program on the criteria of effort and priority. After thirty minutes of discussion, the small groups reported their findings to the larger group. Figure 4.1 shows the kind of grid the committee members made to help them choose two new programs for the coming year. The numbers match the list presented earlier; for example, 1 = immunizations; 6 = nutrition.

Based on the criteria of effort and priority, the committee could recommend an immunization education program and an alcohol information program. The committee felt that it was important to begin with programs that required relatively little effort but were of high priority.

**Priority Level**

|  | | High | | Low |
|---|---|---|---|---|
| **Effort Level** | **Low** | 1, 12, 13 | | 9, 14, 16 |
|  | | A | C | |
|  | | | B | D |
|  | **High** | 5, 7, 8, 10, 11, 17, 18 | | 2, 3, 15, 19 |

**Figure 4.1   Health promotion projects**

SOURCE: Developed by Nancy Gonzalez-Caro, M.P.H., Health Education Coordinator, Santa Clara Kaiser-Permanente Medical Center.

At their next meeting, the committee discussed these two proposed programs on the basis of the questions proposed in Table 4.2. They decided to begin planning an immunization education program. The health educator worked with the committee to identify criteria they could apply for the introduction of new programs.

## Establishing organization-wide services

Between 1975 and 1978, hospitals experienced a dramatic rise in the number of patient education and health promotion departments. In 1978, the American Hospital Association surveyed its 5,000 member hospitals and found that 68.8 percent reported new departments. This represents a growth rate of 64.9 percent in just three years. In recognition of this tremendous growth, the minimum requirements for establishing new health education services are given here for those of you who may be in a position to be the first health educator in a medical care setting.

Of course, even though a formal department or function may not have existed in the past in your organization, some educational services—both informal and formal, planned and unplanned—have probably been offered to some clients for many years. In most cases, health care agencies and organizations have many years of experience offering patient education and health promotion services outside the context of a formal department. Usually, interested clinicians decide to complement their treatment of patients with an educational component especially designed to serve those who have similar health problems. Clinicians usually offer this service as an extension of their special field of interest—such as the pulmonary specialist who offers a stop smoking clinic, the registered dietitian who offers a weight reduction class, or the physical therapist who offers a back care class. It is not unusual for hospitals and clinics to have fifteen or twenty of these services offered by individual clinicians for the people they treat. Moreover, these services are often conducted without the knowledge and participation of administration or other health professionals in the organization. Since most clinicians function fairly autonomously in medical care settings, informal educational services can be offered without much visibility as long as they are part of routine patient care and are reimbursable. Even small- to medium-sized health institutions often have some of their individual clinicians sponsoring diabetes, postmyocardial infarction, preoperative, and prenatal education for years without formal health education departments, formal programs, coordinators, or budgets.

However, this informal mode of education is usually accompanied by variable program results, haphazard attention to educational quality, and a limited ability to serve people—only when surplus time and interested staff are available. Therefore, many hospitals and clinics feel that it is in their best interest to formalize health education functions. In 1974, the American Group Practice Association issued a statement that represents the current interest by hospitals and clinics in formalizing hospital- and clinic-based patient education services:

> Patient education is the process by which patients and/or those responsible for their care (1) are taught their roles in the maintenance of health and the treatment of disease and (2) are motivated to carry out their identified responsibilities.
>     Patient education is an integral part of quality health care.
>     Effective patient education programs are based upon the needs and resources of both patients and health professionals and should consist of directed efforts toward achievement of stated goals. Program objectives must also be amenable to evaluation.
>     These programs, provided by trained patient educators, should be focused on improving health through the cooperative efforts of patients and health professionals.
>     It is the responsibility of health professionals and the institutions and organizations they represent to establish, maintain, and evaluate such services. Appropriate standards for the quality, delivery, utilization and costs of such health care services must be established.
>     Cooperation on the part of the informed patient is also vital. It is recognized that an increase in knowledge does not assure patient cooperation in medical treatment programs. For this reason, it is recommended that educational programs be planned as an integral part of comprehensive health care delivery systems which recognize the informed patient as an essential member of the health care team.
>     Payment for qualified educational programs appropriate to the health needs of the patient is a legitimate part of the health care costs. Recognizing that community education and preventive information are of immense value, it is recommended that financing of such efforts be broadly based through the joint efforts of health care institutions, organizations, foundations, and governmental agencies.*

You will know if the timing is right for health education services to be coordinated organization-wide if you have (1) educational goals that have been adopted by all major departments, (2) trained patient educators, (3) standards for health education practice, (4) educational programs that are integrated to patient care, and (5) reimbursement and other financial sources of support for health education services.

*Reprinted by permission of the American Group Practices Association.

## PREPARING THE WAY

When organizations decide to initiate new patient education and health promotion departments, it is up to the health educator to prepare the way, and the health educator rarely starts from scratch. The challenge for the new health education department head or functional leader is to learn what services existed informally in the past, who the interested pioneers are, and what climate has been created by these prior experiences. Positive prior experiences set the stage for positive future planning; the reverse is, unfortunately, just as true.

Getting started on the wrong foot can cost a new department tremendous losses in time, money, and reputation. As countless burned-out health educators can attest, beginning without the appropriate foundations invites overwhelming frustration. The hope that the future will bring about a realignment of values and a revised mandate usually proves fruitless.

Many institutions initiate patient education and health promotion departments for the wrong reasons. For instance, creating a department simply to enhance the position of the hospital in the health care market, or to seek new sources of revenue, are not strong rationales on their own. These may ultimately become benefits that well-planned, responsive programs reap, but they are not sufficient foundations for new health education programs.

The American Group Practice Association's statement on patient education is an example of a rationale that can provide a strong foundation for comprehensive health education services in a hospital or clinic. AGPA based this statement on evidence that improved health care, better use of physicians' consultation time, less repetitious instruction time for physicians, improved use of ancillary personnel, and increased staff and patient satisfaction are benefits that can be derived from planned health education services. Before your organization firmly decides to establish a health education department, several preliminary steps should be taken.

### Obtain administrative support

To begin with, the administrative team needs to believe that a mandate for a health education function exists and that it is consistent with the organization's goals. Health education must be thought of as an institution-wide function that is integrally tied in to the reason why the institution exists. Those who are responsible for health education services will need to ensure that this integration takes place—but the consciousness for an integrated service must preexist as a mandate. Programs that have tried to survive without this mandate are like plants left out of soil.

Ad hoc efforts, no matter how noble, are doomed to short-lived successes. (Ad hoc efforts are those that proceed in organizations without administrative mandates.) Two classic examples of ad hoc performers are the zealous practitioner and the militant committee.

Zealous practitioners are professional health workers in the health care system who believe in the timeliness and appropriateness of formal health education services, and who set out *single-handedly* to establish these services within their organizations. Such individuals often begin by offering health education services to their clients. Eventually, these individuals write proposals to the administration, to establish more comprehensive educational offerings. When they face weak administrative commitment to allocating resources for educational services, zealous practitioners often fall into the trap of offering to generate volunteers from a cadre of other interested professionals who will give their time to education in addition to their existing tasks. They also offer to seek seed money from outside granting agencies or foundations. Neither alternative offers a lasting solution to limited resources for educational services. Beginning an organization-wide formal health education program without a mandate and without resources is like building a house without a foundation. Moreover, when zealous practitioners leave their organizations, their entire programs crumble.

Zealous practitioners also often band together to form ad hoc health education committees. Such hard-working groups often spend years planning and organizing among themselves, somehow hoping that eventually their efforts will be appreciated or rewarded with visibility and resources. They feel their exuberance and energy are bound to communicate themselves to the skeptical and reluctant among their peers and superiors. They hope that their own commitment will eventually reap tangible results, such as staff time allocations or an operating budget.

Interested individuals will benefit in banding together for mutual support and for setting strategies for gaining an official mandate. But they should not assume that their own commitment is equivalent to administrative support or an organizational mandate.

In general, the type of mandate required for initiating formal health education services is rarely generated by staff demand alone. It is usually earned subsequent to effective lobbying, informed and thoughtful presentations of rationale, and hard evidence of the benefits the proposed program will bring to clients and to the organization. Client demand is often more powerful than staff demand. See Table 4.3 for a sample outline of a proposal to create a health education program in an institution.

During the lobbying phase, the health educator may want to convene an ad hoc committee as a means to gaining institution-wide support and involvement on behalf of health education. The ad hoc committee

**Table 4.3    Proposal to initiate health education services**

1. *Objective*
   A general, but realistic statement of what a health education department could contribute to meeting the needs of clients and of the organization.

2. *Statement of Strategy*
   A brief outline of short-term and long-term strategies for setting priorities, planning, implementing, and evaluating health education services.

3. *Rationale*
   A crisp but compelling narrative of examples of empirical studies that demonstrate the likelihood that Items 1 and 2 are in the best interest of the organization. All claims should be referenced and supported by research data. Exhortations and position papers are best left out of such proposals.

4. *Resource Requirements*
   A budget outlining the personnel costs and operating costs for one year. Attach an organization chart illustrating the reporting relationships.

can be useful as a sounding board while a strong proposal is being written. Members of the committee may want to lobby their constituents while a mandate is being formulated or debated. The committee should not, however, survive a rejection of the proposal.

There are undoubtedly many ways to secure an organization-wide mandate for the provision of planned health education services. One possible approach is to present a proposal, based on the format suggested in Table 4.3, to senior management. You can point to successful services offered at other institutions that are similar to yours, pointing to the opportunities, the need, and the benefits. Another approach is to illustrate the need on the basis of one or more pilot programs. Small successes that showcase potential benefits and minimize negative effects can help you build your case for larger, institution-wide services. In the first approach, the flow of educational services is from the top down, as Figure 4.2 illustrates. In the second approach, the flow of educational services is from the grassroots level, as Figure 4.3 illustrates.

## Obtain decision-maker support

Official mandates for the initiation of a health education service do not arise without the support of those in power. Sometimes the power resides with the administrative team; sometimes it is housed in other decision-making committees, or in the hands of informal leaders who are often unmarked on the organizational chart. If you determine who is really in

**Figure 4.2   Top down mandate**

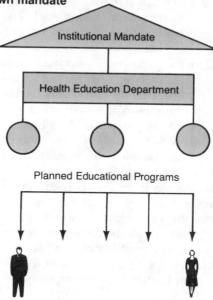

Planned Educational Programs

Providing Direct Educational
Services to Clients

**Figure 4.3   Grassroots demonstration**

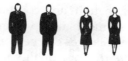

Clients Receive Education
from a Pilot Program

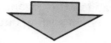

Costs and Benefits Are Documented

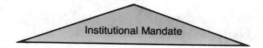

charge, you will greatly enhance plans for generating support. An informal series of discussions with department heads and opinion leaders in the organization generally leads to a consensus regarding which individuals or groups should, at a minimum, be included in the planning and be approached for support. Possible individuals could be the director of nursing, the medical director, or the chief of staff; possible groups could be the board of directors, the board of trustees, a consumer board, or one or more departments in the institution. This list can be quite varied, depending on the organization. In addition to finding out who should be involved in soliciting an approval to get started, it is wise to find out who may be in a position to sabotage the new program if they are not included from the beginning.

These issues—power, inclusion, bargaining for support—are usually (and unfortunately) the last attended to by people seeking to establish new health education programs. These issues are also probably the single greatest contributors to the long-term success or failure of the program. Being adept at generating the confidence and support of decision makers is possibly the best predictor of a person's ability to effectively manage the complexities of an organization-wide health education program.

One caveat is necessary here. Some people have been misled to believe that the simple inclusion of decision makers in the planning process necessarily guarantees their agreement and acceptance. A delicate balance between (1) being prepared—offering a rough scheme or list of options for debate—and (2) presenting a predetermined plan before a committee must be struck. Successful health education programs must necessarily go through the arduous steps of planning; these steps require debate, disagreement, negotiation, and consensus. If a program truly is organization-wide, it must meet multiple and sometimes competing objectives. Meeting such challenges can be done without seriously jeopardizing professional standards for a quality program. It does, however, require that the leaders of the health education program be both professionally proficient and politically effective.

A new health education coordinator may want to meet informally with other department heads in the organization. Here are a few questions that could be asked to begin sorting out who the key personnel are:

**1.** Whom do you ask for advice before you submit an idea to administration for approval?

**2.** Who has the final say on budgets, space, and personnel?

**3.** When there's a crisis in the hospital or clinic, with whom does administration confer to keep operations going and to get advice on the situation?

**4.** If you could only have two people from the organization to testify on your behalf to administration, whom would you choose?

**5.** What people in the organization have a solid track record of getting proposals accepted? How did they go about getting these results?

**6.** Which departments have the most resources? How did their department managers achieve this level of support?

## Obtain a budget

Every operation in a health care agency or institution has a budget. Each year costs and revenues are forecast, and a system for monitoring income and expenses is put into place. Complex systems of payments and reimbursements for health care services ensure that organizations can continue to operate. Despite this reality, some advocates of health education accept jobs as health educators or propose programs with the prospects of running a department or a function without a budget. The axiom that there is no such thing as a free lunch is as true for fledgling health education units as other business or altruistic endeavors. Besides the practical implications of trying to provide a service without funds for staff or materials, being without a budget poses a genuine survival threat that transcends dollars and cents. Like mandates, budgets bring a level of accountability and visibility that signifies legitimacy in organizations. Table 4.4 provides examples of HMO health education staffing and budget allocations.

Although some patient education and health promotion services eventually become self-supporting through direct fees or third-party payments, all services require an initial investment for planning, pilot testing, and quality control. These start-up costs are often greater than the operating costs for the first couple of years. An organization's commitment to health education must be suspect if the organization is unwilling to make an investment of any type in providing such services.

## Arrange for space

Typically, health care agencies and institutions are designed with the objective of providing health care services to individuals. Examining rooms, treatment rooms, laboratories, and provider offices make up the predominant uses of floor space. Few existing health care facilities have special rooms designed for client education. In fact, most institutions have tremendous space limitations and competition for space.

Minimally, health education staff need to be housed so that there is access to all the other staff, as well as to the clients. In addition, appro-

**Table 4.4  Examples of HMO health education and promotion staffing and budgets (June 1981)**

| | Plan | | | | | | |
|---|---|---|---|---|---|---|---|
| | Genessee Valley Group Health Puget Sound (Rochester, N.Y.) | Group Health Cooperative of Puget Sound (Seattle, Wash.) | Kaiser-Permanente Medical Care Program (Oakland, Calif.) | Multigroup Health Plan (Wellesley, Mass.) | Mastercare (Albuquerque, N.M.) | Valley Health Plan Association (Amherst, Mass.) | Rhode Island Group Health Association (Providence, R.I.) |
| Enrollment | 35,000 | 285,000 | 1.7 million | 2,500 | 13,800 | 15,500 | 32,000 |
| HMO type | Group | Staff | Group | Group | Independent practice association | Group | Staff |
| Number of sites | 2 | 15 | 18 | 5 | 280 physicians (100 offices) | 2 | 2 |
| Date of incorporation | 1973 | 1947 | 1946 | 1980 | 1973 | 1976 | 1971 |
| Professional full-time equivalent | 1.0[a] | 8.3 1.25 instructors[a] | 2.5[a] Regional office 15.5 medical | 1.0[a] | .6[a] | 3.0[a] .75 instructors | 2.0[a] |

| Functions[b] | | | | | | |
|---|---|---|---|---|---|
| 1 — | 1 XXX | 1 X | 1 XXX | 1 — | 1 XXX |
| 2 X | 2 XX | 2 XX | 2 X | 2 — | 2 XX |
| 3 XXX | 3 XX | 3 XXX | 3 XXX | 3 XX | 3 XXX |
| 4 XX | 4 XXX | 4 XXX | 4 XXX | 4 XX | 4 XXX |
| 5 X | 5 XX | 5 XX | 5 X | 5 — | 5 X |
| | | | | | 5 X |
| Budget allocation (per member per month) | $.16 (17% of budget generated from co-payments) | $.10 (16% of budget generated from co-payments) | $.08 | $.81 | $.12 (solely charged to administrative costs) | $.40 = Site 1 / .50 = Site 2 / $.17 |

SOURCE: Mullen and Zapka (1982), pp. 39–40.

[a]Other participating professionals not located in health education and promotion cost center are not included. Support staff not included.

[b]Categories are (1) service uses, (2) member participation, (3) self-care and patient education, (4) disease prevention and health promotion, and (5) staff and materials development. This list includes only those functions carried out under the auspices of the health education and promotion unit. Key: XXX = extensive activity; XX = moderate activity; X = limited activity; — = no activity.

priate space for the delivery of educational services must also be available. For instance, if personal intake interviews precede group classes, a private room that ensures confidentiality must be made available.

If clients are to register for a class, the registration station should be convenient to the location of the class. If a group is meeting to provide mutual aid and support, the space should have movable chairs and should provide an environment that is conducive to engendering support. If a class is oriented to the provision of new skills, space should be provided so that participants have the opportunity to practice the new skills. Usually, all these types of space—particularly in the most accessible, and therefore most desirable locations—are at a great premium. All the organizational commitment and resources are meaningless if there is no physical space in which to provide the proposed educational service. Nevertheless, a certain amount of creativity can often be applied to this universal dilemma. Renting nearby community facilities—such as churches, community centers, and schools—sometimes solves several problems (such as space limitations and lack of community visibility). Mobile units, for instance, exemplify a spirit of outreach that counteracts the aloofness the health care system sometimes conveys. Offering services to people where they work, shop, or live may not only be a practical solution to an internal space problem but may also provide a new dimension to the way people define or use health education services.

The critical point at this stage in the development of a health education program is to secure commitment for office and classroom space. It is important that the type of space identified match the philosophy and objectives of the health education program.

## Allocate staff time

The providers of diagnostic, treatment, and health maintenance services also need to be educators. Sufficient time—an agreed-on minimal standard—must be made available so that the educational component can accompany the other services provided. If diagnosis and treatment are allocated to a fifteen-minute visit, another unit of time needs to be added expressly for the educational component. There is no surer way to guarantee that education will not be provided than to expect providers who are used to providing treatment or health maintenance services in fifteen minutes, to then add education within the same time allocation. Something will necessarily be dropped, and it is usually the education.

People at all levels of the health care delivery system already feel stretched to accomplish all that is required of them. Three situations usually occur if staff are asked to provide educational services in addition to all the other tasks demanded of them. One, if they try to accommodate the request, they burn out within a short period of time. Two, they refuse to cooperate, and block all other intrusions on their already overcommitted schedules. Three, they interpret this new request as having very low priority in the organization, and relegate it to those situations when they can squeeze it in. Under these circumstances, education is rarely made available, is inconsistent, and is unpredictable.

In addition to educational services that are integral to care, most treatment procedures and health-maintaining regimens require more than a perfunctory informational session. Coping with illness, managing chronic health problems, providing self-care, and following health-promoting recommendations require complex skills. Most people need practice under supervision, the time and opportunity to transfer other life skills to current health problems, and plenty of support in order to be successful over time. But all these activities do not require intense intervention by highly trained professionals. Peer support and lay leaders often are as effective, if not more effective. In any case, mechanisms to pay for staff time for education-integral care, as well as staff time for education that complements and supplements care, must be assured at the outset of program development.

Formulas for staffing ratios in all direct service departments need to take into account individual and group educational services. For instance, hospital nursing departments can project nursing staffing requirements on the basis of diagnosis, acuity, and learning needs. If two newly diagnosed diabetics are admitted from the emergency room, the nursing floor supervisor can judge the number of nursing care hours those diabetics will need based on a protocol that translates the type of diabetes into hours of nursing care plus hours of education for the patient and the patient's family. Some patients will be too sick for educational services until the second or third day of hospitalization. Some will need more skills before they are discharged than others. All these factors will influence staffing patterns.

In addition, staffing requirements for specialized instructors (such as stop smoking counselors, stress management leaders, diabetic educators, and cancer support group facilitators) need to be forecast and guaranteed early in program planning. Formal health education programs cannot exist on the goodwill of volunteer health professionals who serve after work or come in on their own time to provide educational services. Nor can it be expected that staff will be able to add an educational function to their already overcommitted schedules.

## Write job descriptions

All personnel—whether they are full-time health-care providers or outside instructors hired on a contract basis—must have job descriptions that contain performance standards for their educator roles. Performance evaluations, salary reviews, and merit increases need to be related to that proportion of their jobs that is devoted to education. Any health education program that does not have these mechanisms will not be taken seriously, will not be able to hold people accountable for providing educational services, and will be unable to control for program quality.

## Develop departmental lines of communication

All line functions and most support functions in health care agencies and institutions have one identified person who is held accountable for that service. Committees made up of representatives of other departments cannot be accountable for health education services. One person must be designated as a liaison to administration, as a primary spokesperson and advocate of the unit, and as the individual who is accountable for the successes and failures of the unit. If health education is meant to be a service that cuts across all departments and disciplines—as it is best suited to be—it must not be housed within one existing department. If health education is seen as serving the interests of only one department of the organization—such as nursing, or internal medicine, or obstetrics and gynecology, or physical therapy—rather than as serving the mutual interests of the entire organization, its potential will be severely limited.

Moreover, problems may arise in the future if health education is made a functional subunit of an educational department. The education department has been traditionally seen primarily as an inservice staff or continuing education unit or as a training department for managers or residents. It may not be a suitable location for direct services to clients. Furthermore, health care providers may minimize the role of health education as a necessary aspect of consumer health care because of its secondary location on the organizational chart.

It may be tempting to place health education in an existing department where existing support may be present (such as training or nursing). Nevertheless, such a move prevents the kind of widespread support that fully relevant health education services require. Generally speaking, the most effective arrangement is for health education to be designated as a formal department, with a department head who reports directly to the administrator or to a designee of the administrator, such as an assistant administrator. In the long run, coalitions of independent departments (rather than the subjugation of one function within another) probably best serve the varied interests and needs of these departments. Popular coalitions are composed of nursing inservice, medical education, organization development, education and training, and health education. These coalitions can be powerful advocates of a broad spectrum of educational services in medical care settings. Coalitions can offer mutual support and can prevent the competition for resources that sometimes occurs among departments with similar goals.

## Obtain clerical support

Along with all the other considerations that have been mentioned, it is primary that the health education department be given the support necessary for telephone coverage, correspondence, and preparation of educational materials. The value and the volume of clerical support for an efficient health education department should not be underestimated. It is improbable that a health education department could get off the ground without communications support.

## IS IT TIME TO PROCEED?

Table 4.5 presents a checklist that could assist health educators in determining whether sufficient conditions exist in the organization to merit moving forward with a formal health education program. Before reading

**Table 4.5   "Go/no go" checklist**

The following conditions should be explicitly available before serious action is taken to establish a formal health education program in a health care agency or institution. Check the conditions that you are confident exist. The score card may help you decide to go to the next steps or to continue work on building a more secure foundation. Assign each step one point.

\_\_\_\_\_ Administrative support

\_\_\_\_\_ Decision-maker support

\_\_\_\_\_ Designated budget

\_\_\_\_\_ Assignment of office and classroom space

\_\_\_\_\_ Allocation of staff time for conducting educational services

\_\_\_\_\_ Communications support

*Score card*

      6:   Go.

   4–5:   Continue to build base of support.

Less than 4:   Your organization is not ready. Plan strategy to wait for better circumstances, or continue to build base of support.

the remainder of this chapter, take a few minutes to complete the checklist on the basis of your situation or a hypothetical situation.

If you scored "Go" on the Table 4.5 checklist, you are ready to move to the next steps. For some health educators, particularly those who are not familiar with the complexities of the medical care delivery system, setting time frames for developing a new health education department is frustrating and frightening. The new department head wants to be both responsive and realistic. Generally speaking, many clinicians and administrators are impatient with planning processes and expect that health educators should be able to walk in one day and provide services the next. "Surely," they say, "you should know from the literature, your training, and your own experience, what it is that our providers and clients want and need in the way of educational services." You may in fact know what needs to be done, but don't jump into action before you complete the next several steps.

Because the effectiveness of ongoing health education services depends on the ability of the health educator to be visible and to communicate with representatives of all departments in the organization, it is important to set a precedent for making personal contact early in the tenure of the department. To begin with, individual meetings are important, first with department heads and chiefs of service, and then with their respective departments for dialogue regarding definitions and directions for health education. The health educator must be an accomplished interviewer as well as listener at this juncture. He or she should prepare in advance an interview schedule, with key questions, to elicit information regarding departmental priorities, barriers and resources for future health education programs, managerial style, organizational values, system assets and problems, perceptions regarding unspoken decision-making protocols, organizational climate, informal leaders, and trouble spots for future problem solving. A sample interview questionnaire is given in Table 4.6.

The information gathered through these interviews should be kept confidential. The health educator needs to be seen as trustworthy and contributing to the commonly held goals of a diverse group of people. This information-gathering procedure establishes at first-hand a precedent for cooperation and inclusion. It also helps the health educator to become known to key people throughout the institution; this is a great way to be introduced to names, faces, and places. This interview can be the first step in establishing a support network among colleagues in the organization.

### Establish an advisory committee

Once you have made the rounds of all department heads and departments, you will be able to select from them the key people who represent

**Table 4.6   Sample staff questionnaire**

1. Tell me a little about your department's top priorities for this year.

2. How would a health education service help serve your department's priorities?

3. What should I know about the management style of our organization?

4. What are the values that operate in the organization that support a health education service?

5. What are the values that operate in the organization that might hinder a health education service?

6. What problems should I expect as I try to gain support for health education?

7. How can I keep these problems from surfacing?

8. Who are the key people that I should talk to next? Are there questions I should ask them?

major entities, disciplines, and constituencies from within the organization. The health educator needs to be able to define the mission and functions of the advisory committee, as well as the expected frequency and duration of expected meetings over the subsequent months. Administration and key decision makers should review the list of people to be invited before the invitation to participate is made.

The people selected to serve on the advisory committee are usually already very busy and usually hold positions of significant authority. Therefore, committee members must be made clear on their mission and functions very early and must be prepared in advance for each meeting. Also, the agendas must be relevant, well paced, and lead to productive meetings.

Since this committee is advisory, it is extremely important that the individual members not only represent constituencies, but that a system for gauging the sentiment of these constituencies be established. For example, to what extent does advice reflect the individuals on the committee—their values and personal interests—rather than of the group they represent? If constituencies are to be represented genuinely, then issues cannot be raised, discussed, and decided within a single meeting. In order for the representatives to meet with their constituents, an interval of time needs to separate the introduction of the issue and the discussion of it. When the members return to the committee for the next meeting, then they can accurately report all viewpoints they have been delegated to represent.

### Set policies and priorities

With input from administration and the advisory committee, the health educator should set out a few basic policies that will then guide future planning, implementation, and evaluation of the health education program. To begin, such policies should include (1) a definition of patient education and health promotion, (2) the statement of organizational mandate and purpose for health education, (3) the organization chart with lines of authority clearly identified, (4) the mandate and purpose of the advisory committee, with a list of all members, (5) a protocol establishing how decisions are made for health education services, and (6) a statement regarding the role of the health educator in relationship to other departments.

The following is a sample of statements of goals and objectives for a health education advisory committee.*

*Developed by Pamela Jean Larson, M.P.H., Health Education Coordinator, Oakland Kaiser-Permanente Medical Center.

*Goals*

To improve patient care and member satisfaction with services at the Oakland Medical Center by recommending educational policies and setting long-range and short-term member and patient education goals

*Specific Objectives*

  **1.** To receive, compile, and interpret possible reasons for member dissatisfaction with services offered or obtained

  **2.** To discuss, assess, and recommend possible educational interventions in areas which are actual, or potential, sources of dissatisfaction

  **3.** To integrate such intervention within the framework of existing services with the concurrence of Medical Center administration and involved personnel

  **4.** To develop member education programs for better utilization of services and enhanced preventive care

  **5.** To act as a catalyst, resource, and coordinating body for the development of patient- or disease-oriented educational programs

  **6.** To keep the Medical Center informed of all educational activities in process

  **7.** To evaluate ongoing educational programs and report to medical center administration and staff; [to] establish criteria for an evaluation

  **8.** To promote the concept of member and patient education as an inherent component of health care

  **9.** To set member and patient educational priorities

Table 4.7 is a sample roster of a health education committee. Figure 4.4 is a sample organization chart. These samples come from organizations that have comprehensive patient education and health promotion operations. They are provided here as guidelines for developing departments.

Distinguishing between wants and needs may seem like a conflict of jargon. Before priorities can be set, however, it is important to understand the differences among what the administration wants and needs, what providers and staff want and need, what clients want and need, and what the health educator wants and needs. Services that are wanted by these various groups primarily reflect the groups' interests and values. These services may or may not influence the actual health status of the client group, although they may affect the clients' perception of health status. Services that respond to needs, on the other hand, can be substantiated by evidence of deficits, such as mortality or morbidity data, or other measures of health status such as biomedical measures of blood

**Table 4.7    Health education committee roster**

---

*Ex-Officio*
  Physician-in-Chief
  Administrator

*On Call*
  Reception Supervisor

*Regular Members*

| | |
|---|---|
| Surgery Supervisor | Medical Station—Nurse Practitioner |
| Health Education Assistant | Health Librarian |
| Health Educator | Pediatrics—Nurse Practitioner |
| Anesthesiology Physician | Marketing Representative |
| Communications Supervisor | Registered Dietitian |
| Unit Manager | Physical Therapist |
| Urology—Physician | Patient Assistance Supervisor |
| Public Relations Representative | Pediatrics—Physician |
| Medicine—Physician | Preventive Medicine—Physician |
| Surgery—Registered Nurse | Volunteer—Coordinator |
| Health Education Coordinator | Hospital Nursing Supervisor |

---

SOURCE: Developed by Pamela Jean Larson, M.P.H., Health Education
Coordinator, Oakland Kaiser-Permanente Medical Center.

**Figure 4.4    Health/patient education organization chart**

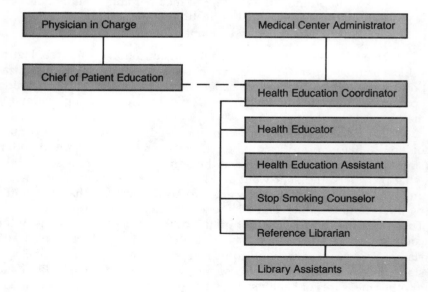

**Figure 4.5   Vicious circle when wants are not distinguished from needs**

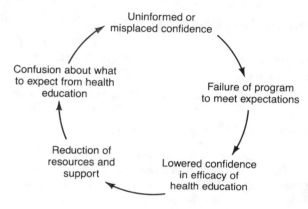

pressure, laboratory tests, or standardized tests of quality of life. A case can be made for setting priorities based either on wants *or* on needs, but it is important to make the distinction first. The pitfall exists when perception of need—rather than genuine need, as perceived by the patient or client—leads to the investment of limited resources in an educational service. When expected outcomes do not occur, rather than faulting the misperception of the service's ability to effect change, most people usually blame the educational service. A vicious circle then ensues: the disappointment leads to the subsequent reduction of resources and support for health education efforts (see Figure 4.5).

Well-intentioned advisory committees sometimes get involved in advocating educational services that best serve the needs of the staff, rather than the needs of the clients. These sentiments are often expressed in terms of saving staff time, ensuring compliance with treatments, promoting kept appointments, and advancing client satisfaction with the care that is given. Although effective health education services often provide these impressive results, it is problematic to set priorities on these end points alone. Medical care organizations are experiencing tremendous competition for access to the health care dollar; this experience creates limited resources for health education. Therefore, it is imperative that priorities be set with an eye to both pragmatism and results. A number of targeted questions can assist in this priority-setting process:

**1.** What are the most pressing health problems the people we serve face?

**2.** In which of these areas are educational interventions most likely to yield results?

**3.** What is the minimum educational intervention required to yield the hoped-for results?

**4.** What are the costs of this intervention, both to the organization and to the client?

**5.** Should these educational services be offered as a component of the health care we offer?

**6.** Should the educational services be a necessary adjunct to the health care we offer?

**7.** Are these services offered anywhere else in the community?

One of the biggest dilemmas in using needs as a qualification for a high-priority service is that there often exists a large gap between perception of need and traditional definitions of need. People often express their greatest needs in areas of life that have the least-known relationship to health status. For example, in one small community in the Northwest a telephone survey of a large random sample of households yielded cleanliness and pollen allergies as the greatest health problems they faced. But the local health department statistics reported venereal disease, drug abuse, and teenage pregnancy as the leading community health problems. If the primary institutional effort were made on behalf of the prevention and treatment of venereal disease, probably very few people from the community would have participated. There is little justification for investing great sums of money on services that few people will use.

## Survey interest groups and the system

Somewhere, in between (1) offering services that many clients will respond to but that will yield little result and (2) offering needed services that few clients will use, is the preferred strategy. Simply asking providers what their clients want, need, or will participate in will not provide a complete picture, either. When provider surveys are matched on the same items as client surveys, great discrepancies often appear. The best approach is to survey a segment of the following interest groups—clients, providers and staff, and administration. Armed with these data and case studies from empirical research found in the professional literature, health educators will be able to (1) establish criteria for setting priorities, (2) establish a method for weighting these criteria, and (3) establish a system for selecting realistic priorities given the resources that are available.

Once the planning roles have been delegated, the health educator should bring together the individuals who will take on the various tasks, in order to conduct an informal organizational diagnosis. The group should systematically identify all the organization's resources that can positively influence the planning and implementation of the educational program. Occasionally, community and outside professional resources can also be identified now. Then the group should identify the possible barriers that may exist in the planning or in the implementation stages. The members should discuss system problems such as delays in getting appointments, the lack of continuity of care, the unavailability of medical records to instructors, and the lack of resources or support. And strategies for overcoming each barrier should be proposed. The group must act on those strategies most likely to be changed by a specific group and make referrals to the other decision and action groups. Since educational programs do not take place in a vacuum, all aspects of the organization that affect the potential educational service need to be mobilized on behalf of the program early in the planning stages.

### Set standards

Before actual planning can begin on a specified educational program (such as diabetes education, back care class, stress management seminars), minimum standards must be set for what is required of the program. For example, the following questions should be answered for the program under consideration:

**1.** Does the proposed program fall within the health education mandate?

**2.** Will the proposed program meet an explicit need for the client population?

**3.** Will the proposed program contribute to the achievement of one or more of the organization's goals?

**4.** Is the primary department affected by the program willing to contribute resources to the planning, implementation, and evaluation of the program (for example, obstetrics-gynecology for Lamaze classes, or physical therapy for back care classes)?

**5.** Are there budgeted funds for the operation of the program?

**6.** Has responsibility for a written protocol for the planning, implementation, and evaluation of the program been accepted?

**7.** Has someone been assigned responsibility for the actual delivery of the educational service?

**8.** Has space been allocated for the proposed program?

**9.** Has a quality assurance mechanism been built into the implementation and evaluation phases of the program?

## Set time lines

Now the framework for planning one proposed educational program has been established. The health educator can now work with the various people who have accepted planning and implementation responsibilities to set realistic time lines for each task. In most cases, these people work nearly full time in one clinical role or another. Therefore, time lines need to be set in the context of everyone's obligations, in the light of the problems that need to be solved, and with the acknowledgment that gaining the cooperation of all people involved usually takes a significant investment of time. It is not unusual for the planning process for a single educational program (for example, six one-hour lectures on stress management) to take more than twelve months in the planning. Table 4.8 provides a sample time line.

As the products of the planning process are being developed (such as the educational protocol and teaching plan), many of the providers

**Table 4.8   Time line for the planning and implementation of a health education program**

| Step | Task | Completion date |
|------|------|-----------------|
| 1 | Gain commitment and acceptance of budget | January |
| 2 | Assessment | February, March |
| 3 | Problem identification and problem solving | February, March |
| 4 | Program planning: Set objectives/define outcomes Staff development Operational definitions List of methods Teaching plans ready | April–August |
| 5 | Implementation | September |
| 6 | Evaluation: Behavioral objectives Instruments designed Validity/reliability Health outcomes measured Benefits tested | April May–July August At class, at end of class, and one year later At class, at end of class, and one year later |

and staff who will be affected by the proposed educational service should be kept in touch with the planning and should have input along the way. Final protocols, teaching plans, and implementation and evaluation strategies should be signed by designated department heads, chiefs of service, and administrators to signify their cooperation and support. If the service is sponsored by a department other than health education (for example, obstetrics-gynecology) the health educator should also sign all planning documents to signify the cooperation of the health education department in the planning process.

## Conduct inservice training

It is quite common for an educational program to be planned by one or two people from a sponsoring department but to be implemented by many more staff personnel. All individuals who have accepted the responsibility of providing an educational service to clients should participate in the inservice training. The amount of inservice time devoted to preparing instructors will vary according to the program. Nevertheless, if the inservice training is divided into thirds, say, one-third should be devoted to the content of the educational service (such as diabetes, hypertension, or stress management) and two-thirds should be devoted to the process (educational methods and tools). Most educational services will be provided for clients in groups. But most instructors are most familiar with educational approaches based on one-to-one encounters. Therefore, many instructors will be tempted to lecture on pathophysiology rather than to provide learning opportunities based on skills practice, discussion, and group support. Moreover, few instructors have seen top-quality health education services in action. Therefore, their skills are limited to their own experiences. Videotapes and role models may be useful aspects of the inservice training. All instructors need to participate in several trial runs of the complete course under supervision before they are actually given access to clients.

New services should be treated as experiments until they have been offered several times and evaluated. Health educators and instructors need to avoid the temptation to conduct massive promotional efforts for untested services. The big productions can be reserved for programs that have proven their worth or their potential. Clients should be informed when they are invited or referred to pilot programs. Their participation in evaluating the outcomes of the service should be solicited. Pilot programs offer the additional advantage that various components of a package can be tested in order to finally arrive at an optimum configuration of educational content and methods.

## Build in feedback systems

Since health educators are ultimately responsible for the quality of educational services targeted to clients of the health care system, you should design feedback systems during the planning, implementation, and evaluation stages. Solicit feedback from those involved in these stages (staff, administration, and clients). Documentation of this feedback is recommended—both for clinical follow-up (in the medical record) and for administrative follow-up (in quarterly reports and project updates). Chapter 7 will give you practical examples and tools that will be useful when you design feedback systems during the various stages of planning. Keep in mind that the guidelines apply both to starting educational services from scratch and to upgrading existing services. Health educators who follow these guidelines for structuring the situation for action are making a valuable investment in the future of the health education service.

Table 4.9 is a checklist that summarizes the steps in getting started. Chapter 5 gives you a sample of an educational protocol that can act as a roadmap for you to follow once you feel that all the items on the checklist have been taken care of.

**Table 4.9   Getting started checklist**

\_\_\_\_\_ Establish an advisory committee

\_\_\_\_\_ Set basic policies and priorities

\_\_\_\_\_ Designate minimum standards

\_\_\_\_\_ Survey interest groups and the system

\_\_\_\_\_ Set time lines

\_\_\_\_\_ Conduct inservice training

\_\_\_\_\_ Build in feedback systems

# EXERCISES

1.  You are working part time in the business office of a 300-bed community hospital while completing a master's degree in health education. You would like to see the hospital provide more leadership in the community, with a positive health image and a formal health education effort. How would you go about raising interest in the concept of an organized health education service within the hospital? List the steps you would take. Write a brief rationale for each step.

2.  You are a health education coordinator in a prepaid group practice that provides both inpatient and outpatient health care services. You have operated a health education department with the same staffing level and same operating budget for three years, in spite of inflation and increasing expectations from providers, administration, and clients for more educational programs. How would you go about generating more support? What specific steps would you take to increase your capability to provide more services?

# RESOURCES

Green, L. W., Kreuter, M. W., Deeds, S. G., and Partridge, K. B. *Health Education Planning: A Diagnostic Approach.* Palo Alto, Calif.: Mayfield, 1980.

These authors present a framework for planning health education services that can be successfully applied to health education services in medical care. Chapter 7 examines the administrative diagnosis phase of the planning framework, which provides a useful approach to assessing organizational problems. Chapter 10 applies the framework to patient care, with special attention given to community health nursing as a model of community health care. Appendix B presents a clinical application of the framework in the context of a hypertension education project.

Madnick, M. E. *Consumer Health Education—A Guide to Hospital-Based Programs.* Wakefield, Mass.: Nursing Resources, 1980.

This book records the experiences of the staff of the office of consumer health education in the Department of Environmental and Community

Medicine at the College of Medicine and Dentistry of New Jersey and the Rutgers Medical School. Chapter 4 offers an administrative perspective that differs from ours. Nevertheless, the attention given to the role of advisory committees and team approaches to planning is valuable. Keep in mind that this resource describes what is, rather than what should be.

Redman, B. K. (ed.). *Patterns for Distribution of Patient Education*. New York: Appleton-Century-Crofts, 1981.

This anthology of program descriptions is especially helpful for nurse educators. Although administrative and political issues are absent, very typical, status quo samples of teaching protocols and nursing care plans are described from actual programs in primarily university-based medical centers. Chapter 3 describes a nursing department's successful attempt to organize a multidepartmental patient education program. The chapter takes the program through its genesis and development and concludes with an analysis of the experience.

Taylor, R. B., Ureda, J. R., and Denham, J. W. *Health Promotion Principles and Clinical Applications*. New York: Appleton-Century-Crofts, 1982.

This book was written for the primary health care provider. Through the use of this book, practitioners should be better able to (1) understand the epidemiological, biomedical, statistical, behavioral, and educational principles of health promotion; (2) determine the health promotion needs of the individual and family; (3) prescribe specific health practices appropriate for each individual's age, sex, health status, and belief systems, and (4) maintain continuing supervision in accord with up-to-date scientific data. Chapter 6 is a rich resource for the health care provider who wishes to integrate health promotion into the medical encounter.

# 5

## Developing protocols and teaching plans

BECAUSE MEDICAL CARE is a field of practice dominated by a prevailing view of autonomous clinical decisions made by health care providers, there has been a growing realization over several decades that quality of care can be assured only when standards of practice can be agreed on by the profession. Physicians and nurses and other health professionals have standards of practice. These standards are yardsticks against which decisions and procedures can be judged. Providers using these yardsticks can make autonomous decisions, but within a range of possibilities that has been agreed on by the profession. When clinical decisions, procedures, and actions are agreed on by a profession, they are usually documented in the form of a protocol.

Appendix 5.1 illustrates the steps in health education planning that are geared to elicit behavior change in clients. This protocol is designed to be used by clinicians as they counsel clients. The protocol highlights benchmarks in the educational process. The educator is assumed to be familiar with educational principles based on theories of health behavior change. Protocols assume that the educator is proficient enough in educational methods and interpersonal communication skills to modify the process for the specific needs, concerns, and objectives of the client.

The maintenance of standards of practice requires that protocols be translated into action plans. Teaching plans are one form of action plan. They are more specific than protocols, and they are designed to meet the unique learning needs of special interest groups. There may be a standard protocol for the management of chronic back pain, for example. Physical therapists, however, may have many plans for teaching back care.

127

In this chapter, we discuss the benefits and limitations of teaching plans and protocols and provide generic guidelines for developing protocols and plans that can be applied to any patient education or health promotion content area.

The model that follows provides the best framework available for the development of educational protocols and teaching plans. The model synthesizes educational, behavioral science, and epidemiological theory and outlines the steps that you should follow to plan health education programs. Because the model is a planning tool, it is introduced here as a foundation to the protocol development process.

## THE *PRECEDE* MODEL

PRECEDE is an acronym for P̲redisposing, R̲einforcing, and E̲nabling C̲auses in E̲ducational D̲iagnosis and E̲valuation. The model is a framework for health education planning (Green et al., 1980). Its utility for the practitioner and clinician is great. It can be used to plan direct educational services for clients, to plan educational programs for special target groups, and to plan institution-wide, comprehensive educational efforts. As you use the PRECEDE model, it will serve to keep you from common pitfalls of educational practice. Figure 5.1 shows the model and notes the four steps that we will now discuss.

### Epidemiological and social diagnosis

When clients present themselves with illnesses, you first need to understand the nature of the disease, the usual course, the effects (such as disability), and the duration. In addition to the individual medical history of the patient, you must understand how the disease has affected patients with the same disease in the past. The aggregated history of the disease in recent years, as well as the specific details of the individual under your care, gives you a better understanding of the health problem under consideration. It is also important to consider the disease's and the treatment's effects on the client's lifestyle, as well as on the quality of life. You should ask, "What demands will the therapy and rehabilitation make on the client and the family? Will the client be able to return to work? What economic impact has this illness had on the client and the family?"

The answers to these questions will help you assess the overall health education goals. In other words, what realistic expectations can you hold regarding the results of your health education interventions? What improvements in health status and quality of life can you antici-

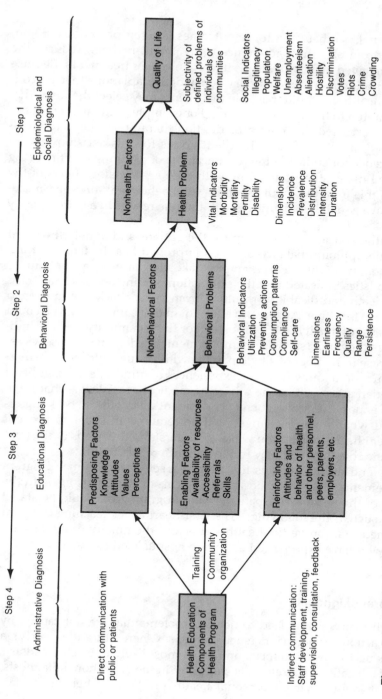

**Figure 5.1   Health education planning model (PRECEDE)**

SOURCE: Adapted from L. W. Green, M. W. Kreuter, S. G. Deeds, and K. B. Partridge, *Health Education Planning: A Diagnostic Approach* (Palo Alto, Calif.: Mayfield, 1980). Reprinted by permission of Mayfield Publishing Company.

pate? The balance between these outcomes is often precarious. Sometimes, for example, strict adherence to treatment regimen reduces the clients' perceived quality of life, as in certain cancer treatments. Because health education requires voluntary behavioral adaptations that are conducive to health, it is quite possible that clients may select therapies that are most suited to their styles of living. For example, a client may choose a severely restricted diet over a medication therapy—if both are medically agreed-on alternatives. The client's basis for this decision may be the preference for enduring the complications of planning and financing a restricted diet, rather than living with the negative side effects of the drugs. In this example, both therapies (one behavioral, one pharmacological) have equal therapeutic benefit, but one results in a better quality of life.

It is the educator's role to lay out the options and to help the client achieve the optimum balance between improved health status and improved quality of life. For example, take the case of a community whose statistics indicated that the population is being adversely affected by early death and disability, resulting from heart attacks, of men aged thirty-five to fifty-five. As a health educator in that community, you could identify a set of quality of life problems for the community and the individuals residing in it (such as unemployment, burden on social services, and increase in number of single parents with young children). Furthermore, you would know from the experiences of hundreds of other heart attack patients, as well as the advice of medical specialists, what rehabilitation is possible, how much of the patient's life will be "back to normal," and what sorts of changes will be required in order to prevent subsequent heart attacks. You will also understand the needs of the family, and the role they will play in the patient's rehabilitation.

The end product of this first step is a set of educational program goal statements that should be stated in terms of client outcomes. In the example of the heart attack patients, the program goal would be stated in terms such as the following: "The post-heart attack teaching program is designed to improve the health status and the quality of life of individuals who have experienced and were hospitalized for heart attack."

## Behavioral diagnosis

Although many factors lead to health problems that are not caused by people's actions or behaviors (such as age, sex, heredity, and poverty), a health educator needs to focus on factors most likely to be changed as a result of education. Therefore, at this point in the educational diagnosis, you must identify which personal health practices or behaviors have contributed to the client's health problem and rank their importance in terms of their impact on health outcomes. In addition to ranking behavioral problems on the criteria of importance, you should also rank them in terms of their potential for change through education.

For example, among individuals who have had a heart attack, the personal health practices that would contribute to subsequent heart attacks include smoking, overeating, too little or too much exercise, uncontrolled hypertension, and inability to cope with stress. A scale might be devised to rank each practice according to relative contribution to future heart attacks (see Figure 5.2). In the same way, the list of personal health practices could be weighted for their likelihood of being changed as a result of a health education intervention. Figure 5.3 shows a changeability scale. (For greater detail on this process of weighting behaviors, see Green et al., 1980, Ch. 4.)

Once each behavior is weighted and given a numerical value, it is possible to rank the personal health practices. Behaviors that are high both in importance and in changeability are the prime targets for health education attention and resources and should rank high on your list. If you had unlimited time, money, and staff to conduct health education services in hospitals and clinics, it might be possible to develop programs to influence all pertinent health behaviors. However, since most of us have limited resources, it makes sense for us to do a good job in areas that are both important and are likely to work.

The end product of the second step is a set of behavioral objectives describing the target population, what behaviors they will accomplish, what change is expected, and how soon all this change will take place. In the example of the heart attack patients, one behavioral objective might be "Twenty percent of the post–heart attack patients who are admitted

**Figure 5.2  Importance scale**

| 1 | 2 | 3 | 4 | 5 | 6 | 7 | 8 | 9 | 10 |
|---|---|---|---|---|---|---|---|---|----|

| Little or<br>no importance | Medium<br>importance | Great<br>importance |
|---|---|---|

**Figure 5.3  Changeability scale**

| 1 | 2 | 3 | 4 | 5 | 6 | 7 | 8 | 9 | 10 |
|---|---|---|---|---|---|---|---|---|----|

| Little or no<br>potential for change | Medium potential<br>for change | Great potential<br>for change |
|---|---|---|

to the Coronary Care Unit will have stopped cigarette smoking within two years after the post–heart attack teaching program."

## Educational diagnosis

By now, many practitioners may feel that they are ready to begin educational interventions. However tempted you are to jump right in and begin educating clients, your data base is still not complete. The richest level of analysis is still waiting to be accomplished. This third step requires homework on the part of the practitioner, the organization development specialist, the medical social worker, the health psychologist, the home health worker, and others in order to understand the factors that preceded and have most influenced the health behaviors under consideration. Your job is to coordinate the collection of this information.

The first category of variables—predisposing factors—includes the patients' knowledge, attitudes, values, and perceptions about their illness or their therapy, the prognosis, the effects of the disease on their lives, and their hospitalization. The second category of variables—enabling factors—includes the availability of resources, the accessibility of services, referrals, waiting times, and the skills that the client possesses. The third category of variables—reinforcing factors—includes the attitudes and behaviors of health practitioners, peers, family, and employers. (This last category differs from the first in that it reflects the attitudes and actions of people who influence the client positively or negatively.) Once these factors have been identified, only those that rank highest should be selected as the targets of the educational interventions. Again, these variables should be ranked on the criteria of importance and changeability.

The product of this third step is a list of learning objectives for each of the high-ranking factors. You need to identify which educational strategy or strategies would be accomplished in order to best influence the predisposing, enabling, and reinforcing factors. One of the most significant results of this step is the realization that a variety of educational methods need to be employed in order to accomplish significant behavior changes. This step, more than any of the others, helps health educators to avoid the temptation to apply simple approaches to complex, multidimensional health dilemmas.

For example, if appropriate exercise is a high-ranking health behavior for preventing subsequent heart attacks, then the factors listed in Table 5.1 might be identified. After weighting these factors on the criteria of importance and changeability (see Figures 5.2 and 5.3), you and your client might identify the top-ranking factors as shown in Table 5.2. Sample learning objectives for each factor are listed in Table 5.3. Sam-

**Table 5.1   Educational diagnosis for exercise after a heart attack**

1. *Predisposing factors*
   a. Client's knowledge of the effect of exercise on the heart and circulatory system
   b. Client's attitudes toward exercise
   c. Client's perceptions of appropriate limits for physical exertion
   d. Client's fears of possible threat of subsequent heart attacks or death as a result of exercise

2. *Enabling factors*
   a. Availability of safe, pleasant walking route near home
   b. Access to the YMCA cardiac fitness and rehabilitation program
   c. Referral by a practitioner to an exercise program
   d. Cost of an organized exercise program

3. *Reinforcing factors*
   a. Having someone at home who enjoys exercise and who will encourage patient to exercise
   b. Being encouraged by peers at work to participate in an exercise program
   c. Being encouraged by the physician and nurse to participate in an exercise program

**Table 5.2   Sample of behaviors identified as important in making an educational diagnosis (cardiac patients)**

1. *Predisposing Factor:* Client's perceptions of appropriate limits of physical exertion

2. *Enabling Factor:* Client's referral by practitioner to exercise program

3. *Reinforcing Factor:* Client's having someone at home who enjoys exercise and who will encourage client to exercise

**Table 5.3   Sample learning objectives for a post–heart attack exercise program**

1. By the end of the post–heart attack educational program, 80 percent of the participants will list ten appropriate activities in which they can engage, according to the individual level of disability.

2. The primary practitioner will refer all post–heart attack clients that have been identified as able, to an exercise therapy program in the community.

3. Eighty percent of post–heart attack program participants will exercise regularly with one other family member.

**Table 5.4   Sample educational strategies for a post–heart attack exercise program**

| Factors | Strategies |
| --- | --- |
| 1. *Predisposing*<br>   Perceptions of exercise limits | • Lecture-discussion of parameters following cardiac stress test<br>• Film demonstrating levels of activity |
| 2. *Enabling*<br>   Nurse referral | • One-to-one discussion of benefits of program<br>• Pamphlet describing exercise program<br>• Discussion of costs of program in relation to benefits derived |
| 3. *Reinforcing*<br>   Family member encouragement | • Home visit<br>• Group discussion<br>• One-to-one discussion with family member |

ple educational strategies for these learning objectives are shown in Table 5.4.

## Administrative diagnosis

Now educational strategies, such as educational support groups, audiovisual, or organization development methods, may have been identified. Yet it is imperative that actual implementation be delayed for just one more, but crucial, step. At this point in educational planning, you need to look at the organization for clues that will allow you to refine the educational intervention so that there is maximum opportunity for success. The administrative diagnosis is critical in planning for one-to-one health counseling, as well as for organized group teaching.

At this stage of planning, you should have an understanding of the characteristics of your organization—such as (1) the assets and limitations stemming from its size, location, financial structure, and degree of complexity; (2) your organization's stated goals and objectives and how the objectives identified by your health education program complement

or challenge them; (3) interdepartmental communication and collaboration patterns; (4) availability of the educational service elsewhere in the
organization or in the community; and (5) the way decisions are made
in the organization and whether those in power support or do not support the educational efforts. These characteristics are important to your
political efforts. By *politics*, we mean the interpersonal, dynamic process
of achieving your goals even when faced with some resistance.

Some of the most educationally sound health education efforts never
succeed because the health educator in charge of them is apolitical and
has failed to ensure that the programs are given the necessary stamp of
approval within the organization. For example, an inservice division of
the nursing department may initiate a patient teaching program in a
hospital or clinic. Usually, in such a case one nurse comes forward who
is especially interested in that educational program. The nurse writes
an outline of an educational plan and then someone in management in
the nursing service gives permission to begin the educational program.
Eventually a committee, usually made up of more interested nurses,
meet together to develop a standard of care and a teaching protocol. Very
often, not until the program is ready to begin is the nurse reminded to
get the key medical staff on board, or to get administrative approval.
Then when the program budgets are refused and space is denied, morale
among the nursing staff drops.

Grassroots planning should first reach out for organizational commitments to patient education and health promotion. Usually, these commitments can be achieved through (1) visible physician support and (2)
well-written proposals ensuring that the health education goals are consistent with the organizational goals. The administrative diagnosis prepares the educator for these requirements. See Chapter 4 for more details
on gaining administrative support.

## WRITING HEALTH EDUCATION PROTOCOLS

Just as standardized protocols exist for accepted medical and nursing
practice, so also should protocols be written for health education practice,
and they should conform readily to the existing process of planning
nursing or medical care, as well as to the adopted format for documenting
and reviewing such care.

Your educational protocols should reflect a genuine integration into
these other aspects of the total health care scheme. The following steps
in a decision-making model can be useful (Bower, 1972): (1) assessment,
(2) problem identification, (3) formulation of plans for action, (4) planning

for evaluation, (5) implementation, and (6) evaluation. They give structure to the education protocol shown in Appendix 5.2 and filled out in Appendix 5.3. The protocol is easily adapted to other planning models. You will recognize the inclusion of the PRECEDE model components with the problem-oriented medical record documentation model.

A number of assumptions embedded in the education protocol presented in Appendix 5.2 should be discussed here:

**1.** Preparing for educational components of patient care takes time. Nevertheless, the quality of preparation (which takes time) is directly related to the successful achievement of stated outcomes.

**2.** Preparation need not take place in a vacuum. Every medical care organization has many content and process experts. Health educators in your institution, as well as from local colleges and universities, can be rich sources of support and assistance. Inservice instructors and staff development specialists are also great resources.

**3.** You need to examine the other likely places within the organization as well as in your community where your clients are likely to receive similar educational services. Linkages among such inpatient, outpatient, and home health services are of the greatest importance. Providing continuity of messages as well as reinforcement of educational messages is the highest level of service you can offer.

**4.** Care must be given to include all the members of the health care team in the preparation, implementation, and evaluation of health education efforts. For example, very often nurses ask physicians to write educational prescriptions for health education provided by nurses and other care providers. Usually, all team members who are affected by the educational intervention or who have the ability to assist or hinder the success of the education should be included at every step of the planning.

**5.** Special efforts should be taken to provide inservice education for all members involved in implementing and evaluating education. They should receive instructions regarding the rationale for the program as well as for the use of the protocol. All potential problems should be discussed, and strategies should be identified, during the course of inservice instruction, for problem resolution.

**6.** Since staff time and departmental resources are being invested in the educational aspects of care, special considerations should be made to ensure that all administrative concerns are addressed. The educational goals need to be compatible with the organization's goals, and a clear mandate must exist for including health education as a viable component of the medical care provided to your clients. Practitioners who take on educator roles should be given incentives. In addition, space, budget, and scheduling need to be arranged for. Even the best designed educational programs will be stunted if the organizational climate is not right.

**7.** Health education should be documented in the client's medical record. This procedure provides not only continuity of educational services but also a data base for future educational audits and peer reviews of the program.

## MAINTAINING ACCOUNTABILITY

How can health educators achieve and maintain their accountability for programs? The *Accreditation Manual for Hospitals* (1976), published by the Joint Commission on Accreditation of Hospitals (JCAH), specifies the scope of health education programs in medical care. The statements relate to the quality of professional services, patients' rights, emergency services, hospital-based home care, medical record services, nursing services, and outpatient services. The manual specifies that "evidence of the quality of patient care provided in the hospital shall be demonstrated by measurement of actual care against specific criteria. . . . Criteria must be explicit and measureable, and must reflect the optimal level of care that can be achieved through current medical and related health science knowledge. . . . Criteria shall include . . . demonstrated knowledge of the patient concerning his health status, level of functioning, and self-care after discharge" (Joint Commission on Accreditation of Hospitals, 1976, p. 22).

One vehicle for establishing the minimum standards against which health education services may be judged is the written educational protocol. Protocols may be developed to standardize criteria for quality educational services at the most general level (standards for planning organization-wide services) to the most specific (standards for educational services targeted to one client group, such as tension headache patients. Since health educators operate on multiple levels in medical care settings, it is possible that you will have a variety of educational protocols and plans. In the end, you must be accountable for your work. These planning tools provide guideposts for all aspects of the educational process, so that you can accomplish what you set out to do. Educational services must meet high standards of practice, and protocols help you quantify these standards so that you can understand how your efforts measure up.

Protocols and plans have limitations. Sometimes educators insist on following teaching plans verbatim instead of simply using them as guideposts. If your participants have a different agenda from your plans', or if their concerns, learning abilities, or cultural biases dictate other approaches, then you must adjust the educational process. The freedom to be flexible and to be totally responsive to client, organizational, or community demands is a by-product of experience, self-confidence, and firm grounding in the theoretical foundations of health education practice. To be accountable for our work, we need to prepare educational protocols and plans; to be effective in our work, we mustn't take them too seriously.

# APPENDIX 5.1

## Health Education Protocol for Client Behavior Change*

| *Client Outcomes* | *Provider Tasks* |
|---|---|
| 1. States health condition | • Reviews objective data with client (such as laboratory test data, physical examination results, age)<br>• Assesses client's health beliefs<br>• Assesses client's perception of vulnerability to health risk or health problem |
| 2. States willingness to change | • Reviews treatment alternatives<br>• Clarifies client and provider roles<br>• Initiates discussion on benefits and costs of making the change<br>• Generates a statement of willingness to change<br>• Clarifies client's intention for the overall goal |

*Modified from the original work of Maureen Dion, M.P.H., and Julie Howard, M.P.H., the Total Health Care Project, the Kaiser-Permanente Medical Care Program, Oakland, California.

| *Client Outcomes* | *Provider Tasks* |
|---|---|
| 3.  Lists factors affecting behavior (both obstacles and support) | • Introduces self-monitoring skills<br>• Helps client identify factors<br>• Emphasizes supportive factors |
| 4.  Acknowledges that change is a long process | • Encourages client to describe previous experiences with change<br>• Explains that change is a gradual process<br>• Emphasizes that realistic expectations regarding the time it takes to change are important<br>• Explores how activities of daily living and priorities affect client's decision to change<br>• Emphasizes the value of coping skills; describes one or two skills; models one |
| 5.  Develops short- and long-term goals | • Guides client to set small steps for gradual change<br>• Prepares client to anticipate challenges to those goals<br>• Encourages client to identify support for goals and rewards for reaching the small steps along the way |
| 6.  Plans for change | • Helps client develop a daily routine that incorporates small steps toward the goal<br>• Rehearses how small steps can be taken each day<br>• Provides written instructions for daily strategies<br>• Emphasizes benefits over losses<br>• Assists client to predict risk situations that may arise |

| *Client Outcomes* | *Provider Tasks* |
|---|---|
| 7. Acts toward change | • Introduces self-management skills<br>• Encourages strategies that involve the client's support system<br>• Asks client to list items in the environment (office, home, club, church) that help or hinder plans for change<br>• Encourages client to establish meaningful rewards for each small success |
| 8. Defines success; acknowledges difference between setback and failure | • Helps client define each step toward the goal as a measure of success<br>• Encourages client to acknowledge the value of a few setbacks<br>• Encourages client to avoid temptation to define setbacks as failures<br>• Prepares for temptations to relapse and for difficult situations<br>• Helps client revise plans if necessary |
| 9. Schedules maintenance of goals and follow-up | • Encourages involvement of an ongoing support system<br>• Collaborates on a follow-up plan<br>• Helps client develop a contingency plan<br>• Prepares client for ongoing self-monitoring |

# APPENDIX 5.2

## Sample Education Protocol*

Health Problem: _____

Program Goal: _____

_____

I. Assessment

   A. What health behaviors are most linked to the health problem and most able to be changed through education? List in ranked order, 1 being most important.

      1. _____
      2. _____
      3. _____
      4. _____

   B. List the predisposing factors that affect the behaviors listed in Item A. List in ranked order, 1 being most important.

      1. _____
      2. _____
      3. _____
      4. _____

   C. List the enabling factors that affect the behaviors listed in Item A. List in ranked order, 1 being most important.

      1. _____
      2. _____
      3. _____
      4. _____

*SOURCE: Developed by Wendy D. Squyres, Ph.D.

D. List the reinforcing factors that affect the behaviors listed in Item A. List in ranked order, 1 being most important.

1. _____
2. _____
3. _____
4. _____

E. Identify the top-ranking factors from B, C, and D that are most significantly linked to the health behaviors and most likely to be changed as a result of education interventions.

1. _____
2. _____
3. _____
4. _____

II. Problem Identification

A. What potential obstacles or barriers may occur in developing the teaching program?

1. _____
2. _____
3. _____
4. _____

B. What potential problems may occur in implementing the teaching program?

1. _____
2. _____
3. _____
4. _____

III. Plans for Action

A. For each of the factors listed in Item I.E, write learning objectives.

1. _____
_____

    2. _____

    _____

    3. _____

    _____

B. In order for these objectives to be accomplished, which educational methods will be employed? Match one or more methods to each of the items listed in Item III.A.

    1. _____

    2. _____

    3. _____

C. For each operational statement in Item III.A, attach a teaching plan. (Use the accompanying form.)

IV. Planning for Evaluation

A. For each of the top-ranking behaviors selected in Item I.A, write a behavioral objective. Describe (1) what the patient is expected to be able to do, (2) the important conditions under which the performance is to occur, (3) the standard for successful performance (Mager, 1975).

    1. _____

    _____

    _____

    2. _____

    _____

    _____

    3. _____

    _____

    _____

B. For each of the objectives listed in Item IV.A, attach an instrument designed to test its accomplishment. (Use the accompanying form.)

# Teaching Plan to Accompany the Education Protocol

A. **Learning Objective**

   Teaching Content

   Teaching Aids

   Guide Questions for Patients

   Teacher's Resource List

B. **Learning Objective**

   Teaching Content

   Teaching Aids

   Questions for Patients

C. **Learning Objective**

   Teaching Content

   Teaching Aids

   Questions for Patients

## Goal Sheet to Accompany the Education Protocol

Date: _____

Time: _____

| *I Want To:* | *I've Reached My Goal When:* |
|---|---|
| 1. | |
| 2. | |
| 3. | |
| 4. | |
| 5. | |
| 6. | |
| 7. | |
| 8. | |
| 9. | |
| 10. | |

C. For each of the objectives listed in Item IV.A, describe the expected health outcome.

1. _____

2. _____

3. _____

D. How will the health outcomes be measured?

1. _____

2. _____

3. _____

E. For each of the objectives listed in Item IV.A, what will be the other positive benefits to the patient, the family, or to the organization, that are a result of the educational intervention?

1. _____

2. _____

3. _____

F. How will the benefits listed in Item IV.E be measured?

1. _____

2. _____

3. _____

G. How can the measurement of the outcomes of the educational intervention be set up to ensure that what was set up to be tested actually was tested and that the results have some implications for other similar teaching situations?

V. Implementation

Attach a time line for the planning and implementation activities—for example:

| Steps | Tasks | Completion Date |
|---|---|---|
| 1 | Assessment | _____ |
| 2 | Problem identification and problem solving | _____ |

3        Program planning:

            Staff development             _____

            Operational definitions       _____

            List of methods              _____

            Teaching plans ready         _____

4        Evaluation:

            Behavioral objectives         _____

            Instruments designed         _____

            Health outcomes determined   _____

            Benefits tested              _____

            Validity/reliability checks     _____

# APPENDIX 5.3

## Filled-in Version of the Sample Education Protocol*

Health Problem: Control/Prevention of Chronic Headaches

Program Goal: To provide knowledge and skills that will enable patient to
use alternate methods of pain control other than prescription drugs.

I. Assessment

    A. What health behaviors are most linked to the health problem and most
able to be changed through education? List in ranked order, 1 being most
important.

        1. Selecting appropriate modality for pain control/prevention

        2. Planning and executing daily relaxation techniques

        3. Eliminating stress-producing elements from diet

        4. Keeping journal for self-monitoring

    B. List the predisposing factors that affect the behaviors listed in Item A.
List in ranked order, 1 being most important.

        1. Willingness to try new methods

        2. Knowledge of purpose and expected results of alternative methods

        3. Knowledge of stress-producing elements in diet

        4. Ability to keep journal

    C. List the enabling factors that affect the behaviors listed in Item A. List
in ranked order, 1 being most important.

        1. Availability of time and space for practice

        2. Financial ability to obtain stress-reducing dietary elements

        3. Financial ability to obtain manuals/equipment

        4. _____

*SOURCE: Information provided by Margaret Winslow, student, University of California,
San Francisco, Patient Education Certificate Program, 1982.

D. List the reinforcing factors that affect the behaviors listed in Item A. List in ranked order, 1 being most important.

1. Availability of advice/support from instructor

2. Willingness of significant others to reduce stress in environment

3. Knowledge of stress-reducing dietary elements by significant others

4. Cooperation and encouragement of significant others in the practice of alternative methods

E. Identify the top-ranking factors from B, C, and D that are most significantly linked to the health behaviors and most likely to be changed as a result of education interventions.

1. Knowledge of purposes and expected results of alternative methods

2. Knowledge of stress-reducing dietary elements

3. Ability to keep useful journal

4. Support of significant others for alternative methods

II. Problem Identification

A. What potential obstacles or barriers may occur in developing the teaching program?

1. Obtaining favorable priority ranking for program from program committee

2. Obtaining administration and staff support for demonstration and instruction of alternative methods

3. Securing qualified instructors

4. Getting adequate publicity

B. What potential problems may occur in implementing the teaching program?

1. Changes in priorities within health education department

2. Inadequate publicity

3. Matching room availability with staff availability

4. Resistance of significant others to participate

III. Plans for Action

A. For each of the factors listed in Item I.E., write learning objectives.

1. By the end of the first session, 75 percent of the participants will have selected an alternative method to use.

2. By the end of the second session, 80 percent of the participants will be able to report correct application of method.

3. By the end of the third session, 95 percent of the participants will be able to identify stress-producing dietary elements.

B. In order for these objectives to be accomplished, which educational methods will be employed? Match one or more methods to each of the items listed in Item III.A.

1. Lecture, demonstrations, self-surveys (evaluation), bibliographies

2. Self-report forms, demonstration, bibliographies

3. Film, flip chart, lecture, handouts

C. For each operational statement in Item III.A, attach a teaching plan. attached

IV. Planning for Evaluation

A. For each of the top-ranking behaviors selected in Item I.A., write a behavioral objective. Describe (1) what the patient is expected to be able to do, (2) the important conditions under which the performance is to occur, and (3) the standard for successful performance (Mager, 1975).

1. Participant will use sign-up sheet for method in class and instructor will verify appropriateness for person, i.e., review time, space, money.

2. Participant will be able to report/demonstrate correct application of method. Self-report chart or demonstration will be verified by instructor.

3.  Participant will be able to identify stress-producing dietary elements at home and work. Self-reporting checklist will be collected.

B.  For each of the objectives listed in Item IV.A., attach an instrument designed to test its accomplishment. (See attached sample.)
    attached

C.  For each of the objectives listed in Item IV.A., describe the expected health outcome.

1.  Fewer or less intense headaches

2.  Better nutrition

3.  Fewer doctor or nurse practitioner visits and fewer prescriptions

D.  How will the health outcomes be measured?

1.  Self-report

2.  Self-report

3.  Number of prescriptions or doctor-nurse practitioner visits

E.  For each of the objectives listed in Item IV.A., what will be the other positive benefits to the patient, the family, or to the organization, that are a result of the educational intervention?

1.  Patient—Better feeling about self and world; more time, energy, and money for positive activities

2.  Family—Better nutrition and more harmonious interaction

3.  Organization—Less sick time and higher productivity

F.  How will the benefits listed in Item IV.E be measured?

1.  Follow-up visit with instructor or other staff with self-report

2.  Chart check for doctor-nurse practitioner visits and prescriptions

3.  Six-month follow-ups for two years

G. How can the measurement of the outcomes of the educational intervention be set up to ensure that what was set up to be tested actually was tested, and that the results have some implications for other similar teaching situations?

V. Implementation

Attach a time line for the planning and implementation activities—for example:

| Steps | Task | Completion Date |
|---|---|---|
| 1 | Assessment | January, February 1984 |
| 2 | Problem identification and problem solving | March |
| 3 | Program planning | |
| | Staff development | April, May |
| | Operational definitions | June |
| | List of methods | July |
| | Teaching plans ready | August |
| 4 | Evaluation | |
| | Behavioral objectives | March |
| | Instruments designed | April |
| | Health outcomes determined | September |
| | Benefits tested | September |
| | Validity/reliability checks | March, September 1985 |

## Teaching Plan to Accompany the Education Profile

A. **Learning Objective** By the end of the first session, 75 percent of the participants will have selected an alternate method to use for headache pain.

Teaching Content Lecture by primary instructor introducing and explaining expected results from biofeedback, acupressure, journal keeping, visualization, and acupuncture as methods for preventing, controlling, or alleviating chronic headache pain. Demonstration by primary instructor or teaching instructor of methods.

Teaching Aids  Biofeedback machine, Body Buddy (relaxation tool), journal. Handouts for self-evaluation, equipment sources, community resources, bibliographies.

Guide Questions for Patients  Contained in self-evaluation forms. Verbal questions that could be included in lecture to stimulate self-evaluation leading to selection of method might be "Which situations are stress-producing at this time of your life? Which foods and beverages seem to result in added stress? How many 'toxic' people do you feel are in your life at this time? Which stress situations do you feel are self-induced and which are other-induced? What kinds of solutions are you currently using for headache pain control?"

Teacher's Resource List  Bibliographies

B.  **Learning Objective**  By the end of the second session, 80 percent of the participants will be able to report or demonstrate correct application of method selected.

Teaching Content  Verification, clarification, and additional instruction where needed during and after self-report or demonstration.

Teaching Aids  Same as in Item A.

Questions for Patients  Are you pleased with your choice of methods? Where are the areas of greatest success or difficulty? What has been the response of your significant others, doctor, or friends? How do you feel about yourself?

C.  **Learning Objective**  By the end of the third session, 95 percent of the participants will be able to identify stress-producing dietary elements.

Teaching Content  Lecture by nutritionist explaining how certain foods and beverages encourage or cause stress through metabolic changes. Showing of film on nutrition (and, if time, on stress). Discussion of film, journal keeping, and exercise.

Teaching Aids  Flip chart, film, journal sample. Handouts of self-check on eating habits, exercise habits. Blackboard.

Questions for Patients  What is your least favorite food? What is your favorite snack? When are you most likely to have it? What is your favorite beverage? How many times a day do you drink some?

## Sample Goal Sheet for Headache Patients

Date: <u>May 27</u>

Time: <u>3:00 p.m.</u>

| *I Want To:* | *I've Reached My Goal When:* |
|---|---|
| 1. Return to work | I'm well enough to begin working at least three days a week. |
| 2. Make love with Bill like we used to | I'm able to enjoy sex without pain. |
| 3. Sleep more soundly | I sleep eight consecutive hours without awakening. |
| 4. Stop taking pain pills | I can throw all my medications away. |
| 5. Drive a car | I can drive by myself to Don's school. |
| 6. Go to a movie | I can sit in a crowded theater comfortably for two straight hours. |
| 7. Go to a nightclub and dance | I can stand the loud noises and dance without pain. |
| 8. Not have to depend on doctors | I can stop seeing Dr. Carlton. |
| 9. Travel to see my sister. | I can visit Martha in Oregon at Christmas. |
| 10. Climb stairs more quickly | I can climb 20 stairs, one right after the other. |

# APPENDIX 5.4

## Patient Education Program Plan

Title of Program: _____

1. Need:
   - What is the need identified?

   - How was the need determined and by whom?

2. Standards/outcomes for patient education program:

3. Program goals and objectives:

4. Target group (inpatient, outpatient, family members):

5. Program outline:
   - Content:

   - Method:

   - Instructor:

   - Time:

6. Facilities used:

7. Time and frequency of offering program:

8. Publicity methods:

9. Evaluation methods:

10. Immediate follow-up:

11. Cost
    - Time of employees' teaching:

    - Time of education coordinator:

    - Supplies:

    - Audiovisual materials:

    - Food

| | Estimated Cost | Actual Cost |
|---|---|---|
| | | |
| Totals | | |

12. Sources of funding:

13. Comments and evaluations:

_____

Education Coordinator's Signature

# EXERCISES

1.  The following is an example of headings used in a teaching record that is to become part of a client's medical record. It is designed to record the educational encounter. Given your understanding of accountability for quality in health education practice, identify the strengths and weaknesses of this format. Using a concrete example, suggest ways in which to correct or modify the weaknesses.

**Teaching Record**

| Diagnosis: | | | | | | |
|---|---|---|---|---|---|---|
| Item to be taught | Date started | Patient's understanding (Good, Fair, Poor) | Reinforcement | | Patient verbalizes understanding | |
| | | | Needed | Given | Yes | No |

2.  For one educational program in patient education or health promotion, complete the outline of the program plan suggested in Appendix 5.4. Once you have completed the plan, suggest three or more ways to improve on the format.

# RESOURCES

American Hospital Association, *Implementing Patient Education in the Hospital*. AHA no. 1488. Chicago: American Hospital Association, 1979.

> This manual is a loosely organized compendium of materials from hospitals all over the country. Chapter 8 is devoted to designing a patient education program for specific patient populations. Many samples of teaching plans are included, for a variety of health problems and from a variety of hospitals.

Bressler, R., Bogdonoff, M.D., and Subak-Sharpe, G. *The Internists' Compendium of Patient Information*. New York: Biomedical Information Corporation, 1983.

> To encourage internists to educate their clients, the publishers of the *Compendium of Drug Therapy* have compiled this companion resource book. Multiple tear sheets are provided on thirty-two of the most common problems seen by primary-care physicians. The topics cover a span from angina

to valvular disease. Each sheet is a summary of information on the health topic of interest, followed by space for individualized instructions. The tear sheet is designed so that the primary-care physician can augment patient counseling with this summary of the information sheet. The emphasis is on pathophysiology. By using these information sheets, physicians can feel free to spend more of the counseling time on psychological and social issues. The compendium editors do not suggest this advantage, nor do they help physicians go beyond simple information dissemination with these educational aids.

De Joseph, J. Writing Educational Protocols. In W. Squyres, *Patient Education: An Inquiry into the State of the Art.* New York: Springer, 1980, 45–112.

De Joseph presents an extensive teaching plan for nurse educators in coronary care units and medical units in hospitals who teach coronary rehabilitation programs. This plan was developed at the Stanford University Hospital and is used widely in the West. The plan includes (1) references for nurse preparation, (2) suggested content, (3) teaching aids, (4) guide questions to ask patients, (5) a knowledge assessment questionnaire, (6) a physical assessment form, (7) a psychological survey questionnaire, and (8) a teaching progress sheet for inclusion in the medical record.

Freedman, C. R. *Teaching Patients: A Practical Handbook for the Health Care Professional.* San Diego: Courseware, 1978.

The original version of this manual was designed in conjunction with the San Diego Lung Association to help health care professionals to sharpen their patient education skills with chronic obstructive lung patients. In its current form, the manual is intended to be used in any type of teaching situation in a medical care setting. The skills orientation—both for participants and for educators—is a welcome addition to the literature. The manual is written in a workbook style and includes a format for and samples of teaching plans.

McCormick, R. D., and Gilson-Parkevich, T. (eds.). *Patient and Family Education: Tools, Techniques, and Theory.* New York: Wiley, 1979.

The authors summarize educational theories and give practical suggestions (and many examples) for preparing teaching plans and teaching aids. They include more than seventy patient education aids for pediatric and adult services that are currently in use at Children's Hospital in Columbus, Ohio. Chapter 2 summarizes educational theory and offers two formats for writing health education teaching plans.

One shortcoming of the models offered is the emphasis on knowledge acquisition rather than on skill development. Participants may verbalize information correctly, but may not know how to take action—or may even choose to not take action. Checklists that document the dissemination of information do not answer the critical question "Did my educational efforts work?"

Pritchett, S. *Patient, Family and Community Health Education: Design and Management of Hospital-Based Programs.* Atlanta: Pritchett & Hull Associates, 1977.

This workbook is designed for people who are new to designing and coordinating hospital-wide health education services. Pritchett wrote the workbook for health educators in "average community hospitals." The workbook takes the reader through the steps in developing a hospital-wide program for patients and families, and includes community outreach education aimed at disease prevention and health promotion. After working through the 85-page book, the reader will have an action plan for implementing hospital-wide health education services. A sample format for teaching plans for specific programs is also included.

Zander, K. S., Bower, K. A., Foster, S. D., Towson, M. C., Wermuth, M. R., and Woldum, K. M. *Practical Manual for Patient-Teaching.* St. Louis: Mosby, 1978.

The authors of this manual are members of the Retrospective Audit Committee of the Department of Nursing at Tufts-New England Medical Center Hospital. The committee felt that the problem-oriented medical record method of charting was too cumbersome for recording the detailed content of every teaching session. They believed that nurses would not use a system that was too elaborate, time consuming, or repetitive, so they produced a system that is easy to use. The manual is a compilation of teaching plans that can serve as a reference for the nurse educator. The plans provide a format that can be placed in the patients' medical records.

This reference will be useful for hospital-based nurse educators. However, the plans suffer from overzealous objectives and from an emphasis on content rather than on educational process. If nurse educators have had little training in the educational process, these plans will not help them create a bridge between the content and the learner objectives as they are stated in each plan.

# 6

## Selecting educational methods

IN THE EDUCATIONAL protocol which is provided in Chapter 5, section IIIB requires the educator to match educational methods with the learning objectives. Chapter 6 further elaborates on the PRECEDE model by classifying methods in ways that will help you develop sound teaching plans and conduct educational programs that match your clients' needs and expectations. Four major teaching methods are highlighted. This chapter also offers criteria for selecting educational methods.

### GETTING READY TO DECIDE

Are you ready to tackle the problem of selecting the best educational methods for the services you are planning? Take a moment to answer the following questions, which will test your readiness:

**1.** Do you already have a written statement of the health problem that your educational program is designed to ameliorate or prevent?

**2.** Have you already determined the actions that your clients must take (individually or collectively) on their own behalf in order to prevent or manage their health problem?

**3.** Have you already identified client factors (such as clients' knowledge, attitudes, beliefs, and cultural dispositions) that may affect the likelihood that these actions will be taken?

**4.** Have you already listed the physical, economic, or system barriers that might help or hinder clients in their efforts to take action?

**5.** Have you already determined the extent to which your clients' peers, family, and health providers influence the likelihood that these actions will be taken?

**6.** Have you examined your clients' learning patterns and preferences? (For example, do they like to read information more than they like to hear health messages? Do they prefer participation in groups to individual counseling?)

If you answered yes to these questions, you are ready to think about which educational methods are best suited to meet the needs of your clients and are best suited to meet the objectives of your educational effort. If you answered no to any of these questions, reread Chapter 5, and complete the "Educational Diagnosis" section.

Educators often employ a favorite educational method, regardless of the factors that influence their clients' behavior. But the methods suggested by an educational diagnosis vary, based on the clients' characteristics and health problems, on the actions the client is being asked to take, as well as on the environment of the community and of the organization serving the client. For these reasons, employing educational methods contraindicated by a diagnosis, or in the absence of a diagnosis, may lead to program failure. Programs fail when they cannot meet their objectives.

Instead, you may find it useful to conduct an analysis on three levels—individual, programmatic, and institutional—before deciding which methods are best for the goals you have in mind. First, look at your clients' needs, learning styles, cultural orientations, values, beliefs, and language ability. Second, analyze the educational program—its objectives, time frames, and relationship to other educational services available in your organization and in your community. Third, look at your institution—space available, budget, organizational climate, and political milieu. Analysis at all three levels will give you information that can guide your selection of educational methods.

Before we proceed to the selection process, let us make an important distinction between method and technology. The greatest boon and trap for education in the twentieth century is, undoubtedly, technology. Educational technology capable of matching client and program needs can enhance learning and health behavior change. However, sometimes health professionals hope that technology (such as closed-circuit television, printed information, or movies) can substitute for a formal, planned educational process. This hope is not supported by research and leads to ineffective programs and frustrated clients. Educational methods are not substitutes for the educational process—they are simply tools that help the client to learn in the context of a more complex learning/teaching effort.

Moreover, educational methods are often adopted before programs are planned. For example, movies are purchased, videotapes are produced, or pamphlets are printed before a formal program is even conceived. Hospitals install bedside televisions with in-house broadcasting capabilities, without understanding how to apply this method. It is inappropriate to create an educational program as an embellishment to a preexisting film, for instance, simply because the film is available. The competition for limited resources for all educational services, and the challenge to set priorities that best serve clients, call for a more systematic process of integrating methods into other aspects of educational planning. Figure 6.1 shows the steps that precede and follow the selection of educational methods.

Educational services offered in medical care serve a wide range of client goals. For example, a growing number of educational programs are geared to providing social support for the hospitalized, chronically ill, or grieving. These services can provide a much-needed buffer against the isolation and fear that pervade such clients' experiences. In emotional and social support groups, clients may not be expected to do anything but participate. At a time when clients' personal internal resources are so depleted, the support group can provide a place where people can simply be accepted as they are and be refueled to go on with their lives. Methods such as active listening, discussion, and praise and encouragement are useful in such settings.

Most other educational services, however, have as an intermediate goal a change in clients' habits or activities that will improve or protect their health. In such cases, clients must take certain steps to meet their goals.

**Figure 6.1   Health education planning steps**

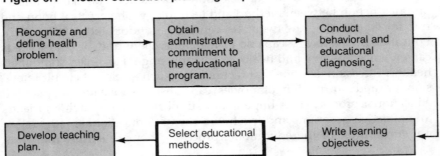

**Table 6.1 Two sample health education programs: Behaviors and methods**

---

### Patient education program: Back care class

| *Target client health behavior* | *Educational methods* |
|---|---|
| Daily back exercises | • Demonstration |
| | • Practice |
| | • Lecture |
| | • Questions and answers |
| | • Audiovisuals |

### Health promotion program: Stop smoking class

| *Target client health behaviors* | *Educational methods* |
|---|---|
| Quit smoking cigarettes | • Discussion |
| Begin physical exercise program | • Lecture |
| Design personalized strategies that will prepare for tempting situations that come up | • Worksheets |
| | • Audiovisuals |
| | • Questions and answers |
| | • Role playing |
| | • Values clarification |
| | • Self-instructional guides |

---

Table 6.1 takes a sample of two health education programs from a medical care setting and describes target client health behaviors and educational methods used to stimulate the change in behavior. This example is not meant to exhaust all the possible client behaviors to be modified or added, nor does it list all possible educational methods. The table shows the relationship between targeted health behaviors and educational methods.

For example, if you are teaching a class on back care that recommends to its participants that back exercises be done every day, then you may want to emphasize these points in a lecture, lead a question and answer period, do a demonstration of the exercises, and then conduct a session where participants actually do the exercises under supervision with feedback. In this example the methods were chosen for their ability to contribute to the goal of encouraging clients to do daily back exercises after the class is over.

## CRITERIA FOR SELECTING EDUCATIONAL METHODS

The Committee on Educational Tasks in Chronic Illness of the Public Health Service, Health Resources Administration suggests the following criteria for selecting educational methods:

**1.** *Effectiveness.* This criterion indicates the extent to which an activity achieves the stated goal. An educational method is considered highly effective if it attains the goal.

**2.** *Efficiency.* This criterion indicates the amount of resources used to attain the goal. Efficiency takes into account the variables of payroll costs, productivity, and operating costs.

**3.** *Adequacy.* This criterion indicates the degree to which an educational activity or method can achieve the goal. One educational method by itself is usually inadequate. However, when the method is combined with another, a synergistic effect occurs that allows a program to achieve its goal.

**4.** *Appropriateness.* This criterion indicates the relevance of the method in achieving the goal with respect to the culture and environment of the client.

## CLASSIFYING METHODS

There are many ways to classify methods. This section begins by following the steps of the educational diagnosis recommended in Chapter 5: listing methods in the context of (1) predisposing, (2) enabling, and (3) reinforcing factors.

### Predisposing factors

Predisposing factors are the clients' personal preferences—such as their knowledge, attitudes, beliefs, values, and perceptions—that either support or inhibit targeted health behaviors (Green et al., 1980). The following educational methods are most likely to influence a client to make positive health behavior changes:

- Audiovisuals
- Lecture
- Mass media
- Individual instruction

- Simulations and games
- Group facilitation
- Role playing
- Computer-assisted learning
- Interviewing
- Programmed learning

These methods are well suited to conveying health information to clients. They can be used effectively to influence or clarify clients' attitudes, beliefs, and values. Although health information alone rarely leads to long-term health behavior change, after receiving a sound rationale for making a commitment to take action, many clients do so. Also, as people practice the skills required for health behavior change, they often want more information so that they can feel more motivated to go on to the next level of skill.

If you choose to disseminate information, what medium should you choose? Hecht (1978, p. 4) offers the following questions, the answers to which may guide you in selecting the most appropriate medium:

**1.** Must the program use a visual medium, or could it achieve the same goals in a printed format or as an audiotape?

**2.** If it requires visuals, is motion essential to get across the most important ideas? If so, a film or videotape might be indicated. If motion is not essential, a slide program may be most appropriate.

**3.** Will the program need frequent content changes to update it? Such needs may affect the choice of medium. For example, slide programs are easier and less expensive to revise than films or videotapes.

**4.** Will the program be used primarily by individuals, small groups, or large groups? If the answer is "large groups" and if the program requires a motion medium, film may sometimes be more appropriate than videotape, depending on the availability of film equipment and the set-up of the rooms where large groups convene.

Table 6.2 can help the educator make wide media selections. Also, see the Resources section at the end of this chapter for a review of educational methods using media.

## Enabling factors

Enabling factors include the skills and resources that your clients will need to take action. The educator may employ the following educational

**Table 6.2   Matching media capability with media type**

| Capability | Type |
| --- | --- |
| 1. Learning objectives | |
|    a. Knowledge | • Slides<br>• Motion picture (film and videotape)<br>• Television<br>• Audio recordings<br>• Programmed instruction<br>• Textbooks, brochures, pamphlets<br>• Oral presentations<br>• Computer-assisted programs |
|    b. Skills | • Motion pictures (film and videotape)<br>• Demonstration |
|    c. Attitudes | • Motion pictures (film and videotape)<br>• Television<br>• Audio recordings<br>• Programmed instruction<br>• Demonstration<br>• Printed materials<br>• Oral presentations<br>• Computer-assisted programs |
| 2. Portability (use at home, etc.) | • Videotape<br>• Audio recordings<br>• Slides<br>• Printed materials |
| 3. Large room (conventions, ballrooms) | • Large-screen televisions<br>• Multiple TV monitors<br>• 35 mm film |
| 4. Conference room | • 16 mm film<br>• Videotape<br>• Filmstrips<br>• Sound on slide<br>• Chalkboard<br>• Chartpad |
| 5. Individual/one-to-one | • Print materials<br>• Flip charts<br>• Computer-assisted instruction |

methods to ensure that clients are able to follow through on their decisions to engage in positive health behaviors:

- Audiovisuals, educational television
- Behavior modification
- Individual instruction
- Practice sessions
- Modeling
- Role playing
- Simulations and games
- Community organizing
- Organizational development

Injecting insulin, for instance, is a behavior that requires proper technique and the ability to meet certain performance standards. One or more of the methods listed could be used to teach the necessary skills for successful insulin injections.

The most powerful method for building or improving skills is to get the client into action. Practice under supervision and with feedback is the best possible method to use when you are helping clients build their skills. The more passive methods of having the clients observe someone else performing the skill (modeling, audiovisuals) are not as effective as the trial and error benefits of doing it themselves. Coaches of professional basketball teams wouldn't think of sending their basketball players on a court against another team after only having them watch a film of other players making baskets. Even after a number of film showings, the team could not become proficient without actual practice. Yet many educators assume their clients will be able to gain new skills or sharpen old ones simply through exposure to audiovisuals or demonstrations. We set unrealistic expectations when we select a single educational method that is not powerful enough on its own to influence the targeted behavior.

The basic ingredients of a good practice session are as follows (Freedman, 1978, p. 123):*

1. Select practice opportunities which match the objective and which are as much like what the patient will do (or does) at home as possible. Write a brief description of what the patient should do in each situation. (Often this will be little more than a restatement of the objective.)

*Reprinted with the permission of Courseware, Inc., San Diego, California. All rights reserved.

Try to match the task and the conditions (materials, setting, etc.) that the patient will actually be faced with at home. This lets both of you be more sure that the patient will be able to do the task when he's out of the hospital setting. If the hospital conditions are too different, the patient may not be able to translate what has been practiced to the home setting.

**2.** If the patient needs to use the objective in a variety of circumstances, describe the various opportunities you will allow for practicing each circumstance. It is especially important for the patients to practice doing objectives in the various circumstances where they will be used, both to make their use a habit for the patients, and to enable you to see if they have difficulty performing in any of the different circumstances.

For instance, when teaching breathing with body mechanics [as for chronic obstructive lung disease], it would not be very beneficial to confine patients' practice to a small set of limited activities like sitting down and getting up from a chair or simply pushing a broom. The patient should also be given a chance to practice one or more situations which involve reaching, lifting, pushing, bending, etc. Furthermore, these situations should be taken from things the patient is likely to do throughout the day (done in the morning, afternoon, evening). Your description of the practice should specify the situations to be included.

**3.** Consider the kinds of common errors that a patient might make, and
   a. Be sure that your practice will give the patient a chance to make these errors. . . . Patients frequently make [at least] two errors:
      • Mistakenly recognizing the circumstances for a particular decision or action so that (1) he makes the decision or takes action when he shouldn't, or (2) he doesn't make the decision and take action when he should
      • Being unable to follow steps or do calculations in complex situations
   It's important to provide patients with practices that show you (and the patient) whether he has fully mastered the objective or whether he's likely to make mistakes.
   b. Think of several ways of pointing them out and correcting them, while still reinforcing the positive aspects of the patient's overall performance. For instance, when teaching a patient to perform bronchial drainage who has difficulty staying in a position long enough, you might comment on his ability to assume the positions well, cough properly, etc., and then tell him that patients often have difficulty telling how long they have been in a position and when they have been there long enough. You might then suggest

that he look at his watch for the next position to keep track of time.

Certain behavior modification strategies, such as goal setting, contracting, self-monitoring, and self-reward, are excellent methods to employ in conjunction with practice. These methods are covered in detail in other texts mentioned in the Resources section of this chapter.

Enabling methods also include rerouting resources or changing faulty systems. For instance, it is very valuable to reduce waiting time for appointments, make transportation more accessible, and make options economically feasible. Nevertheless, these methods usually require major investments of time and energy on the part of the educator, in concert with others. Organizational deficiencies often cause very real barriers for clients who are struggling to make positive health behavior changes. Common examples are long waiting lists for classes, difficulties in making appointments, inaccessibility of classrooms, class times that meet the scheduling needs of the staff but not of the clients, discontinuity of care, and difficulty in documenting educational services in the client's health record. These dilemmas may not be in your power to solve. Nevertheless, you are often in the best position to initiate organizational change by bringing these matters to the attention of decision makers and to stimulate interdepartmental problem-solving meetings.

Very often, there are very real economic and physical barriers in the community—such as lack of outdoor facilities for physical exercise in inner cities, racial discrimination, or widespread economic deprivation (such as job layoffs in the automobile and airline industries, which leave people without a source of income). Under these conditions, the educator could refer clients to community services, if such services exist. However, where social action is required, you need to be involved in the community, to act as a catalyst for social change on behalf of your clients. Recognition of the complete profile of your clients—their psychological needs and characteristics, their social networks and affiliations, and their physical environment—allows you to influence your clients' health potential in the most powerful way. As an educator, in recognition of this dynamic relationship, you can act as an advocate for the client on as many levels as are feasible.

## Reinforcing factors

Reinforcing factors determine whether your clients' health actions are supported by others. The sources of support include the clients' parents, spouse, children, other relatives, friends, neighbors, fellow workers, the boss, health providers, or medical care system staff. The reinforcement may be positive or negative. The challenge for the health educator is to develop strategies that (1) include several key people in the clients' lives, as participants in the educational program, and (2) help the clients expand their own skills in generating support and coping with negative reinforcement.


## MAJOR TEACHING METHODS

Educational methods that you may employ to reinforce your clients' positive health behaviors are, for example, (1) group facilitation, (2) role playing, (3) interviewing, and (4) simulations and games.

### Group facilitation

Group facilitation is a process whereby the educator brings clients and members of their families or support networks (such as friends or neighbors) together in order to discuss issues relevant to reinforcing positive client health behaviors.

  In these discussions, clients must feel free to raise issues and concerns about their willingness or ability to follow through on the actions they need to take. The educator structures the discussion in such a way as to increase the participation of clients, their families, and their friends in defining obstacles to action. The facilitator sets an environment where clients are able to ask for help and are able to participate in mutual problem solving with their support group. As problems are raised, the educator resists the temptation to give solutions to these problems. Throughout the group discussions, the educator makes sure that the environment in the group is conducive to client and family problem solving. As clients hear others in the group express concerns or solutions, they learn that they are not alone in their experience. At the same time, clients expand their repertoire of solutions. Chronic health problems, such as arthritis, cancer, and diabetes, are most amenable to such group work.

  Many educators in the medical care delivery system are clinicians by training; they are used to dispensing advice and to working directly with clients on a one-to-one basis. Because there is a growing recognition of the value of mutual aid and support in the therapeutic process, and because of their efficiency, groups have become a more important form of medical education. Group facilitation skills can be learned and refined by all health professionals. We strongly recommend that all educators who have not had formal training in group facilitation do so before actually acting in this role with clients. Many hospitals and clinics and universities offer continuing education classes and workshops on group facilitation skills for health professionals.

## Role playing

Role playing is a method that can be adapted to meet the objectives of an educational group or that can be a part of a one-to-one educational session. Through role playing, clients can learn how to effectively ask for support or to deal with social situations where they may encounter negative reinforcement. Either the educator or the client can design a hypothetical situation for the role play. For example, what does a drying-out alcoholic say to the friend who offers a drink? Clients can be given the opportunity to play several roles during the session (as themselves, as their spouse, and so on). In this way, through rehearsal, clients become more comfortable with situations as they actually come up in daily life. The role-played situations should approximate clients' life experiences—otherwise clients will feel that this exercise is trivial or a waste of their time. The role plays should be structured and given a defined time limit, and at the end of the session there should be time to discuss clients' reactions to their role-playing experience.

## Interviewing

Interviews are another educational technique for reinforcing positive health behaviors. You can interview clients and their families or peers in order to shed light on their issues and concerns. Interview data also can suggest realistic strategies for solving problems.

It is important to keep in mind that the main purpose of one-to-one interviews is to generate information, not to dispense advice. Special attention should be given to structured yet open-ended questions that encourage clients to describe their experiences and concerns and that encourage the significant people in their lives to listen and to express their willingness to help the client toward a goal.

Interviewing as a technique has some drawbacks, however. Conducting interviews is much more labor-intensive than leading or coordinating educational groups. Moreover, as rich as one-to-one interviews are as a source of data, they do not compare to group experiences. Educational groups give participants an opportunity to learn from each other.

## Simulations and games

As educational methods, simulations and games are very similar to role playing. Instead of using a real-life situation (as in role playing) simulations use analogies that teach skills rather than teach reactions to specific situations. Simulations and games try to build on a process, such as steps in making a decision or steps in solving a problem, regardless of the situation. For instance, clients and their families may be asked to play an abbreviated game of Monopoly. There is usually a point in the game where one player attempts to negotiate for land or property. The players learn that tradeoffs in all areas of life are usually much like these nego-tiations. After the game, the client and a family member could be led through a discussion that summarizes the skills they used in the nego-tiation process. Eventually, the educator challenges the client and family member to extrapolate the application of those same skills from the game situation to any other situation where the client must negotiate (such as asking for help). Clients may suggest simulations for practice; educators may devise simulations and games for their clients. There are health-related games commercially available. One such game is called "Hold the Salt." The purpose of this game is to help schoolchildren and their families to become aware of the importance of reducing sodium in their diet. This board game conveys information about high and low sodium intake and gives children practice in keeping track of sodium intake in order to keep within the recommended dietary range for middle school. Figure 6.2 shows how the board is set up for this game.

Table 6.3 summarizes the various educational methods that may be used to influence factors that will help or hinder your clients' abilities to take positive actions that will contribute to their own health. It may be helpful to refer to Chapter 5 if you need to review educational diagnosis and definitions of the factors listed in Figure 5.1, step 3.

## PRINCIPLES FOR SELECTING METHODS

These following seven principles can serve to guide the selection of ap-propriate educational methods:

**1.** Choose educational methods only after the educational and be-havioral diagnosis has been completed. You should already know what you and your clients hope to accomplish from the educational program and have a list of health behaviors that the client wishes to improve or change.

**2.** For most educational programs, choose at least three different methods, as a rule of thumb, and choose methods that can influence predisposing, enabling, and reinforcing factors.

**3.** Make sure that all methods you select stimulate client, family, and friend participation in the planning, implementation, and evaluation

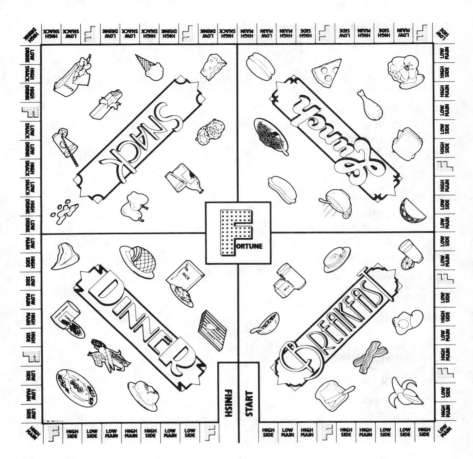

**Figure 6.2   "Hold the Salt" game**

To win in the "Hold the Salt" game, a player must move a marker around a board divided into quarters (breakfast, lunch, dinner, and snack), acquiring the fewest number of salt units. If the player lands on a "low-sodium" main dish for breakfast, he or she picks from the low-sodium stack of cards and could draw a card for a hard-boiled egg or for cereal cooked without salt. If the player lands on a high-sodium board space and picks from the high-sodium stack, he or she might pick pancakes or dry breakfast cereal flakes. (High-sodium tallies for foods that do not taste salty always raise players' curiosity and interest.) Fortune cards, which teach sodium reduction strategies, such as "Change canned vegetables for fresh vegetables," are drawn if the player lands on a "Fortune" board space. Players record the sodium units collected for each meal on a "Salt Tally." "Hold the Salt" board game sets and program guides may be obtained by contacting Health Skills, Inc., 101 East Melbourne Avenue, Silver Spring, MD 20901; phone (301) 567-4659.

SOURCE: Reprinted with the permission of Health Skills, Inc.

**Table 6.3   Educational methods**

| Method | Predisposing | Enabling | Reinforcing |
|---|:---:|:---:|:---:|
| Group facilitation | | | |
| • Peer group discussion | x | | x |
| • Mutual aid and support | x | | x |
| • Problem solving | x | | x |
| Role playing | x | x | x |
| Modeling | | x | x |
| Behavior modification | | x | |
| Skill practice | | x | |
| Simulations and games | x | x | |
| Community organizing | | x | |
| Mass media | x | x | |
| Audiovisuals | x | x | |
| Lecture | x | | |
| Individual instruction | x | x | |
| Programmed learning | x | | |
| Computer-assisted learning | x | | |
| Interviewing | x | | x |

*(Factors spans Predisposing, Enabling, Reinforcing columns.)*

of the health education program. Educational methods that require only passive involvement of clients do not adequately prepare clients for all the changes they need to make.

**4.** Take into account such client factors as age, level of disability, literacy, and cultural biases when choosing educational methods. Every educational plan for group approaches needs to include referrals or contingencies for clients who have special needs.

**5.** Select methods with which you feel comfortable. Become proficient in each method you choose. Simulations and role playing are useful strategies for updating your own skills. It is also very useful to videotape yourself in action and then to play back the tape for self-analysis.

**6.** The more complex the behavioral problem, the more educational methods you should employ. For instance, a lecture on its own, or a pamphlet on its own, is not sufficient to prepare a client for something as complex as losing twenty pounds of body weight. Weight-loss programs often employ such educational methods as food diaries, daily weigh-ins, group support, monetary incentives, and relapse prevention techniques.

**7.** If the educational program is designed to influence long-term behavior change, you will need to choose methods that influence predisposing, enabling, and reinforcing factors. Methods that influence predisposing factors have the shortest-term effects. Methods that influence reinforcing factors have intermediate-term effects. For example, smoking cessation programs that provide information on the health effects of nicotine will do little to motivate people to quit smoking. Many people are encouraged to quit when family members have stayed off cigarettes for years with success. Others sign up for classes when their health care providers refer them. Most people who choose educational groups participate in role playing, simulations, and other problem-solving techniques as a way to prevent relapse. In this combination of methods, there is greater likelihood that participants will maintain their stop smoking states over time.

These seven principles are a summary of conclusions derived from the PRECEDE model as they apply to selecting educational methods. These guidelines are meant to demonstrate that the selection of methods is an integral part of the planning process and not an arbitrary decision.

## BEYOND DIRECT SERVICE

The aim of this chapter is to prepare you to select educational methods while planning health education. We have made the direct provision of educational services to clients the focus of the planning process. Nevertheless, health educators have a variety of roles and responsibilities in medical care settings. Providing educational service to clients is only one of these many roles.

Health education coordinators are resource people to instructors and to groups of interested health professionals. Coordinators advise on the planning of specific health education programs. As a resource person, you must select from a repertoire of educational methods. You will need to choose methods best suited for working with committees and individuals. Sometimes health educators provide continuing education programs for interested health professionals on the educational planning process, on educational methods, or on health education content areas. The objective of continuing education programs is provider knowledge, attitude, and behavior change. Your challenge is to use the principles mentioned in this chapter for selecting educational methods that will help you meet the course objectives of continuing education programs, too.

Situations regularly arise where institutional policies, management style, or interdepartmental conflicts interfere with health education department goals and objectives. In these instances, health educators must rely again on their repertoire of educational skills so that they can act as an agent for positive organizational change. Educational techniques such as group facilitation, interviewing, negotiating, mediating, resolving conflicts, and problem solving can be employed with decision makers, administrators, and department heads.

One further challenge that health educators face is to ensure that their own skill levels in a variety of educational methods are kept upgraded and updated. Educational methods are the main tools of practicing health educators—whether their practice takes them into the direct delivery of educational service, into program planning, or into management.

# EXERCISES

1.  For each of the following health education programs, project which
    client behaviors may be expected to change as a result of the edu-
    cational process. List the educational methods that may help clients
    make the necessary behavior changes. Be prepared to explain your
    choices.

| Patient education | Client health behaviors | Educational methods |
| --- | --- | --- |
| Breast self-examination | | |

| Health promotion | Client health behaviors | Educational methods |
| --- | --- | --- |
| Stress management | | |

2.  The following list of roles and functions was taken from job descriptions of health educators in medical care settings. List four or five educational methods that you think health educators in each role will be required to use proficiently.

|                               | |
|------------------------------|-|

*Roles*                                     *Educational Methods*

a.  Coordinating and             a. _____
    planning health
    education services           b. _____

                                 c. _____

                                 d. _____

                                 e. _____


b.  Consulting and training      a. _____
    for other departments
                                 b. _____

                                 c. _____

                                 d. _____

                                 e. _____


c.  Facilitating organiza-       a. _____
    tional change
                                 b. _____

                                 c. _____

                                 d. _____

                                 e. _____


d.  Providing health educa-      a. _____
    tion services
                                 b. _____

                                 c. _____

                                 d. _____

                                 e. _____

|            *Roles*                     | *Educational Methods* |
|----------------------------------------|-----------------------|

e. Advocating goals and
   needs of the health education department

a. _____
b. _____
c. _____
d. _____
e. _____

f. Managing the health
   education function

a. _____
b. _____
c. _____
d. _____
e. _____

g. Auditing programs and
   assuring quality for
   programs

a. _____
b. _____
c. _____
d. _____
e. _____

# RESOURCES

Bartlett, E. Selection of Educational Strategies. In L. W. Green, M. W. Kreuter, S. G. Deeds, and K. B. Partridge. *Health Education Planning: A Diagnostic Approach*. Palo Alto, Calif.: Mayfield, 1980, chap. 6.

This chapter gives the reader an excellent review of health education strategies, including many key methods from individual instruction to social action. It features a guide for linking educational methods to diagnostic categories. The classifications include (1) those relating to the health problem, (2) those relating to the desired health behavior, (3) those relating to the target group, and (4) those relating to administrative factors.

Lazes, P. (ed.). *Consumer Health Education Handbook.* Germantown, Md.: Aspen Press, 1979.

Lazes's book has three chapters related to educational methods. One chapter, "Using Media in Hospitals," devotes attention to the milieu within which audiovisual and graphic media can best be put to use, and presents guidelines for selecting such media. The author also gives an in-depth look at programs in hospitals that have used media as an action tool for health behavior change. Another chapter, "Media for Community Health Promotion," details how mass media can be used to promote health in the community setting, and presents a case study of the use of media in a program aimed at reducing heart disease risk factors. The third chapter, "Simulation and Gaming in Health Education," introduces the reader to a variety of simulations that are available to health education specialists who wish to employ these techniques in their work.

Rees, A. M. (ed.). *Developing Consumer Health Information Services.* New York: Bowker, 1982.

This book was prepared to help librarians and other health information providers develop and manage consumer health information services, programs, and networks. The first two parts of this book are of significant interest to health educators in medical care—particularly those who are establishing health information centers in their hospitals or clinics. Part One defines the changing social environment that initiated and supports the consumer health information movement, discusses the nature of medical consumerism and the need for lay health information, and outlines the role of the library in meeting this need. Part Two summarizes the design and essential characteristics of the seven principal library-based consumer health information programs in the United States and Canada—including hospital, HMO, and academic medical center libraries.

Spiegler, M. D. *Contemporary Behavioral Therapy.* Palo Alto, Calif.: Mayfield, 1983.

Spiegler discusses behavioral therapy in terms of how it functions and what it accomplishes; he wrote the book for readers with diverse backgrounds and interests. The author summarizes the available research evidence and evaluates each method. In addition to the section on behavioral assessment, you will be interested in the author's treatment of modeling therapies, cognitive behavioral therapies (such as self-talk and self-instruction) and self-control therapies (self-monitoring, self-reinforcement, and problem-solving therapy).

Squyres, W. D. Closed-Circuit Television: The Promise and the Problems. *Promoting Health* (American Hospital Association), (January–February, 1981), 2(1).

In this article Squyres presents the issues related to the question "Is CCTV a worthwhile investment?" She summarizes the problems and advantages of running an in-house closed-circuit television system.

# 7

# Evaluating educational services

We HAVE DISCUSSED setting up programs (Chapter 4), developing plans and protocols (Chapter 5), and selecting educational methods (Chapter 6). In this chapter, we will explore how to evaluate educational services.

Programs are evaluated to find out how well they work and how to improve them. But if you say the word *evaluation* in a roomful of health educators, eyes roll upward. Pained expressions appear. People grumble, "We had to beg, borrow, and steal to get the money to run our shoestring programs. Now they want us to evaluate them too!"

These health educators are not trying to avoid knowing if their programs are effective or how to improve them. Instead, the pressure to prove the worth of patient education programs is intense, and these health educators feel it. Hospital administrators, legislators, and third-party payers (insurers, for example) see patient education as a new service, and they want to see evidence that it is effective (D'Onofrio, 1980). Perhaps because the field is relatively new and because the body of empirical evidence that justifies it is modest, practicing health educators are often asked both to manage programs and to gather evidence to justify their existence. Many of us resent this dual mandate because it seems to require massive data gathering, sophistication in research methodology and statistics, and finances and staff we do not have. The concept of evaluation itself is discomforting because the process itself often signals the end rather than the improvement of a program.

Few health educators recognize how much they rely on evaluations in their day-to-day work. For example, we rely on evaluations published in the epidemiologic literature when we decide to offer a stop smoking program instead of one on stress reduction. We evaluate theories of learning when we decide to use certain techniques in a diabetes education course. We use the formal steps of the evaluation process when we make certain managerial decisions. At the time, we may not formally label what we do as evaluation. Nevertheless, we are actually more competent at evaluating than we give ourselves credit for.

In this chapter, we discuss evaluation from a practical standpoint. We believe that to do useful evaluations health educators can use many of the skills they already have. This chapter is guided by the following premises:

**1.** Evaluation is an important process. You need to know if your programs are working and how to improve them.

**2.** Every evaluation is conducted in a political context. It is important to know who will use your findings, and for what.

**3.** Evaluations should not be conducted without a clearly defined purpose. They should be designed to provide information that is not already known and important to have.

**4.** Compromises in research design are often necessary. Although scientific rigor should be a goal, controlled experiments are not the only way to produce useful evaluations.

This chapter covers a range of more informal approaches to evaluation that will help educators find out what worked and what didn't in their educational efforts.

Program evaluations are often done to help people make the following decisions:

**1.** To improve the ways a program operates

**2.** To decide how to allocate funds and resources among different programs

**3.** To add or drop specific program components, strategies, and techniques

**4.** To initiate similar or different programs elsewhere

**5.** To continue or to discontinue a program

**6.** To accept or reject a specific program's approach or theory

This list summarizes the decisions that the evaluation process helps you make. As you can see, a range of opportunity would be missed if evaluation were omitted or overlooked during the planning and implementation of health education programs. The rest of this chapter discusses each of these opportunities and recommends ways to match evaluation strategies with these purposes.

## DO OUR PROGRAMS WORK?

Basically, we evaluate programs to see if they work, but "work" can mean different things to different people. For example, consider an abortion counseling program. The women who receive the counseling, the counselors, the program coordinator, the administrators of the clinic where it is offered, and community groups may all have different criteria for judging the effectiveness of the program (Weiss, 1972, 1973).

Consider what might be going on in the mind of a single woman who has just been told that she is pregnant. She might really want the child but has no means to support it. She is uncertain about what to do, so she makes an appointment with an abortion counselor at the local community clinic. The woman hopes that the counselor can help her decide whether or not to have an abortion. During the counseling session, the woman sorts out the consequences of her different options. She leaves with a decision that feels comfortable to her and a knowledge of the medical procedures that will be used during the abortion she has decided to have. She thinks that the abortion counseling program at the clinic is very helpful. She indicates her satisfaction on a questionnaire asking her to rate the program.

Now, take a minute to identify with the abortion counselor who later sees that questionnaire and is very pleased with the information. When the counselor originally designed the program, she had the feelings of her clients foremost in her mind. When the counselor drew up the original goals and objectives for the program, she had to choose the most appropriate focus for the counseling; for example, to help women come to terms with their decisions, to understand the abortion procedure itself, to learn the most effective birth control measures, or some combination of all of these. The positive comments on the questionnaire convince the counselor that she made the right decision. The program coordinator is also pleased as she wraps up a hundred questionnaires with "satisfied" ratings and takes them to the administrator of the clinic to demonstrate the effectiveness of her program.

Now, try to see the situation from the administrator's perspective. The administrator has recently been told to cut out programs that are perceived as frills because the clinic is "over budget." The administrator thinks that abortion counseling programs are worth their cost only if it can be demonstrated that they reduce the number of women who have repeat abortions. The administrator may be personally sympathetic toward programs that give people emotional support, but she feels that unless it can be shown that such programs accomplish more than that, they do belong in the frills category. She looks at the satisfied responses on the questionnaires, but they do not persuade her. The administrator continues to wonder if the program's funds and resources might not be better spent on primary care services. In addition, the administrator is concerned about the effect of such a program on public opinion. For example, if antiabortion groups are well organized in the community and word got out that the local clinic runs an abortion counseling program that helps women feel better about having abortions, those groups might organize to get some of the clinic's public funding rescinded. The administrator may ask the program coordinator for information relevant to her own concerns. First, to stave off the antiabortion groups, she may require data that demonstrate that the counseling program is not proabortion but neutral, and that many of the women who are counseled decide against having abortions. And to justify funding for the program, she may want data showing that women who are counseled have fewer repeat abortions than women who are not counseled.

Each of the people in this example has different interests and therefore different questions about the abortion counseling program. True, everyone wants to know if the program is effective, but there are vast differences among the definitions of effectiveness. When planning and conducting an evaluation, it is important to understand the interests both of the people involved in the process and of those affected by the outcome. Some important objectives are those of the organization or medical center offering the program, the program administrator, the funding source, the public, and the evaluator (Shortell and Richardson, 1978). Table 7.1 summarizes the different objectives served by evaluations.

The interests of these parties are different and often not compatible. There is also no automatic hierarchical order of interests that an evaluation should serve. We recommend that, before you begin to evaluate any program, you systematically consider who asked for the evaluation, for what purpose, who else is interested in the findings, and how they will use the data. Then clarify your own interests and make the best choices you can, knowing that no one evaluation can possibly answer everyone's questions or serve everyone's interests.

## TYPES OF EVALUATIONS

Evaluations may focus on the process of implementing a program, on the short-term impact of the program on the participants, and/or on the long-term outcome for the participants (Green, 1979). In a process eval-

**Table 7.1 What are the different objectives served by evaluations?**

| Interests | Organization | Program administrator | Funding source | Public | Evaluator |
|---|---|---|---|---|---|
| 1. Demonstrate program effectiveness and benefits | x | x | x | x | x |
| 2. Demonstrate program efficiency | x | x | x | | x |
| 3. Justify past or projected expenditures | x | x | | | |
| 4. Gain support for expansion of program | x | x | | | |
| 5. Determine subsequent actions | x | x | | | |
| 6. Understand broad impact of a program | | | x | | |
| 7. Demonstrate programmatic impact in a political context | | | x | | |
| 8. Create opportunity for increased community participation | | | | x | |
| 9. Contribute to the field of health education | | x | | | x |
| 10. Advance professionally | | x | | | x |

uation, information is gathered on the actual operation of the program—that is, qualifications of the staff operating the program, actual services offered, content of classes, audiovisual materials used, educational techniques, and so forth. The main question addressed in a process evaluation is this: Does the program operate up to a standard, set either by the professional community of health educators (general) or by the program planners (specific)? The professional community evaluates program process through peer reviews, audits, accreditation, and government or administrative monitoring of contracts and grants (Green, 1979). Program planners set minimum standards for the successful operation of a program.

In an evaluation of a program's impact, information is gathered on the immediate effect of the program on the knowledge, attitudes, and behaviors of those who come into contact with it (Green, 1979). In this type of evaluation, information is gathered from and about the participants in the program. The main question addressed in an impact evaluation is: What effect does the program have on the knowledge, attitudes, and behaviors of the participants? For example, "Can patients who take a breast self-exam course perform the examination according to a set of standards?" Table 7.2 gives you an opportunity to test your understanding of the types of evaluation described so far. Take some time now to do this matching exercise.

Evaluations of long-term outcomes involve studies of morbidity and mortality. These require the observation of (1) large numbers of people over (2) long periods of time. Health educators practicing outside a research setting can rarely fulfill either condition. When trying to determine if it is more worthwhile in the long run to offer programs that address one particular risk factor over another, rather than conduct your own study, it is best to consult complete reviews of the epidemiologic literature that include all current findings about the relationship between particular behaviors and diseases. For example, if you are interested in the effect of diet on coronary heart disease, you might consult an article by Hulley et al. (1980). When trying to design or improve a program already in operation, look at how the program operates and at its short-term effects. Health educators practicing in medical settings can and should undertake these kinds of studies.

In this section we have identified the various types of evaluation; in the next section we discuss how to select programs to evaluate.

**Table 7.2   Types of evaluations**

Match the type of data with the type of evaluation it represents.
Place a check in the appropriate space.

| Type of data | Process evaluation | Impact evaluation | Outcome evaluation |
|---|---|---|---|
| 1. Number of lessons given to weight control group on how to choose a low-calorie meal in a restaurant | \_\_\_\_\_ | \_\_\_\_\_ | \_\_\_\_\_ |
| 2. Number of low-calorie meals actually consumed by weight control group | \_\_\_\_\_ | \_\_\_\_\_ | \_\_\_\_\_ |
| 3. Proportion of group experiencing a reduction in blood pressure | \_\_\_\_\_ | \_\_\_\_\_ | \_\_\_\_\_ |
| 4. Number of pounds of body weight lost or gained | \_\_\_\_\_ | \_\_\_\_\_ | \_\_\_\_\_ |

Note: Check your answers.   Answers: (1) process, (2) impact, (3) outcome, (4) impact.

## CHOOSING THE FOCUS OF THE EVALUATION

Last year, the administrators of a multiinstitutional health center asked their patient education coordinators to choose one health education or health promotion program to evaluate. In the beginning, many coordinators ambitiously wanted to evaluate programs such as weight control, diabetes education, and prenatal care. But by the end of the year, most had decided to evaluate their stop smoking programs. Why? First, their stop smoking programs were the most expensive programs to run, and many of the health educators felt under pressure to justify them. Second, most of the programs consisted of small group counseling sessions, which meant that, at best, they reached only a few hundred people a year. Were such groups cost-effective? Other considerations related to the evaluations themselves: (1) people who run stop smoking programs agree somewhat on what the indicators of success are (reduced smoking or complete abstinence one year after the program), and (2) because of the strong link between quitting smoking and improved health, stop smoking programs may not be viewed with the same skepticism as stress reduction courses, for example, where the benefits are not as well documented.

There are many questions to ask when choosing a program to evaluate. Several are related to what you want to know about one particular program. Some questions will be more important to you than others. The following questions can help you decide if a particular program is a good candidate for evaluation:

**1.** Are there adequate funds to run the program?

**2.** What about the staff—are the people running the program performing competently?

**3.** What about the techniques being used? Are there other techniques that might be more effective?

**4.** Are enough people being reached by the program, and are they the ones who really need it? Do the referral mechanisms need to be changed?

**5.** Do you need evidence of success so that more people will use your program?

**6.** Are you or the administration questioning the need for the program altogether? Maybe there are other programs operating within the hospital or clinic that are doing the same thing. Maybe there are very successful programs in the community, and your efforts would be better spent on referring people to them.

**7.** Is the reputation of your department on the line? Does the administration want to see something effective come out of your efforts?

Maybe if you focus on your most successful program, and publicize the results of your evaluation, your department will gain more credibility.

**8.** Do you think your program is so effective that you want to gather conclusive evidence so that other hospitals or clinics will adopt it?

The questions just given are designed to be asked about a particular program that is a candidate for evaluation. There are general factors to consider when you are selecting one program to evaluate from among several specific candidates. The factors are

**1.** The importance of the program for improving health

**2.** The cost of operating the program

**3.** The amount of effort required to reach the target population

**4.** The need and potential for improving the program

**5.** The importance of the program to the administration

Programs that are important for health, are expensive, require many resources but reach few people, need improvement, or are important to the administration should be the highest priorities for evaluation. The general factors to consider when you must choose a program to evaluate are as follows:

**1.** *Importance of the program for improving health.* A stop smoking program may be more crucial to evaluate than a nutrition program to prevent heart disease, because studies indicate that quitting smoking may reduce the risk of lung disease and heart disease, while the evidence on the reduced risk of heart disease from changes in diet is less substantial.

**2.** *Cost.* Other things being equal, the more expensive the program the more it needs to be evaluated.

**3.** *Number of people reached.* Programs that reach few people but require enormous expenditures of effort—such as one-to-one stop smoking counseling programs—need scrutiny.

**4.** *Room for improvement.* Programs that you and your staff suspect have the most potential for improvement are important to evaluate.

**5.** *Importance to the administration.* Programs most important to the administration have high priority for evaluation.

## A CASE STUDY: SELECTING A PROGRAM TO EVALUATE

A health educator chose for evaluation a class taught to newly diagnosed hypertensives. The class is taught by nurse practitioners. The educator selected the program for several reasons.

Several concerns about the class had been voiced around the hospital. Some of the physicians felt it was a waste of valuable nursing time. They would have liked to see it discontinued.

The health educator herself believed that a one-session class is not enough to teach people what they need to know about hypertension, and not enough to provide the support necessary for the participants to quit smoking, lose weight, or make any of the other recommended changes in their lifestyles. The health educator wanted to have more class sessions, but she was in a difficult position. To obtain administrative support for increasing the number of sessions, she would have to demonstrate that the participants benefited at least a little from one class session and would benefit more from several sessions.

The health educator was also concerned that the class focused too much on the physiology of the disease and did not give the patients time to talk about what it means to them to be told that they have hypertension. She thought that patients need a place to say that their illness makes them angry or afraid, if that is how they feel.

The instructors knew that some of the physicians wanted to discontinue the class. The instructors were concerned about their jobs and about the future of the class. They believed it was a necessary program for patients.

Obviously, several people would be affected by this evaluation.

The first step taken by the health educator was to identify who would use the results of the evaluation and how they would be used. The administrator requested the evaluation. She was interested in a justification of the program before guaranteeing its longevity or authorizing any expansion of it. The physicians who felt it was a waste of time might have used any findings that indicated that the class was not effective to pressure the administrator into giving the nurse practitioner instructors different responsibilities. The health educator planned to use the findings to improve the class content and to demonstrate the need for more classes if the findings pointed in that direction.

The next step, if taken early in any evaluation, will save many headaches later on: the health educator identified the personnel who would be affected by or involved in the evaluation, and she let them know that their comments and suggestions were wanted.

To implement this second step, the health educator contacted all the medical center personnel who would be affected by the evaluation and asked them to attend several lunch meetings to discuss it. These personnel included the class instructors, the supervising nurse practitioner, the physician chief of the hypertension clinic, the physician chief of the department of preventive medicine, the physician patient education chief, and two internal consultants on evaluation. In addition, two hypertensive patients who had already taken the class were invited. The stated purpose of the meetings was to discuss what the evaluation should focus on, what questions it should answer, what the research design should be, who would actually do the work, and what the findings might be used for. Some of the unstated, but important, purposes of the meetings were to reduce the anxiety the class instructors felt about the evaluation and to gain their support for doing it.

## Developing a plan

After several meetings, the group reached some consensus about the need for the evaluation and its possible uses. A proposal was drafted that included the questions to be addressed, the rationale for doing the evaluation, sample size and selection procedures, methods for data collection, a timetable, and a draft of a telephone interview for current participants. The group wanted to know if newly diagnosed patients with hypertension who attended the class were more likely than those who did not attend to

**1.** Keep their first appointment with their physician or nurse practitioner after they were told in the screening clinic that they had high blood pressure

**2.** Know the high blood pressure medication and the dosage they were supposed to take

**3.** Accurately remember their last blood pressure reading taken at that medical center and know whether it was in the normal or high range

**4.** Try to lower their blood pressures with nonpharmacological means such as reducing salt in their diets, increasing their exercise, and making efforts to reduce stress

These categories of information were chosen because all the members of the group agreed that they tried to focus on these items in the class.

To address directly the class instructors' fears that the evaluation results would result in the discontinuing of the class, the uses of the data were specifically stated in the proposal: "The results of this evaluation will be used to make improvements in the existing class. For example, greater emphasis might be placed on the importance of keeping follow-up appointments or on giving patients referrals to weight control, nutrition, and stress reduction programs. The results of the evaluation will not be used as justification for discontinuing the class." There is never any guarantee that the results of an evaluation will not be used to discontinue a program. However, directly addressing the issue in the evaluation proposal can reduce the possibility of discontinuation.

The group agreed that the information they wanted could be gathered most easily through telephone interviews with patients, half of whom attended the class and half of whom did not. Patients would be asked questions about their visits to their physician or nurse practitioner, their medications, blood pressure levels, diet, exercise, stress, and the reasons they did not attend the class or, for those who did attend, their suggestions for improving it. Information on blood pressure levels, provider visits, and medications prescribed that was received during the telephone interviews would be checked against information in the patients' medical records for validation.

## Obtaining cooperation

The health education coordinator who was planning the evaluation knew that any real improvements in the class as a result of the evaluation would have to be implemented by the class instructors. Therefore, she made every effort to involve them and other hospital personnel in the design phase. Her inclusion of two patients who had attended the class during the planning of the evaluation was also important. They made suggestions for questions to be asked during the telephone interview, and they volunteered to do some of the interviews.

The evaluation would also address the interests of the physicians and administrators. It would focus on actions that the physicians and administrators would agree were important for patients with hypertension to take: keeping appointments, knowing medications and dosages, remembering if the last blood pressure reading was high, trying to lower their blood pressure nonpharmacologically. If the evaluation showed that more of the patients who attended the class did these things than patients who did not attend the class, the physicians and administrators would be more likely to support the program.

The coordinator knew that by obtaining everyone's cooperation early in the planning stage and by choosing a design and method that everyone thought would yield credible information, many fears about the evaluation process and its results would be alleviated.

## DOCUMENTING PROGRAM OPERATIONS

Whether or not elaborate evaluations of programs are conducted, a comparison is needed between the actual operations and activities of a program and the operations and activities originally intended by those who designed the program. It is difficult to decide whether a program is a success or a failure unless what is being done is clear; it is difficult to know what has been done long after the fact. Imagine asking a class instructor what topics he covered in a hypertension education class six months after he taught it. Would you believe that his description was complete? The actual operations of a program must be documented while the program is in progress. Many programs fail not because they were poorly conceived but because they were poorly implemented (as shown in the documentation).

## Sources and types of information to document

There are four general sources of information for documenting program operations: (1) direct observation by the evaluator, (2) service records, (3) information from the program staff, and (4) data from the program participants and their associates (Rossi and Freeman, 1982). For example, direct observation of diabetes education classes taught by several instructors can tell you if each instructor covers all the appropriate topics in each class. Service records can tell you how many of the people who inquire about a program actually sign up for it. The program instructors can tell you if they are unable to cover the necessary information in the time allotted for the program. The participants can tell you if it was difficult to get information about when and where the program was given.

Some kinds of information (and sources) that it is important to document on the day-to-day operations and activities of your program are listed as follows. (Examples of data collection forms are included in the appendices to this chapter.)

**1.** *Goals of the program.* Why the program exists and what you hope it will accomplish.

**2.** *Personnel.* The number of paid and unpaid staff who operate the program, and the qualifications (both necessary and actual) of each staff member. This means the number of FTEs (full-time equivalent employees) needed to run the program, and the education and job experience required for each. This information can be obtained from job descriptions, time cards, and budgets.

**3.** *Services offered.* The number and type of services offered. They can include classes, group counseling sessions, lending of audiovisual equipment, and providing answers to reference questions about diseases. This information can be obtained from printed descriptions of services, course outlines, publicity flyers, and the observations of classes by participants and evaluators.

**4.** *Materials.* The number, type, and titles of materials given to people who participate in the program. Materials include books, pamphlets, packets, workbooks, and anything else given to participants. This information can be obtained from purchase orders, bibliographies and references used by instructors, as well as from questionnaires given to participants.

**5.** *Means of referral.* The ways people may be channeled into a program and the number and proportion of people referred in each way— that is, the number of participants referred by a physician, a friend, a flyer, and so on.

**6.** *Participants.* The special characteristics that define the target population, and the characteristics of the actual participants. For example, all newly diagnosed patients with diabetes might be the target population of a diabetes education program, and the participants are the people who actually attend. The evaluation may show you that most of the participants have had diabetes for more than five years. It is important to know the age, sex, and education of the participants so that the program can be adjusted accordingly. Some sources for this information are preprogram registration forms, profile and intake forms, visit records, medical chart entries, appointment schedules, attendance sheets, and questionnaires administered to participants.

**7.** *Participant satisfaction.* This factor refers to participants' subjective assessment of the program—its content, its methodology, the appropriateness of materials such as pamphlets and films. This information can be gathered informally from critique sessions held during the program sessions or classes, the notes of observers of the program, interviews with participants, and questionnaires to participants.

**8.** *Staff satisfaction.* This factor refers to staff (program instructors and assistants) assessments of how well the program is going. Comments from staff are important to obtain on an ongoing basis because the first signs of trouble in a program are often recognized by the staff. Evaluations often validate the hunches of instructors who run programs. This information can be gathered informally through meetings with instructors. At regular times during a program, instructors can be asked to describe what is happening in their classes and what they think about their program. For example, a stop smoking counselor might be asked to sum up her experiences with each group she runs. She might be requested to comment on the group dynamics, whether or not the people she expected to quit smoking actually did, and anything else she thinks led to successes and failures in the group.

**9.** *General personnel satisfaction.* This category refers to comments made by other hospital or clinic personnel, particularly those who refer people to the program, or the administrators. It is important to get information on how a program is seen by others in your hospital or clinic. The best thing to do is to keep a file of informal conversations by program. This way you can maintain a perspective on the various groups of clients you serve.

**10.** *Costs.* The cost of running a program; also any information on the cost of the service before it was under the auspices of the health education department. For example, if physicians taught patients with diabetes how to inject insulin on a one-to-one basis before a group program run by nurses was developed, it would be important to document the cost of the old program compared to the cost of the new one. This information can be obtained from budget reports, monthly expenditure ledgers, and the records of hospital or clinic cost centers, which often show the costs of specific services. Often, though, such costs will have to be extrapolated from informal time and salary estimates of relevant personnel. Remember, you have to weigh the cost of measuring a program's success against the cost of delivering the program.

**11.** *Program impact.* This term refers to any changes in the knowledge, attitudes, behavior, and environment that occur among participants, instructors, staff, administrators, physicians, nurses, or anyone else affected by the program. Information on impact may take more effort to get than information on the other areas. But end-of-class questionnaires asking participants about their smoking habits at that time, for example, are not too difficult to administer or tally and would be worth having. Wherever possible, longer-term impact should be assessed to determine whether the program has any lasting effects. A mailed questionnaire six months later, for example, may provide insight into a program's effectiveness that was not visible at the end of the original program.

## The sample forms in the Appendices

Examples of forms that have been used to obtain information on some of the preceding items are shown in Appendices 7.1–7.6. They include the following:

**1.** The stop smoking program attendance sheet (Appendix 7.1) is filled out by the program group leader. It serves as an easy way to keep track of which sessions participants attend and who drops out of the program.

**2.** The stop smoking program intake form (Appendix 7.2) is filled out by the leader during an initial individual interview with each participant. It provides baseline information on the participant that is used during the course of the program and later, after the program has ended, to show how much a participant's behavior has changed. For example, a participant may have been a two-pack-a-day smoker before the program and may manage to cut down to ten cigarettes a day one year later. This may represent a greater improvement than that for the participant who cuts down from ten cigarettes a day to five cigarettes a day.

**3.** The medical chart entry in Appendix 7.3 is an example of what program instructors might put in a participant's medical record to inform the physician of the participant's progress.

**4.** The librarian gives the health library visit record in Appendix 7.4 to each person entering the library. Tallies of the sheets indicate who uses the library and which services they use most often.

**5.** The television survey in Appendix 7.5 is given to hospital inpatients to see if (a) they know about the hospital's cable TV station, which shows health education programs; (b) they watch any of the programs; and (c) they find the programming to be interesting.

**6.** The physician survey in Appendix 7.6 is distributed to all the physicians in the hospital. It is used to promote awareness of the health library and to see how physicians use the services and whether they are satisfied with them.

If records are kept on the preceding items as part of the day-to-day operations of a program, the program will be easier to run. Informed day-to-day decisions will also be easier to make, and evaluation will be relatively straightforward.

## METHODS FOR CONDUCTING IMPACT AND OUTCOME EVALUATIONS

The information you gather in a process evaluation should provide an accurate and reliable sense of what you are doing. The information you gather in evaluations of outcome and impact should show the results of what you are doing. To understand the impact or effect of your health education program, you need to know what would have happened if it had never been offered (Fitz-Gibbon and Morris, 1978). You must therefore compare the experiences of the group of people who received your program to those of a group of people who did not. This second group (known as a *control*) should be identical to the first in all ways except that it did not receive your program (Rossi and Freeman, 1982).

Such a comparison would allow you to say that whatever differences exist between the two groups are really due to your program (Anderson et al., 1980). Unfortunately, the people in the two groups are rarely identical. Therefore, if the people in your program lost more weight or smoked fewer cigarettes than the individuals who were not in your program, you will never really know whether your program made the difference or whether there were other differences between the two groups. For instance, the people in your program may have been more highly motivated to lose weight or stop smoking to begin with.

Many of the discussions in the literature on research design describe techniques, all varying in effectiveness, that can minimize the differences between (1) the group of people receiving the program, or the treatment group, and (2) the group that does not, or the comparison or control group (Suchman, 1967; Rossi and Freeman, 1982; Campbell and Stanley, 1966; Cook and Campbell, 1979).

## Random assignment

The best technique for minimizing differences is randomly to assign people to one group or the other (Campbell and Stanley, 1966). To assign people randomly means to use a method for placing people into the two groups that gives each person an equal chance of being placed in either group (Anderson et al., 1980). For example, you could assign each person to a group by tossing a coin: heads, the person is in the treatment group; tails, in the control. Thus, neither any characteristic of any individual (such as greater motivation) nor the opinions of the investigator could influence the composition of either group. The primary virtue of random assignment is that it provides the greatest assurance that the two groups will be similar with respect to the characteristics that can affect the behaviors under observation, whether these characteristics are known or unknown to the investigators conducting the study (Anderson et al., 1980).

Suppose you are planning to evaluate a weight control group. You have decided that the effectiveness of the program will be determined by how much weight the people in the group lose after six months in comparison to the amount lost by a group that does not have the program. You want to be sure that the two groups do not differ in any ways that are related to the likelihood that they will lose weight. If most of the people in the weight control group are very obese and highly motivated to lose weight, but most of the people in the other group are thin and do not want to lose weight, it would be difficult to consider the program a resounding success if the participants lost more weight than the controls. Since attitude toward losing weight and actual weight at the start of the program can influence the outcome under observation—weight lost—neither group should have too many highly motivated or very obese people at the beginning. Random assignment is the best way we know to ensure that the groups are balanced. A note of caution, however—even random assignment may not be enough to ensure similarity between the two groups. It is important to make sure that no important differences exist by looking at distributions of different characteristics—such as age, sex, and weight—in the two groups.

Although evaluations that employ random assignment represent conventional theory about how to design evaluations, many evaluators cite difficulties they have encountered when trying to use it in action settings (Weiss, 1972; Cronbach and Associates, 1980). Some of the main criticisms are that random assignment

**1.** Cannot be used when the program being evaluated has already begun or has ended

**2.** Often means withholding treatment that might be beneficial from those who need it

**3.** Is problematic because it is impractical to have empty places in programs when there are people who wish to participate in them

**4.** Is often time consuming and expensive.

There has been much debate on the ethics of withholding treatment. A question often posed is "How can we really know if the treatment is beneficial unless we test it with a group that does not receive it?" (Weiss, 1972). Some solutions are to allow the people in the control group to participate in the program at a later point in time or to allow them to participate in a less expensive, less time-consuming version of the program or in another program directed at the same goal (Fitz-Gibbon and Morris, 1978). Thus, treatment that might really help people is not withheld merely for the purposes of evaluation.

## Matching the comparison group

Identify the important characteristics of the people in the treatment group and choose a comparison group that matches the treatment group on these characteristics (Rossi and Freeman, 1982; Weiss, 1972). Suppose 500 people have signed up to participate in a stress management class offered at your clinic, and 100 of them have attended the first session. You could choose the other 100 from the remaining 400 on the waiting list who most closely match the 100 who have begun the program on age, race, sex, amount of stress in their lives, or any other characteristics that might determine their reaction to the class. You would then have two similar groups to observe, one receiving the program and one not.

The main weakness of this technique is that you can match only on known characteristics. If some unknown factor influences the outcome you are measuring and the two groups differ on that factor, it may affect your findings in ways for which you are unprepared.

## Statistical adjustment

To adjust statistically for known differences in the treatment and comparison groups, you would use statistical methods to account for differences in important known characteristics such as sex, race, age, education, and severity of disease. The main weakness of this technique is the same as that for matching: you can account only for known differences between the two groups. See Rossi and Freeman (1982) for a detailed discussion of this technique.

## Before-and-after comparison

A before- and after-program comparison using only the group receiving the program (Campbell and Stanley, 1966) might be a reasonable choice if you are evaluating, for example, a diabetes education class in which the participants are taught home glucose monitoring (Cronbach and Associates, 1980). You test the participants right before the class and establish that they do not know the technique. You test the participants after the class and find that over half of them can now do the monitoring. You can be reasonably sure that the class accounts for the change in skill level from before and after the session. However, you will not know whether another teaching method would work better. The main disadvantage of this technique is that it allows you to find an effect, but in most situations you cannot conclude that the effect was due to your program.

## Using established norms

Observe the effect of a program on a group and compare those effects to established norms about typical changes that occur in similar groups receiving similar programs (Rossi and Freeman, 1982). For example, if published findings on smoking cessation programs indicate that most programs can get 20 percent of their members to quit, you might offer your program and decide that unless you can achieve greater than a 20 percent quit rate, you will discontinue your program and do referrals to other programs instead. The disadvantage to this method is that published studies often describe programs being offered to people who are very different from the individuals in your program, and there are other kinds of differences for which you cannot account.

## QUANTITATIVE AND QUALITATIVE DATA

A division is often made between "quantitative" and "qualitative" data, as though an evaluation could be comprehensive and yet omit one or the other kind of information. We do a disservice to health education when we think this way. Both kinds of information are needed to describe the effects of a program and why those effects occur.

Quantitative data are obtained with standardized means of measurement such as scales, machines that record physiologic responses, and questionnaires with a finite number of specified response categories. They are expressed numerically—number of pounds lost, number of millimeters of mercury that blood pressure is reduced, number of months a person has not smoked, percentage of participants who quit smoking, percentage of participants who have had heart attacks, and so on. Quantitative data about a program's effects on an individual can be obtained from questionnaires, medical records, and government records. Similar data can be obtained on a program's effects on the organization that offers it through questionnaires to the hospital staff, visit records of different services, and accounting records. Quantitative data are used to answer questions such as "Has an educational program decreased the number of broken appointments or unnecessary hospitalizations?"

Qualitative data consist of detailed descriptions of situations, events, people, and observed behaviors as well as direct quotations from people about their experiences, attitudes, beliefs, and thoughts. The qualitative approach to measurement relies on what people themselves say in their own words (Patton, 1980). Case histories, open-ended narratives, and parts of letters are examples of qualitative data. The main sources of these data are in-depth interviews and direct observations. Other sources are open-ended questions on a questionnaire, such as "Do you have any suggestions for improving the weight control program?" Quantitative data can give you broad information about large numbers of people. Qualitative data can add depth and detail to your understanding of a situation.

The need to include both qualitative and quantitative data in articles describing program evaluations was illustrated by two articles that appeared in the *American Journal of Public Health.* One was a report entitled "Five-Year Blood Pressure Control and Mortality Following Health Education for Hypertensive Patients" (Morisky et al., 1983); the other was an editorial questioning the plausibility of the Morisky findings (Kirscht, 1983). The five-year study was a controlled, randomized trial. It showed that after five years, the patients who received counseling and education were better at keeping appointments, controlling their weight, and controlling their blood pressure. They also had a lower hypertension-related mortality rate than the patients in the control group, who received no counseling or education.

The Morisky study is important because it employed the kind of research design that is credible to all audiences (a randomized, controlled trial) and showed that health education programs could actually improve health. Because many formal, scientific evaluations of health education programs have shown little impact on behavior, use of health services, morbidity, or mortality (Alogna, 1981; Mazzuca, 1982), this is precisely the kind of finding that proponents need to show to those who are skeptical of health education's merits. The writer of the editorial questioned the plausibility of the results: "The results [of a] five-year follow-up of hypertensive patients suggest the effectiveness of an educational program. Seldom is such information available. . . . I am both skeptical and intrigued by the results" (Kirscht, 1983). Kirscht raised several questions about the appropriateness of the data analysis. However, his main skepticism could not be eliminated by more appropriate data analysis because it came from his not being able to understand how a few brief counseling and education sessions could so greatly affect patients. (This concern is ironic, because hospital administrators and funding agencies often view health education programs as worthwhile only if they can inexpensively solve the two most long-standing and difficult problems in the delivery of medical care—too frequent use of health services and unhealthy lifestyles.)

What is striking about both articles is their failure to acknowledge that some qualitative data, possibly direct quotes from the participants of the study about how the counseling and education affected them, might have explained why the patients in the treatment group did so well. Interviews with the patients might have revealed that counseling got the patients' family members directly involved in their care. While the counseling sessions may have been short, the family members who went to them may have given the patients the encouragement and support they needed to do whatever was necessary to keep their blood pressure under control. The addition of this kind of qualitative information to the original report might have addressed the critics' chief concerns.

## EVALUATIONS AND THE SOCIAL IMPACT OF PROGRAMS

Selecting the questions that an evaluation should answer is often difficult. It requires a clear understanding of how your own interests—first as a health educator, second as a health educator in a medical setting—fit with those of the others affected by the evaluation.

In many ways health education can be seen as part of a broad social movement, the goals of which are to remove "health" from the sole province of the "professionals" (the doctors) and put it in the hands of the "patients" themselves. The movement strives to give people more information on how they can take care of themselves if they are sick—

for example, diabetes or hypertension education that stresses self-management—and how they might prevent disease by using information and gaining skills that help them to stop smoking, improve their diet, lose weight, or exercise to lower their risk of cancer and coronary heart disease.

The health educator in the medical care delivery system is an organizer and a consciousness raiser of participants in the programs, health providers, and administrators who staff the hospitals and clinics. If a health educator works in a private hospital where often the goal is to increase use of health services, and patient education programs are seen mainly as good public relations, the health educator should think about making evaluations that demonstrate that patient education programs can have a positive effect on people's lives and are more than good public relations. If a health educator works in an HMO with a fixed budget and a desire to decrease use, the health educator should demonstrate that health education programs are good practice and not worthwhile only if they decrease use. If lowering use were the most important reason for having health education programs, then few health educators would be health educators. As a health educator, you need to figure out how to make evaluations that are useful both to you as an organizer of a movement to promote health and to the institution in which you work.

Suppose you run a stop smoking program at a hospital, and your administrator has asked you to evaluate it. You have reviewed the studies in the field, and they show that roughly 20 percent of the people who participate in organized stop smoking programs quit smoking after one year. Should you do another study that asks who has quit after one year, and is a 20 percent quit rate enough to justify a program?

Here is where your conception of your part in a social movement to promote health is crucial. First, you want to increase the number of people who are committed to not smoking. It is therefore important to document any increase in interest. Keep records of how many and what sorts of people call about your stop smoking program. Last year maybe only a few hundred people called, and most of them were of the same age, sex, and social class. This year, you find that twice as many people have called. Many of them heard about the program from people who had participated during the previous year. These new people might be a more diverse group. By knowing something about these people, you can judge if your message is getting across. Your program should not only help people become ex-smokers but should also make organizers of them. That is how small, intensive groups can have broader impact. While it is important to ask people a year after their program ends whether or not they are smoking, it is equally important to get other information:

**1.** Did they get enough information and learn enough of the skills necessary to quit smoking so that, even if they were not successful this time, they will have the resources to do it some time in the future, if they again decide to quit?

**2.** Did they help anyone else to quit smoking? Did they refer anyone else to the program?

**3.** Did anything else in the community help them in their efforts to quit? Did your program direct participants to those resources?

## QUESTIONS TO ASK

There is a minimum number of questions on which to focus—for, say, a stop smoking program—that will help you achieve your program and administrative objectives. For instance, the following questions indicate the minimum questions that a health educator might ask about a stop smoking program. With just a little additional thought you can adapt these questions so that they are applicable to any patient education or health promotion program dealing with any chronic or acute condition or any other lifestyle change.

**1.** How are the participants referred to your program?

**2.** How many people inquire about your program?

**3.** How many people get into your program?

**4.** What are their demographic characteristics?

**5.** What percentage of your participants were referred by other program participants?

**6.** What percentage had quit smoking by the time the program ended?

**7.** What percentage were still not smoking one year after the program ended?

**8.** What percentage of the participants (whether or not they quit) had enough information or skills to quit on their own at a later, more opportune time?

**9.** What percentage went out and tried to help other people quit smoking?

**10.** What percentage referred their friends and family members to the program?

**11.** How many people did they refer?

Those eleven questions should be asked of all stop smoking program participants, and they should be asked in a consistent manner so that different groups conducted over different time periods can be compared. The questions may or may not be on the agenda of the hospital administrator, but they should be on yours.

You will want to ask two other kinds of questions: those that suit the purpose of the hospital administrator, and those that focus on action. When it comes to stop smoking programs, administrators want the following questions answered. With few modifications, you can use them for other patient education and health promotion programs as well.

**1.** Does the program affect use of other health services? That is, does participating in a stop smoking program result in more outpatient clinic visits (because patients have become more attuned to their bodies), or fewer visits (because patients have quit and have fewer health problems)?

**2.** How much does the program cost to operate?

**3.** Are the most effective and least costly methods being used?

**4.** Are there other methods that might work better?

**5.** Are the people who participate in the programs pleased with them?

**6.** Do the people who quit smoking actually have lower blood pressures, fewer heart attacks, and lower incidence of cancer?

**7.** Does this program do well when it is compared to others of the same type?

**8.** Is it worth the cost and time to run a program at the hospital or clinic, or would referrals to community programs be equally effective and less time consuming?

Interest in Question 8 would greatly depend on whether the setting was a prepaid or fee-for-service operation. In a prepaid system, referral to community programs might be more appealing because it would not take so much staff time and other resources. On the other hand, because the administrators of a fee-for-service institution might be trying to encourage use, they may think that it is important to have a program of their own. A fee-for-service hospital or clinic administrator may offer more support to programs that reach many people than to those which are more effective but reach smaller numbers. Administrators in either setting may want their stop smoking programs to reach as many people as possible so that the hospitals have good reputations in the community.

It is important to know whether smoking cessation programs can be cut to fewer "program" sessions and have added maintenance sessions. Would a scaled-down version of the program be just as effective? In other words, can a cheaper program succeed with less effort by participants and less investment by the medical care facility? Answers to some of these questions may be better acquired through a review of the literature than by analysis of your own data. Remember, when consulting the literature, make certain that the findings are relevant to the people you serve.

## UNEXPECTED RESULTS

One phenomenon that is active in medical care settings is the "Hawthorne effect" of evaluation, whereby the evaluation itself seems to have positive effects on the quality of a program. For example, we did an evaluation of a diabetes education program at a medium-sized suburban hospital. The evaluation involved interviewing the physicians about their perceptions of the diabetes education program. We were particularly interested in the physicians' expectations for such a program. The interviews resulted in increased referrals to the program even before they were finished. Ironically, the evaluation had one other unexpected outcome. Since the patient education chief initiated the evaluation, the other physicians in the department assumed that he was an expert in treating patients with diabetes. They began to refer all their difficult diabetic patients to him. Without the interviews, these effects would not have occurred in that hospital. They were positive, unplanned side-effects of the evaluation process.

## SUMMARY AND CONCLUSION

Evaluations of health education programs tell us whether or not programs are effective and what changes should be made to improve them. Patient education is a relatively new health service, and hospital administrators, legislators, and third-party payers want to see evidence that it is truly beneficial. When designing evaluations of health education programs, it is important to be sensitive to the differing concerns and priorities of all interested parties: the organization offering the program, the people who participate in it, and the staff who operate it. No one evaluation can satisfy the diverse interests of all the people involved. It is therefore important to understand the potential consequences of choosing one focus for your evaluation over another.

Health educators should strive to offer programs of the highest quality. To do this requires the gathering of both qualitative and quantitative information on how programs operate and how they affect people.

Health educators have to be skilled at developing inexpensive ways of obtaining this information, as funds for evaluations are not always readily available. How much of each type of data it is necessary to gather depends on the potential audience and uses of the information. To understand how programs operate, complete records must be kept. To understand how programs affect people, comparisons must constantly be made between what is offered and possible alternative approaches. There is no one recipe for making these comparisons. Selecting the appropriate questions to ask, and the research design that can help you answer them, demands creativity and ingenuity. Health education programs have broad social impact. They raise people's consciousness as well as teach them skills. Evaluations should reflect this impact.

While virtually all health educators would agree that evaluation is a key element in high-quality health education practices, many deemphasize it, preferring to organize and manage programs. This is unfortunate. If patient education services are to gain the support necessary for continuation and expansion, more attention must be paid to quality, not quantity. Evaluations can no longer be considered optional. Health educators have no choice but to do them, and in the most thoughtful ways they can.

# APPENDIX 7.1

**Stop Smoking Program**

Group No. _____
Date _____
Leader _____
Location _____

| Name | Phone Numbers | Sessions Attended | | | | | | | | | | | | | | |
|------|---------------|---|---|---|---|---|---|---|---|---|---|---|---|---|---|---|
| | | 1 | 2 | 3 | 4 | 5 | 6 | 7 | 8 | 9 | 10 | 11 | 12 | 13 | 14 | 15 |
| | W -<br>H - | | | | | | | | | | | | | | | |
| | W -<br>H - | | | | | | | | | | | | | | | |
| | W -<br>H - | | | | | | | | | | | | | | | |
| | W -<br>H - | | | | | | | | | | | | | | | |
| | W -<br>H - | | | | | | | | | | | | | | | |
| | W -<br>H - | | | | | | | | | | | | | | | |
| | W -<br>H - | | | | | | | | | | | | | | | |
| | W -<br>H - | | | | | | | | | | | | | | | |
| | W -<br>H - | | | | | | | | | | | | | | | |

# Stop Smoking Program Attendance Sheet

| | | | | | | | No. of attendees | No. of cancellations | No. of no-shows | No. of drop-outs |
|---|---|---|---|---|---|---|---|---|---|---|
| W -<br>H - | | W -<br>H - | | W -<br>H - | | W -<br>H - | | W -<br>H - | | W -<br>H - |

# APPENDIX 7.2

## Stop Smoking Program Intake Form

### Entry Questionnaire—Stop Smoking Group

Name _____

Age _____    Height _____    Weight _____    ( ) Male  ( ) Female

Occupation _____ Marital Status _____

1. Circle highest completed school grade: 1 2 3 4 5 6 7 8 9 10 11 12
   College: 1 2 3 4 +

2. Number of people living in your household (include yourself) _____

3. Number of people living in your household who smoke (include yourself) _____

4. How many packs of cigarettes per day do you usually smoke? _____

5. How many years have you been smoking cigarettes? _____

6. How many different times have you made a serious and deliberate attempt to stop smoking? _____ ( ) None

7. What's the longest period of time you've stayed off cigarettes? _____

8. Do you have, or have you ever had, any smoking-related health condition, such as the following:

   ( ) Heart condition     ( ) Bronchitis     ( ) Emphysema
   ( ) Other disease     (Specify) _____

9. Who is your regular doctor? _____

10. Do you now have, or have you ever had, a problem with alcohol or any
    other drug? _____ None ( )

11. Is this a good time for you to stop smoking?
    Yes ( )   No ( )   Not Sure ( )

12. How many of your friends smoke?
    All ( )   Most ( )   Some ( )   Few ( )   None ( )

13. Do you usually smoke on the job? _____

14. How many of the people you work with are smokers?
    All ( )   Most ( )   Some ( )   Few ( )   None ( )

15. What is the possibility that five years from now, you will be a cigarette
    smoker?          Definitely no ( )        Probably yes ( )
                     Probably no ( )          Definitely yes ( )

16. How did you hear about the Stop Smoking Clinic? _____

# APPENDIX 7.3

## Medical Chart Documentation of Patient Education Program

### Patient Progress Record

| Patient's Name (Last, First, Middle) | Stamp membership card below. |
|---|---|
| Address (No., Street) | |
| (City) | |
| Birthdate | Phone | Code | Group | |

- Patient registered for the Stop Smoking Clinic, group no. _____,
on _____ (month, day, year).

- Patient attended _____ (how many?) of the 15 meetings.

- At the last day of class, patient (check one)
  ___ had stopped smoking.
  ___ had not stopped smoking.

_____
Signature
Health Education Group Leader

# APPENDIX 7.4

## Health Library Visit Record

1. OPERATION:

   1 ☐ Calendar mailing

   2 ☐ Ext Setup

   3 ☐ Letter        1 ☐ Individual    ☐ 1st visit  2 ☐ Return

   4 ☐ Outreach      2 ☐ Group

   5 ☐ Phone

   6 ☐ Pick up A/V     Females ☐☐

   7 ☐ Return A/V      Males   ☐☐

   8 ☐ Visit           Total   ☐☐☐

   Date: _____

   Name: _____

   Birthdate: _____

   Sex: _____

2. WHO:     1 ☐ HMO member  2 ☐ Health professional  3 ☐ Private patient, etc.  4 ☐ Staff

   5 ☐ Other (Specify) _____  ☐

3. REFERRED BY:   1 ☐ Dr. _____ ☐☐☐☐  2 ☐ Friend/Family member

   Name

   3 ☐ N.P. _____ ☐☐☐  4 ☐ Reception  5 ☐ R.N.  6 ☐ Self  7 ☐ Other _____  ☐

   (Specify)

4. REFERRED FROM:   1 ☐ Central medical  2 ☐ Other facility _____ ☐☐  3 ☐ Other

   department                         (Specify)

   1 ☐ Allergy   2 ☐ Class (specify) _____ ☐☐   3 ☐ Derm   4 ☐ ENT   11 ☐ Nurs

   5 ☐ Eye   6 ☐ Fam Plan   7 ☐ Gyn   8 ☐ Med   9 ☐ MCH   10 ☐ Neuro   18 ☐ Urol

   12 ☐ Nutr   13 ☐ Ortho   14 ☐ Pedi   15 ☐ Prenatal   16 ☐ Psych   17 ☐ Surg

   19 ☐ Other (specify) _____ ☐☐

5. VISITOR/BORROWER PURPOSE:   ☐ Consult       ☐ Eval Audio/Equip   ☐ Fam/Friend Med Care

   ☐ General Interest   ☐ Own Medical Care   ☐ Teach/Educ

   ☐ Other (specify) _____  ☐

6. RECEIVED/DIRECTED TO:   ☐ Audiov   ☐ Books   ☐ Equip   ☐ Exhibits

   ☐ Head Libr   ☐ Libr   ☐ Pamphlets   ☐ Rm Reservation   ☐ Sales Shop

   ☐ Other Med Ctr Staff/Dept. (specify) _____

   ☐ Other Facility (specify) _____

   ☐ Other Resource (specify) _____

7. ITEMS (AUDIOVISUALS, EQUIPMENT, ETC.) VIEWED/HEARD/BORROWED/RETURNED:

   _____ ☐☐☐☐   _____ ☐☐☐☐

   _____ ☐☐☐☐   _____ ☐☐☐☐

   _____ ☐☐☐☐   _____ ☐☐☐☐

   ☐ Reference question asked: _____

   _____ Ans.?   1 ☐ Yes   2 ☐ No

   ☐ Inadequate libr. resources—subject(s): _____

   Library staff member: _____

# APPENDIX 7.5

## Television Survey

---

**Survey for Closed-Circuit Hospital Television**

Room no. _____

Dear Patient:

Would you please answer the following questions?

1. Were you told about the closed-circuit hospital television programs on Channel ____?
   No ____ Yes ____ How were you told? _____

2. Did you watch any of the programs on Channel ____?
   Yes ____ No ____ Why? _____

3. If yes, which programs did you watch? (Please list them by name or subject.) Did you find them interesting?

|  | Yes | No |
|---|---|---|
| _____ | ☐ | ☐ |
| _____ | ☐ | ☐ |
| _____ | ☐ | ☐ |
| _____ | ☐ | ☐ |

Please return to the volunteer.                    Thank you.

# APPENDIX 7.6

## Physician Survey: Evaluation of the Health Library

### Physician Evaluation of Health Library

Dear Dr. _____:

1. To what extent does the health library improve the quality of patient care?

   1 ☐ Significant    2 ☐ Moderate    3 ☐ Minimal    4 ☐ None

2. Has the health library helped save you time?

   1 ☐ Yes    2 ☐ No

3. Do your patients find the health library helpful?

   1 ☐ Yes    2 ☐ No    3 ☐ I don't know

4. How frequently do you refer patients to the health library?

   1 ☐ Often    2 ☐ Sometimes    3 ☐ Rarely    4 ☐ Not at all

5. For what purposes do you refer patients to the health library? (Please check all that apply.)

   To augment your own instructions    ☐

   To obtain information on specific conditions or diseases    ☐

   To obtain information on general health    ☐

   To facilitate self-care    ☐

   Other: _____    ☐

6. How well does the health library do the following?

|  | Very well 1 | Moderately 2 | Minimally 3 | Poorly 4 |
|---|---|---|---|---|
| Augment your own instructions? | ☐ | ☐ | ☐ | ☐ |

Dispense
information on
specific conditions
or diseases?          ☐              ☐              ☐              ☐

Dispense
information on
general health?       ☐              ☐              ☐              ☐

Facilitate self-
care?                 ☐              ☐              ☐              ☐

Other: _____      ☐              ☐              ☐              ☐

7.  Please check all the health library services you or your
    patients find helpful:

    ☐ Providing audiovisual aids    ☐ Distributing pamphlets

    ☐ Stocking books for loan       ☐ Offering books for sale

    ☐ Answering reference questions  ☐ Referral to other
                                        resources

8.  Would the health library be a more effective resource if changes
    were made in any of the following:

|                                                     | Yes 1 | No 2 |
|-----------------------------------------------------|-------|------|
| Services offered                                    | ☐     | ☐    |
| Quality of information dispensed                    | ☐     | ☐    |
| Subject areas covered                               | ☐     | ☐    |
| Types of materials (e.g., films, books, pamphlets)  | ☐     | ☐    |
| How materials are chosen                            | ☐     | ☐    |
| Staffing                                            | ☐     | ☐    |
| Location                                            | ☐     | ☐    |
| Physical setup                                      | ☐     | ☐    |
| Hours open                                          | ☐     | ☐    |
| Publicity about it                                  | ☐     | ☐    |

If you have answered yes to any of the above or have any other suggestions for improving the health library, please explain here:

_____

_____

_____

_____

9. How long have you been working with this medical center?

   1 ☐ Under 2 years

   2 ☐ 2 to 5 years

   3 ☐ Over 5 years

10. Do you have any other comments about the health library or this questionnaire? (Please use back of page for additional comments.)

_____

_____

_____

Please return this questionnaire in the enclosed addressed envelope. Thank you.


# EXERCISES

1. Think of yourself as the health education coordinator at a large urban private hospital. Your administrator has asked you to evaluate the abortion-counseling program offered at the hospital. The administrator has not indicated why the evaluation is necessary.
   a. List some of the reasons why the administrator may want the evaluation conducted.
   b. List all the people (including yourself) who may be affected by the evaluation.
   c. Indicate the different questions that each of these people might want the evaluation to address.

2.   You have just replaced a health education coordinator at a medium-sized outpatient clinic. Several health education programs are already being offered at the clinic. You want to know if they are operating efficiently.

   a. What kind of information would you request from the program staff?

   b. What kinds of records would you ask the program staff to keep on an ongoing basis?

3.   You are the health education coordinator at an urban medical center. You have been asked by the physician liaison for patient education to make a presentation to the local patient education committee on how to choose a program to evaluate.

   a. Make an outline of the topics you plan to cover in your presentation.

   b. What issues will you recommend that the committee consider before choosing a program to evaluate?

4.   You are trying to determine if your smoking cessation program is "successful."

   a. How could "success" be defined?

   b. What kinds of questions would you ask, and who would you ask them of, to find out if your program is successful?

5.   You are evaluating a stress management program offered at your medical center. How can you determine if the program is effective in helping participants reduce tension in their daily lives? (Be specific. Try to think of all the possible sources of information that you might use and how you would interpret this information.)

# RESOURCES

Campbell, D. T., and Stanley, J. C. *Experimental and Quasi-Experimental Designs for Research.* Chicago: Rand McNally, 1966.

   This book is an essential classic in the research methodology literature. The authors cover the fundamentals of research designs for laboratory and for various "real world" settings.

Cronbach, L. J., and Associates. *Toward Reform of Program Evaluation.* San Francisco: Jossey-Bass, 1980.

   This provocative assessment of the evaluation research field emphasizes the political context within which evaluations occur. Although not specifically oriented toward health education, it provides many informative examples of program evaluations in large bureaucracies. The book offers an interesting complement to *Evaluation* by Rossi and Freeman.

Davis, J. A. *Elementary Survey Analysis.* Englewood Cliffs, N.J.: Prentice-Hall, 1971.

Davis's analysis is a good source for learning how to examine and interpret relationships among psychosocial and demographic variables; for example, how does patient education affect blood pressure level, holding the variables of age and sex constant?

Dillman, D. A. *Mail and Telephone Surveys: The Total Design Method.* New York: Wiley, 1978.

Dillman offers a holistic approach to the nitty-gritty details of designing and implementing mail and telephone surveys. The book covers important material often slighted in general research design texts, such as wording, order, and layout of questions in a survey. An extremely helpful "how to" manual, it emphasizes the importance of careful planning and personal attention to respondents to ensure collection of useful data.

Fitz-Gibbon, C. T., and Morris, L. L. *How to Design a Program Evaluation.* Beverly Hills, Calif.: Sage, 1978.

One of eight slim volumes in the Program Evaluation Kit developed at the Center for the Study of Evaluation (University of California at Los Angeles), this book delivers what its title promises at a level suitable to the novice program evaluator. Liberal use of illustrations lends clarity and concreteness to presentations of steps in research design, study implementation, and interpretation of results.

Green, L. W., Kreuter, M. W., Deeds, S. G., and Partridge, K. B. *Health Education Planning.* Palo Alto, Calif.: Mayfield, 1980.

A brief but important chapter in this recent health education text outlines several evaluation designs, ranging from simple record keeping to full-scale research projects, while arguing that assessments of the immediate behavioral impacts of health education programs are most useful at this time.

Leaverton, P. E. *A Review of Biostatistics: A Program for Self-Instruction.* Boston: Little, Brown, 1978.

This is a good introductory review of biostatistics with helpful exercises.

Mazzuca, S. A. Does Patient Education in Chronic Disease Have Therapeutic Value? *Journal of Chronic Disease,* 35 (1982):521–529.

Mazzuca reviews thirty experimental studies reporting the effects of patient education on compliance with a regimen, progress toward a therapeutic goal, and long-range health outcomes. Patient education programs that were given a behavioral, individually oriented emphasis produced greater beneficial effects than did didactic programs that emphasized improving patients' knowledge about their diseases.

Patton, M. *Qualitative Evaluation Methods.* Beverly Hills, Calif.: Sage, 1980.

This book is a readable, entertaining, informative treatment of nonquantitative data gathering and analysis methods. Excellent chapter on qualitative interviewing techniques. As in his earlier *Utilization-Focused Evaluation* (Beverly Hills, Calif.: Sage, 1978), Patton advocates evaluation designs that match appropriate methods ("how to find out") to desired outcomes ("what to find out") so that evaluations can be used to inform rational decision making. Patton cautions that "an evaluation not worth doing is not worth doing well."

Rossi, P. H., and Freeman, H. E. *Evaluation: A Systematic Approach.* 2nd ed. Beverly Hills, Calif.: Sage, 1982.

This book is the most comprehensive, up-to-date textbook on evaluation research. It is one of the best introductions to the field for the beginning student, and a valuable reference tool for the professional evaluator. In neatly designed, well-written chapters, the authors provide lucid definitions of key concepts, informative discussions of research design problem points, and many examples of evaluation studies.

Suchman, E. A. *Evaluative Research: Principles and Practice in Public Service and Social Action Programs.* New York: Russell Sage Foundation, 1967.

Suchman's work is seminal in the evaluation field; written from the classical experimental research design perspective.

Weiss, C. H. *Evaluation Research: Methods of Assessing Program Effectiveness.* Englewood Cliffs, N.J.: Prentice-Hall, 1972.

This concise, sensible treatment of how to do program evaluations offers a straightforward presentation of several research design strategies. It is one of the earliest works to focus explicitly on the organizational and political constraints within which most evaluation studies are implemented and their findings are disseminated.

# PART THREE

# INTERVENTION SKILLS AND METHODS

# 8

# Educational assessment as intervention

INFORMATION ALONE SELDOM changes behavior. Unfortunately, during health education sessions many health care providers and educators continue to emphasize the physiological aspects of the disease process. But other health educators are challenging the assumption that information and fear tactics should be the primary methods for changing client behavior (Leventhal, 1965; Janis, 1968). Growing numbers of consumers and health care providers believe that education requires more than the traditional focus on physical aspects of disease and pharmacological approaches to treatment.

In this chapter we present an educational assessment process that can be a significant component of behavior change interventions. This process links physical assessment with (1) psychological, social, and behavioral issues affecting the client's health status; (2) adherence to treatment plans; and (3) health promotion efforts. Health care providers can use this approach to emphasize behavior change rather than health information. This assessment process assumes that the client is a valuable source of expertise. We present extended examples to illustrate the application of the assessment skills discussed. Finally, we discuss how health educators can gain acceptance of educational assessment by administrators, providers, and health education instructors.

This book reflects the position of its authors that health educators in medical care settings are more than just consultants and planners. They also provide direct service. This chapter will help health educators who work directly with clients. For health educators who provide inservice and continuing education seminars for health professionals, this chapter provides the basis for teaching clinicians how to use educational assessment as a part of the medical office or hospital visit and encounter.

Let's start with a closer look at our clients' needs as they are presented to the medical care system. As noted in Chapter 2, the major health problems in this country have shifted from infectious diseases with identifiable causes and cures to chronic diseases with a host of contributing factors and often few specific cures. In addition, reported stress-related symptoms such as headaches, gastrointestinal dysfunction, insomnia, and back pain have increased. Epidemiologists have identified our lifestyle and environment as the major sources of our health problems; yet the medical care system continues to rely primarily on medication and surgery, which have little if any effect on these predisposing factors. Most medical treatment plans require patients to follow a specified medication regimen and to provide self-care at home. Both increased social pressure and legal mandates are guiding the medical care system to provide informed choices to its consumers. This dynamic often creates an adversarial relationship between clients and health care providers.

## THE ASSESSMENT PROCESS

In medical care assessment the health practitioner must systematically gather data to gain a full picture of the situation, to make a diagnosis, and to determine appropriate treatment. It is usually a one-way process of questioning, testing, and examination of the client by the medical provider. The rationale, details, and outcome of the assessment may or may not be shared with the client. One process of medical assessment and documentation widely used in the medical care setting is SOAP (Subjective data, Objective data, Assessment, Plan), developed by Lawrence Weed (1968). Educational assessment uses this same process. Table 8.1 explains the SOAP process. The data gathered according to Table 8.1 are documented in the medical record, are the basis for future discussions with clients on return visits, and can help clients and their providers track behavior changes over time.

### The Goal

The educational assessment process presented in this chapter can be integrated into the medical assessment process and can be formulated in much the same way. However, while medical assessment focuses on the *provider*'s role in gathering data, the primary goal of educational assessment is to foster client *self*-assessment. The purpose is to increase

## Table 8.1   The SOAP process

| | |
|---|---|
| **S** (<u>S</u>ubjective Data) | Gather historic data from questionnaires, and find out the client's view of symptoms and history of the problem. |
| **O** (<u>O</u>bjective Data) | Collect findings of tests and examinations related to the problem. |
| **A** (<u>A</u>ssessment) | Check the health care provider's interpretation of the data and definition of the problem. |
| **P** (<u>P</u>lan) | Obtain further data to define the problem and specific treatment plans. |

both the provider's and the client's understanding of the wide range of influences on the health problem as well as of the factors affecting the client's health behaviors.

This change in orientation sets the tone for a therapeutic partnership between provider and client that supports the influence and expertise of both parties while clarifying the client's role in healing and health action. During this process, the client learns assessment skills that can then be applied to other health problems and behavior change situations. In this way, *the assessment process becomes intervention.* In addition to helping clients acquire new skills, this approach is a particularly useful way for the health practitioner to deal with the clients' too-high expectations of cures and overly simple answers to complex problems.

One creative adaptation of the SOAP method to health education has been developed by a primary care clinic at the University of Vermont Medical School. The clinic staff adapted SOAP as an educational technique by giving their clients copies of their medical records. The records are written in a form that nonmedical people can understand and include a clear statement of problems and plans to emphasize self-help and client responsibility. The staff have evaluated their work and report favorable results—such as lower client anxiety about health, increased client responsibility, more treatment plans developed by providers directed toward client actions, and improved relationships between clients, physicians, and paramedical staff (Tufo et al., 1977). Additional preliminary results show a reduction in smoking behavior among their clients, too.

## Quality assurance

Now, let's look at another way to integrate an educational perspective into the SOAP process. The following outline shows peer review standards for an expanded assessment and intervention process developed by a health educator and medical staff of a primary care clinic.

### Subjective

**1.** Ask for the client's assessment of the problem and of the self-care approaches already tried.

**2.** Obtain psychosocial information on the client's support system, work, family, major worries, and life concerns.

**3.** Review the client's lifestyle and health behavior influences.

**4.** Address client concerns identified on any questionnaires, in subjective notes, treatment plan, or a note on the questionnaire itself.

### Objective

**1.** Have client present his or her health problem.

**2.** Consider the client's type of participation in the assessment and interview—for example, statements of acceptance of problem, recall of experiences, identification of means to change behavior.

**3.** Review written records kept, such as food diary, smoking log.

**4.** Note changes in health status tests regarding behavior change areas such as weight, blood pressure, or cholesterol level.

### Assessment

Obtain the health practitioner's assessment of the situation, including psychological, social, environmental, and behavioral aspects; the client's readiness to change, understanding level, and strengths and weaknesses for making health behavior changes.

### Plan

**1.** Get the patient's agreement to behavior changes.

**2.** Give an individual referral or provider consultation with health education staff to members with two or more cardiovascular risk factors (such as family history, hypertension, elevated cholesterol, low exercise level, obesity, smoking).

**3.** Record health education interventions.

**4.** At first visit have all members view film on introduction to services.

These standards are used as an element of the clinic's quality assurance program. An interdisciplinary group of a physician, nurse practitioner, health educator, and psychologist form a peer review committee that meets monthly to review medical charts to assure quality of care and adherence to the standards for medical record documentation of the educational aspects of the office visit, as well as other medical and psychosocial standards.

## BASIC ASSESSMENT TECHNIQUES

Two basic assessment techniques form the foundation of provider educational assessment skills: (1) questionnaires and (2) listening and questioning skills. These techniques are useful in a variety of settings, including individual client interviews, group sessions with clients, or problem-solving sessions with other departments.

### Assessment questionnaires

Questionnaires are used widely in medical care practice. They are useful ways to collect objective information on such topics as family and medical history, current medications, and symptoms. Traditionally, few questionnaires focus on subjective data such as the clients' areas of interest and their own perceptions of their psychological, social, environmental, lifestyle, and health information needs.

Questionnaires can be designed to be useful both to clients and to staff. For example, a well-designed questionnaire can be an educational tool in a complete health evaluation. It can guide clients through a review of their health and assessment of their situation. For staff, it can provide a useful review of a large amount of information that could be time consuming to obtain verbally. And it can tap important subjective data. Clients' perspectives on their health provide insights for further discussion and assessment.

The Health Improvement Questionnaire in Appendix 8.1 was developed by a health educator and psychologist in a community health clinic (Flanagan, 1978). It supplements a traditional medical questionnaire and is completed by clients who are obtaining complete health evaluations. Flanagan based the format and text on other questionnaires, on input from the clinic staff, and on the results of two pretests with 100 clients each.

Notice that the questionnaire explicitly states to clients the goal of fostering a therapeutic partnership and an expanded view of the many influences on health. Take a look at Section I of the questionnaire, entitled "Health Promotion and Information." This section allows clients to identify their needs for health information and their desire for health behavior change. Section II, entitled "Important Life Areas," identifies clients' psychological and social concerns. And Section III, entitled "Overall Health Review," is designed to illustrate the interaction between physical, psychological, social, environmental, and lifestyle factors.

A few clients refuse to complete such questionnaires. They may feel that doing so is not directly applicable to their health or that the approach is too personal. In this case, the educator can do the assessment verbally. It is important to help clients to identify those areas they feel *do* affect their health. This may be a good time to assure clients of the confidentiality of all medical questionnaires and documents.

The Health Improvement Questionnaire has proven to be a useful tool for both clients and staff to support an expanded assessment process and to develop health improvement programs with specified health behavior change plans. Training sessions and case studies help teach the staff to feel more comfortable in using their clients' answers as a beginning point for the office visit. Most clients report that they gained insight from a process that encourages them to take a larger view of what constitutes health. Herein lies the power of educational assessment as an intervention.

## Listening and questioning skills

The basic skills essential for effectiveness as an educator that are discussed in this chapter are

- Attending to the client's communications
- Asking open-ended questions
- Asking closed-ended questions
- Offering third-party opinions
- Encouraging
- Clarifying statements
- Making statements of feeling

Most people already use these skills regularly to some extent. Self-assessment and practice can help you to further develop and sharpen them.

The following review of the key concepts in listening and questioning is only an introduction to an extensive area of literature. If you intend to use these skills for individual counseling work with clients, you need additional training. Check with the psychology or education department of your college or university about course offerings in these areas.

Attending behaviors let your clients know that your attention is focused on them. Maintain eye contact, without intensive staring, while talking and listening directly to them. Since much communication is non-verbal, posture is important. Face your shoulders toward the client or group, and lean slightly forward to communicate your attention. To take the nervous anticipation out of a visit, prepare clients with an overview of the session. Be careful to accept the client's pace; moments of silence are natural and help to set a tone of mutual respect and problem solving.

*Open-ended questions* are used most effectively to determine the client's view of the situation without directing or suggesting answers. Such questions actively involve clients in the process by asking their feelings, opinions, and assessment of their situation. These questions usually begin with the words *what* or *how*. For example, how do you feel about taking this medicine three times a day? To bring closure to an interview, formulate an open-ended question asking clients to summarize (1) what has or has not been useful during the discussion and (2) what actions they will take—for example, "We've talked about a number of possible choices to reduce your back pain. Could you summarize the most important changes, if any, that you plan to make?"

*Closed-ended questions* require a simple "yes" or "no" answer. They are useful in obtaining factual background information that does not require subjective interpretations. Answers to them do not require much thinking and thus can sometimes serve as a gentle ice breaker to get a conversation started. If used repetitively, however, they set a tone of one-way interrogation and dependence on the practitioner unless a transition is made to open-ended questions. Be careful not to use questions that may seem factual but are actually quite subjective. For instance, the reliability of answers to the question "Do you know how to take your temperature?" is quite low. It would be better to ask, "When you take your temperature, how do you do it?"

*Third-party opinion* questions combine a statement and a question. They can set clients at ease and allow them to express difficult feelings. This is done by relating common feelings and reactions that others have and then asking clients about their own feelings. For example, one might ask, "How do people you know feel about exercise as a way to lose weight? What is your opinion?"

Compare the effects of the three types of questions in the following situation. A patient who recently had a myocardial infarction returns for a follow-up visit with his physician after starting a new medication. The physician says,

- *Open-ended:* "What has it been like taking the new medication, Inderal, for your heart?"

- *Closed-ended:* "Have you been taking your medication?"
- *Third-party opinion:* "Many people find that they miss some of their medication on busy days or cannot remember when they took it last. What has it been like for you?"

In this situation, the open-ended question would be a good starting point, and the third-party opinion question would be useful for stimulating further discussion. The closed-ended question has little reliability in this context, because it only elicits "yes" or "no" answers and does not check out related issues.

Many clients need to be encouraged to express themselves fully. Simple words, phrases, or gestures can encourage clients to elaborate on their feelings or thoughts. A nod of the head, saying "Mm," and asking for more details are often very useful.

Clarifying statements let the clients know that you understand their concerns. You interpret what the client has said, but using different words— for example, "You're saying that you feel the new pill schedule cramps your style." This allows clients to reflect more completely on their own thoughts, correct their misunderstandings, and often invites them to expand on their ideas. Clarifying statements can be useful throughout the assessment process as a means of assuring that both the provider's and the client's communications have been clearly understood by each other.

Responding to the feelings and emotions of clients can help them develop further self-assessments and understanding. These statements go beyond clarifying statements and reflect both clients' verbal and non-verbal feelings. They often begin with statements such as, "You seem to be feeling . . . ," "Sounds like you're feeling . . . ," or "I sense you're . . . ." The following sample dialogue uses the active listening skills just discussed. A client has been discussing her decision about stopping smoking with a health educator:

Client: I'm just not sure if I can do it.

Health Educator (*encouragingly*): Tell me a little more about that.

Client: Well, when I feel pressure at work, smoking helps me relax.

Health Educator (*clarifying*): You're wondering, if you take the smoking away, if the work pressure will just keep building up?

Client: Yeah, I get all wound up, my mind running in all directions, and smoking a cigarette really helps me calm down.

Health Educator (*with feeling*): Sounds like you're feeling a bit scared that you won't be able to calm down at all without a cigarette.

## INFLUENCES ON INDIVIDUAL BEHAVIOR CHANGE

An educational assessment includes identifying the variety of influences on behavior that exist in a given situation, including lifestyle influences. Often the large range of influences can seem overwhelming when working with individual clients or with groups. The use of client self-assessment questionnaires and open-ended questioning skills can help you identify the critical factors that support or impede the change process and the health problem. One physician made it a routine practice before each visit to give his clients a handout that listed the most common reasons people didn't follow their treatment plans. He then used this handout as a basis for discussion during the visit on how to overcome common barriers. The major influences that should be considered in the educational assessment process are as follows:

*Daily routine:*  Regularity of existing routine and ability of clients to identify means to integrate new behavior into a daily schedule

*Support system:*  Presence of involved and supportive family members and/or friends and co-workers to assist in making the change and to discuss concerns; role models that practice new behaviors already

*Health belief system:*  Acknowledgment of relationship between behavior and health conditions or risks, perception of vulnerability, belief in effectiveness and benefits of behavior change, conflicting information or folk healing beliefs

*Experience with medical care system:*  Resolution of residual anger or mistrust from previous unsatisfactory experience with the medical care system, previous noncompliance with successful results, medical needs of a higher priority

*Environment:*  Physical work and home environment conducive or adaptable to change, skills to evaluate media or television input regarding health problem

*Previous experience with change:*  Recognition of generalizable skills from previous behavior changes (for example, clients' skills used in stopping smoking five years ago may be useful to changing diet now)

*Self-management skills:*  Observation of behavior patterns, identification of cues and alternative response patterns, development of self-reward system

*Stress coping skills:*  Presence of some positive means of coping with stress, willingness to explore new means

*Readiness to change:*  Presence of satisfaction with some aspects of major life areas (home, work, personal relationships), conflicting priorities and needs not excessive, client expressed interest

The preceding list describes various factors that are aspects of a person's experience that have influence on his or her health decisions and actions. This list can be used as a basis for interview questions with clients during the educational assessment process. Appendix 8.2 gives a summary assessment form that can be used to rate the client's status in each health behavior influence area. This form can help providers (1) approach educational assessment in a systematic manner; (2) review the influences with clients, asking them to rate themselves in each area; and (3) document the educational assessment (as a medical record form).

## TWO EXAMPLES OF EDUCATIONAL ASSESSMENT AS INTERVENTION

Now let us present two examples that show how to apply educational assessment as an intervention. The first example focuses on the individual level of health education services. A clinical health educator (let us call her Laura Quinn) in a primary care clinic provides direct individualized services for patient education and health promotion. Notice the lack of primary attention to the content or health information aspects of health education in this new direct service role for health educators. The second example involves a health educator (Joe Wadia) who uses educational assessment as an intervention at a programmatic level by providing continuing education workshops for instructors of health education programs. This example illustrates (1) how Wadia responded to an institutional policy that required department managers to develop quality assurance standards and (2) how important it is for health educators to recognize the difference between the programmatic and organizational levels of their coordinator roles.

### The clinical health educator

In Little Rock, Arkansas, a primary care clinic serving approximately 12,000 members in a health maintenance organization setting has established a clinical health educator role. The overall goal of the clinic is to optimize the health of all members by providing sick- and well-care services that integrate health education and mental health counseling. There are ten clinical staff positions, including physicians, nurse practitioners, a psychologist, and a health educator—Laura Quinn.

As the full-time health education coordinator, Quinn spends approximately one-third time on direct clinical services, one-third on consultation with staff regarding their patients, and one-third on administration and program development. Clients for clinical health educator services are primarily referred by other clinical staff for assistance with behavior change as it relates to a particular health problem or general health promotion. Treatment needs involving medication, lifestyle change, and/or home self-care have generally been established by the clinical staff prior to referral.

Health education appointments with new clients are scheduled for 45 minutes. Follow-up appointments range from 30 to 45 minutes, depending on client need, frequency of follow-up, and complexity of client's health problem(s). The most commonly seen clients are hypertensives, diabetics, headache patients, people with low back pain, and clients desiring general health promotion skills in areas such as smoking cessation, stress management, and health risk reduction. Consultation with medical staff occurs as needed throughout the day and in monthly group consultation sessions.

An overall assessment takes place at the initial appointment. This visit also may include health information, referral to other resources, and introductory techniques for decision making and behavior change. The following outline summarizes the educational assessment process used by the health educator:

**1.** Review medical chart for significant diagnoses, review client-identified concerns on assessment questionnaires, consult with the medical provider for questions or concerns

**2.** Introduce yourself to the client, name, role of the clinical health educator, and overview of the appointment goals (assessment, client questions, future plans)

**3.** Check the following client assessment areas:
   a. Perception of current health status, clinical diagnosis, and reason for scheduling appointment
   b. Beliefs regarding relationship between health improvement and behavior change, current health habit review
   c. Knowledge about problems
   d. Support system and stressful life events
   e. Experience with behavior change, perceived barriers to change
   f. Questions (to be encouraged)
   g. Daily routine review
   h. Identification and integration of new activities and changes
   i. Overall readiness for change (supplemented by health educator's perceptions)

Once the assessment has been conducted, the client works with the health educator to identify reasonable alternatives for action. The following variables should be considered in developing a health action plan:

- Client's choices, interest, and self-assessment
- Medical risk level (that is, seriousness or presence of disease complications or high cardiovascular risk factors)
- Other psychological and medical needs identified during visit
- Available health information and library resources
- Group and community resources available
- Level of support in system (for example, spouse unsupportive of patient's need for dietary restrictions)
- Self-management and coping skills (for example, daily eating routine established, with good observation of eating influences and identified ways to deal with stress)
- Comfort of health educator in addressing client's needs

Individualized agreements are then made regarding intensity of follow-up, short- and long-term goals, and use of available resources. As the relationship with the client progresses, continuing assessment, decision making, and self-care techniques are integrated into each visit. The average client makes three visits over the course of one or two months.

As health educators become more involved with direct clinical services, they need to become familiar with common abbreviations and medical shorthand. Table 8.2 reviews some common symbols and abbreviations and can help you read Figure 8.1, which is an example of the SOAP documentation of an educational assessment done by a clinical health educator at an initial client visit.

**Table 8.2  Common medical abbreviations**

| | | | |
|---|---|---|---|
| hx | History | PE | Physical exam |
| dx | Diagnosis | BP | Blood pressure |
| rx | Prescribed | WNL | Within normal limits |
| tx | Treatment | Wt | Weight |
| ↑ | Increase | NAD | No acute distress |
| ↓ | Decrease | RTC | Return to clinic |
| HA | Headache | prn | As needed |
| BID | Two times a day | QD | One time per day |
| TID | Three times a day | HS | Before bed |

## Figure 8.1   Example of SOAP assessment

### SUBJECTIVE (S)

A 37-year-old black female administrator referred by Long, M.D., reports 6 mos. hx of headaches (HA) 2-3x/wk and ↑ neck/left shoulder pain. Dx as functional problems. Health habit review indicates irregular eating often skipping lunch due to ↑ work pressures, ↑ desk work/writing. On phone many times throughout day. Sleep poor, difficulty relaxing. Feels good about stopping smoking 2 yrs. ago but feeling ↑ cravings again. Alcohol 1-2/day. Coffee/colas 6-8/day. Satisfied w/marriage of 5 yrs, considering pregnancy but stress seems overwhelming. HAs come primarily in afternoon, aspirin gives little relief. Rxed Tylenol with codeine for HA w/some relief. Neck/shoulder pain ↑ as day goes on. Heat gives some relief. Occas. recreational activ. w/spouse or friends, but less now due to ↑ work pressures, HA & tiredness. HA/neck pain ↓ during 1 week vacation 2 mos. ago. No hx of other health problems.

### OBJECTIVE (O)

PE done 3 mos. ago WNL
Poor Fitness Test   Wt = 135; BP = 120/74
Pt. specifically states relationship between work stress, poor health habits, and HA/pain and willingness to change.

### ASSESSMENT (A)

- Functional HA, neck & shoulder pain.
- Poor health habits, ↑ caffeine, skipping lunch, poor fitness and body mechanics.
- Situational stress with moderate support system.
- Recent experience with stop smoking positive, possible recidivism now.

### PLAN (P)

1. Eat lunch daily away from desk. Include protein, carbo, veg or fruit.
2. Review time management materials, consider class.
3. ↑ water and noncaffeine beverages. No caffeine after 6 pm.
4. Keep headache journal including food, activity, feelings and headaches, discuss with husband to analyze.
5. Schedule 3 additional appointments over next 6 weeks. RTC 1 week.
6. View headache film. Read headache article and insomnia materials.
7. Call prn.
   (Discuss relaxation exercises, ↑ exercise, neck, & work activities at next appt.)

Over the year and a half of practice, Laura Quinn has continued to work with staff to clarify the process-oriented role of the position; that is, the role to diagnose and treat behavior change problems regardless of the particular medical problem. Acceptance of the role has grown as the medical staff has come to understand that the clinical health educator does not develop a completely new treatment plan with the client but instead builds the client's skills to carry out the treatment plan prescribed by the medical staff. For example, the medical staff no longer primarily refer for weight reduction counseling, but refer for a variety of patient education and health promotion needs.

The continually rising cost of health care raises further issues that open the way for the clinical health educator. Third-party payers and individual clients themselves are identifying less costly, more appropriate approaches to meet client needs. As a result, larger roles for other non-physician personnel are also growing, such as nurse practitioners and physician's assistants. In addition to the central role the clinical health educator plays, a health education assistant staffs a health education resource center with educational resources for health information, combined with personalized discussion and triage.

The word *triage* is used to describe a decision-making process whereby the clinician decides what spectrum of procedures and services the patients should be given in order to resolve their health problem. For example, a physician may refer a patient with hypertension for information on a low-salt diet and help in taking regular hypertensive medication. The health education assistant makes sure the patient has the appropriate information and understands the treatment plan, and discusses how to integrate these changes into the patient's daily routine. Further medical, health education, or mental health concerns may arise during the discussion; if so, the health education assistant consults with the medical staff, clinical health educator, or psychologist and directs the patient to the most appropriate resource.

Referring patients to a health education assistant allows increased use of the teachable moment (which is often bypassed due to clinical time constraints) without a high-cost investment. That is, a health education assistant can work with clients to develop behavior change skills instead of allowing longer appointments with a physician. (The teachable moment is the period of time when the circumstances are such that the client is more ready for an educational experience than usual. For instance, if a person's body weight is complicating a current health problem, that person might be more willing to begin a weight loss program than if the complication did not exist.)

Clinical health education offers staff and clients an additional resource for meeting today's changing health care needs, both by providing direct individualized services as well as by working with other providers to increase the effectiveness of their skills as educators. In clients' medical records, the additional emphasis on behavior change through direct service and consultation is reflected in greater documentation of health behavior change and of psychological and social issues by all providers.

Clients respond positively to these additional services by changing their goals and orientation.

However, the health educator faces issues of territoriality and role confusion in this clinical position. Nurses, physicians, and mental health staff may feel that this clinical role belongs in their domain. With time, such resistance may decline as roles are clarified and trust builds up. The clinical health education role is still evolving and offers the opportunity for health educators to apply their skills in an area where resources are needed. This new role can bridge the gap between isolated health education classes, clinic visits, and the daily life of clients. The clinical health educator brings skills to the medical care setting that can enhance provider behavior change skills and sustain client health actions.

Not only can health educators provide educational assessment services as part of their clinical role, they can also convey these skills to other clinicians. The next example demonstrates how one health education coordinator provided these skills to instructors through a training course.

## The instructor-training role

St. Luke's, a large urban 340-bed hospital with outpatient services in Cincinnati, offers programs in patient education and health promotion.* The forty health education instructors include nurse practitioners, registered nurses, licensed vocational nurses, and health educators. The patient education programs are based in the related medical departments (for example, hypertension classes in the internal medicine department) and receive consultation from the hospital's health education coordinator, Joe Wadia. The general health promotion classes are based in the health education department and are directly supervised by the health education coordinator.

The hospital administration identified the need for an instructor-training program in a number of ways. Recently the administration requested all hospital department managers to develop quality standards. In the process of developing quality standards for health education programs, it became clear that some of the programs did not meet these standards. Wadia had held the health education coordinator position for four years; many of the programs and instructors had been in place for five to ten years. He felt that the teaching styles, which were limited to lecture and content, were not effective. Few clients had actively developed behavior change skills. Now, although Wadia did not have

*This example is based on an interview with Pamela Johnson, M.P.H., Health Education Coordinator, Kaiser-Permanente Medical Care Program, Oakland, California, February 8, 1983.

direct responsibility for the instructors, the organization policy requiring departmental quality standards for health education supported his attempt to improve instructors' skills.

Wadia and instructors held informal discussions, which revealed that the instructors had very little training in health education. They seemed unable to integrate behavior change techniques with the content of many of their programs. A luncheon with instructors was held to further test their openness to examining issues of quality. Many instructors were pleased to receive the coordinator's recognition and thanks for their work; they were interested in further training and networking with other instructors as well as in receiving resources from the health education department.

The health education coordinator proposed an all-day workshop for instructors. The administration provided release time from nursing responsibilities. Wadia gave nursing continuing education units, which are required for license renewal, to all participants. The health education coordinator distributed a pretraining assessment questionnaire to all instructors (see Appendix 8.3 for a sample questionnaire). A review of the completed questionnaires made clear that a great variety of skill levels were represented in the group. Also, through the questionnaire and individual discussions the health education coordinator had with instructors, the instructors revealed a fear of losing control over programs to the health education department and to clients. Building on this assessment and on adult learning theory, the following decisions were made about how the workshop would be structured:

**1.** Begin gradually to gain acceptance of integrating the behavior change process with the content.

**2.** Start with general educational issues, and ask instructors to begin an ongoing self-assessment process.

**3.** Combine content with practice of skills, and make the practice sessions more comfortable by allowing rehearsal.

**4.** Use an outside consultant skilled in education and training to work with the health education coordinator. Ask the consultant to enhance the credibility and objectivity of the workshop, facilitate communication among participants, and model educational assessment techniques and interventions during the workshop.

The following list shows objectives for an instructor-training workshop. Participants will be able to

- Analyze an audience in order to adapt class plans and teaching methods to meet the needs of each group

- Maximize client participation by practicing different teaching methods and by discussing the advantages and disadvantages of each method
- Use instructional media and materials to promote learning
- Gain a better understanding of the overall role of the health education department, and identify ways that the department can better support instructors and their class or program
- Identify and discuss methods to evaluate their class or program
- Develop an action plan that specifically outlines future changes in their class or program

During the all-day training workshop, the leaders modeled group open-ended questioning techniques. Group members were given the opportunity to discuss their needs while being kept on focus by the leaders. The instructors' prior experience with clients served as the basis of a discussion on client empathy and influences on behavior change. Rehearsed practice sessions helped reduce the instructors' fear of trying new teaching methods. Small groups of instructors participated in the practice sessions and gave each other feedback on teaching effectiveness. The group then spent time generating ideas for ongoing self-assessment to improve the quality of health education programs. The workshop closed with instructors evaluating the day and their program's needs. The health education coordinator distributed an Instructor Self-Assessment Form (see Appendix 8.4) as a summary of the skills needed to integrate the content and skills of behavior change into their educational programs. Plans were made for future discussion of the self-assessment.

During the training program, the health education coordinator was careful to separate institutional issues from programmatic training issues. The following institutional issues were identified by the instructors and coordinators:

- Programs were fragmented due to lack of time available for coordination between instructors and the health education department.
- Budgetary cutbacks at the hospital threatened the continuation of health education programs.
- Many programs did not have regularly assigned instructors, because work responsibilities varied.
- Territorial issues between departments further complicated needs to reduce duplication and increase coordination (for example, the dietary department and health education departments both offered hypertension programs, with overlapping content).

- The health education coordinator had no direct authority for instructors or programs; involvement depended on the relationship with the direct supervisor of the instructor, yet the health education coordinator was responsible as a department manager for meeting quality standards for all health education programs in the hospital.

- The organization was more committed to short-term goals of volume (high attendance at programs) and accessibility (availability of the program to clients within a reasonable waiting time) than to more long-term goals of sustained behavior change.

The Wadia and Quinn examples emphasize educational assessment as an intervention tool for educators and clinicians. Health educators can work within their organizations to build a climate so that educational assessment is an acceptable practice by all professionals who choose to adopt these skills.

## REDUCING ORGANIZATIONAL BARRIERS

As change agents within the medical care system, health educators must recognize organizational barriers and must approach them strategically. In doing so, the first principle of change is an essential starting point; *the first principle is to assess the client perspective.* In this case, the clients are medical care administrators and other providers. Then, using their perspectives and needs as a starting point, new ideas and strategies to meet the changing health care needs of consumers can be gradually introduced. In addition to the principles of successful program planning, particular strategies can enhance collaboration between medical providers and health education staff.

### Talking the same language

As relative newcomers to the medical care setting, health educators are often viewed as outsiders who provide nonessential services. A critical first step to foster collaboration and build credibility is to reduce the language barrier. The language of health education and of medical care can be quite different. Health educators must become familiar with basic medical terminology and procedures. An in-depth understanding is not necessary, but some commonality in language improves communication. Health educators should minimize their use of jargon and their emphasis on educational terminology.

Medical and nursing schools have taken steps to reduce the language barrier as well as to improve provider educational skills by adding behavioral scientists and educators to their faculties and by making curriculum changes (see the syllabus put out by the Department of Preventive Medicine and Community Health, University of Texas). Conversely, many health education training programs would benefit from recommending to students additional coursework in counseling, medical treatment and terminology, and content areas such as nutrition, stress reduction, exercise physiology, and behavioral medicine. Further attention by medicine and nursing is evidenced by a review of medical and nursing journals, which frequently contain articles on compliance, behavioral diagnosis, and patient education. Familiarity with journals such as *The Journal of the American Medical Association (JAMA), The New England Journal of Medicine,* and *Journal of Nursing Research* can help educators keep abreast of current medical research and expand their vocabularies (see Resources section for journal addresses).

## A comparison of medical and educational assessment

Another organizational barrier is the fact that many health professionals do not understand how complex behavior change is. Comparing medical assessment and educational assessment can be a useful way to help providers recognize both this complexity and the need to identify a series of opportunities to intervene. Health educators should be conversant with specific examples of integrating educational assessment into a clinical perspective. The ultimate goal is to view educational assessment as one component of the providers' overall medical assessment.

**Client adherence.**   Providers know that some clients do not adhere to their treatment plans. Most providers, though, do underestimate the actual degree of adherence problems. The word *adherence* is used to replace the common medical term of *compliance*. This reflects the transition from client obedience (implied by the term *compliance*) to a therapeutic partnership in which the clients adhere to treatment plans developed with their involvement.

For example, a forty-three-year-old woman has been under treatment for hypertension for one year. She takes hydrochlorothiazide 100 mg two times a day and Inderal 250 mg two times a day. Her blood pressure remains under control at 132/84. Her physician does not know that at refill times she usually has one-third to one-half of each prescription remaining. The client feels embarrassed to say that her initial, well-intentioned efforts to reduce her salt consumption and increase exercise have gone by the wayside. In addition, she experiences periodic high-stress reactions when she has a deadline to meet at work.

This example illustrates the problems of (1) undetected nonadherence to a medication treatment plan and (2) the common setbacks that clients face in making long-term behavior changes. This provider is unintentionally supporting three *detrimental* educational experiences. First, the provider is teaching that clients do not need to completely adhere to a treatment plan and still get the results (such as controlled blood pressure). Second, the provider is teaching that medication is the most important treatment for hypertension. And, third, the client has learned that she has failed to maintain lifestyle changes and that she is weak-willed.

**Disease model versus growth model.** The following example illustrates the results of applying an expanded educational assessment model that recognizes the range of factors influencing blood pressure in addition to the factors of organic disease and medication. Although both the traditional and expanded approaches achieve normalization of blood pressure, the expanded assessment process clearly yields an increased quality of life and less sick-role identity as well as cost savings for the client (Miller, Ramen, Barbour, Nakles, Garrell, and Miller, 1975).

A fifty-year-old white man presents with a history of dizzy spells. His physical exam is negative except for a blood pressure of 150/100. The diagnosis of essential hypertension is made. Laboratory orders include a routine CBC, SMA 6/60 and 12/60, urine, EKG, chest X-ray.[1] Special workup includes a hypertensive IVP, 24-hour urine for VMA, sodium and plasma renin assays. In the following year, while on Chlorothiazide B.I.D., he makes six office visits and is given five electrolyte panels to monitor potassium. Prescription additions include KCL, D.C. Chlorothiazide, and Aldactazide. The patient is assessed as having chronic hypertensive disease, and his blood pressure is satisfactory at 130/85. (Both the patient and his physician regard the treatment as successful—the blood pressure is normal.)

The same patient was taken to a culturally sensitive physician, one who believes that "If you listen to the patient, you will begin to understand the meaning of his illness."

This physician asked, "Why does he have dizzy spells? Are there other factors in his life that cause this symptom?" (The doctor presumed that the blood pressure was not sufficient to cause them.) The doctor thus uncovered a recent business failure, some marital problems, compulsive eating, drinking, and smoking, and poor sleep cycles. These stress factors could produce reactive hypertension and dizziness.

---

[1]The following explanations may be useful: CBC, complete blood test; SMA, extensive blood chemistry; EKG, electrocardiogram; IVP, intravenous pyelogram; VMA, 24-hour urine test, vanilmandelic acid; B.I.D., twice a day; KCL, potassium chloride; D.C., discontinue.

The doctor offered this interpretation to the patient in order to actively involve him in treatment. The doctor also ordered a routine laboratory survey, but deferred the special tests for exotic hypertension factors. When the patient changed his lifestyle, his dizzy spells disappeared and his blood pressure returned to normal. Two follow-up visits corroborated the normalizing of his blood pressure. No further laboratory tests were necessary, nor were drugs ordered (with their potentially harmful side-effects and the need for physician monitoring). Both the patient and the doctor regard the problem as closed; the patient perceives himself as being well.

Both approaches resulted in normal blood pressure. However, when the disease model was applied strictly, as in the first approach, the patient became a "normotensive" person who saw himself as sick with a chronic illness, a reduced life expectancy, a limited potential, a dependency on doctors, and continuing drug therapy. In the second approach, the patient perceived himself as a well person who had control over many aspects of his life.

Moreover, if one charts the two approaches, a dramatic difference in cost is evident. Table 8.3 presents a cost analysis of the disease model versus the growth model. This table shows that the growth model is not only more powerful as a positive educational experience, but also less expensive.

**Table 8.3    Cost analysis of disease and growth models**

| | | |
|---|---|---|
| Patient: | Male, age 50 | |
| History: | Dizzy spells | |
| Physical Exam: | Negative except BP 150/100 | |

| *Diagnosis:* Essential hypertension | | *Diagnosis:* Nervous tension | |
|---|---|---|---|
| First exam | $ 50 | First exam | $ 50 |
| Lab | 206 | Lab | 88 |
| Drugs | 100 | Drugs | 0 |
| Follow-up visits | 90 | Follow-up visits | 30 |
| Additional lab | 52 | Additional lab | 0 |
| | $498 | | $168 |
| *Result:* Chronically ill person | | *Result:* Well person | |

SOURCE: Reprinted from *Medical Self-Care* Magazine, from a review written by John-Henry Pfifferling, Ph.D., on "A Comparison of the Disease and the Growth Model," by Allen Barbour, M.D. [in S. Miller, N. Ramen, A. Barbour, M. A. Nakles, D. Garrell, and S. Miller, *Dimensions of Humanistic Medicine* (San Francisco: Institute for the Study of Humanistic Medicine, 1975)], Fall 1980, Issue no. 10, p. 56. Copyright 1980 by Medical Self-Care.

The growth model sounds easy to apply; and if it were, one would think doctors should readily adopt it. But that does not appear to be the case. Doctors find it difficult to embrace the growth model because they have not seen much modeling of that kind of practice, have not seen statistics to validate its success, or have not been willing to work at activating patient responsibility. And patients find it difficult to embrace the growth model because they have few patient or physician role models, feel the loss of approval if their physician rejects their efforts to participate, and also hesitate to assume responsibility. In any case, taking responsibility runs counter to the authoritarian model of health care most patients have experienced.

## Dealing with common educational fallacies

Changes in the quality of the encounter between providers and their clients come slowly due to the fact that there are many fallacies about the nature of education in medical care. We'd like to present some of these misconceptions here so that when you are faced with expressions of them in practice, you will be better prepared to respond to them.

Formal and informal discussions of health education and patient care with providers and administrators offer you opportunities to identify and assess common misconceptions while reorienting their perspectives. Your skill in translating learning theory and current research into practical issues can help reduce organizational barriers. Often the most common educational fallacies found in the medical care system can seem excessively obvious. But the health educator must make a concerted effort to be patient yet persistent at refuting these fallacies in order to gain staff understanding and acceptance of an educational perspective. The following eight common quotes from a variety of providers, administrators, and staff reflect common educational fallacies. Preparing for them ahead of time can certainly be useful for health educators.

- "Patients know little about how diabetes affects the body; the best approach is to give them a good foundation to understand it."
- "Because of the complexity of medical care diagnosis and treatment, the staff knows best what treatment plan to choose and how to carry it out."
- "It takes too long to do educational assessment, and the cost is too high."
- "The health care system is the client's major source of advice and information."
- "Everyone who seeks medical advice wants to get well."

- "The client's frame of reference and lack of understanding distort communication."
- "The medical care process is based on scientific evidence, whereas patient education is a subjective experience that usually doesn't make any difference."
- "So what if I do find out that they have problems with their boss? What can I do about it?"

## Interdisciplinary resources

As an educator in medical care, you will have the opportunity to create an environment in your organization that is conducive to educational assessment by building coalitions with other health professionals. The medical care system contains rich resources in the various staff disciplines that provide a creative environment for change in medical care organizations. Unfortunately, barriers of interdisciplinary conflict and issues of territoriality can impede this creative process. Building support through networks and coalitions around common provider needs can be useful ways to overcome these barriers. In the process of building coalitions, educators must resist the tendency to blame the organization or administration for problems. Although blaming can be a powerful technique to obtain group solidarity as adversaries to administration, the resulting sacrifice of administrative involvement and support can prove costly to the long-term integration of innovation. Besides, these adversarial relationships are often superficial; in practice, administrators and practitioners need each other and exist in a relatively symbiotic relationship.

## Dealing with difficult clients

The staff of an organization must often deal with difficult clients. Health care providers are sometimes not inclined to want to conduct an educational assessment with a client who they perceive is difficult. As an educator, you can help other providers to develop useful strategies with these clients so that they, too, will have access to the benefits of the educational assessment process. Many such clients have health problems with no clear etiology or no simple cure, such as insomnia, headaches, low back or neck pain, obesity, and smoking. Additional client characteristics may include low motivation, anger toward providers, and resistance and nonadherence to treatment. Most of these people do not have serious mental health problems, and they lend themselves well to the model of assessment presented in this chapter. Some clients find this approach helps them feel more in control over their symptoms, rather than feel victimized by them.

One caution here concerns the issue of efficacy. Once health educators become available to work with difficult clients, the health education programs can become a dumping ground for very difficult ones. And a lack of success with some clients can be used against you to weaken your credibility. Adjusting goals and expectations for client outcomes in this situation is particularly important for two reasons: (1) to prevent provider burnout, and (2) to enhance health education program credibility. You can prevent burnout if you support the client while identifying small, realistic educational outcomes. The health education program's credibility is also enhanced when educational outcomes reflect a broader view of the client's problem or symptom.

For example, the outcome of an educational program with a client with chronic stomach pain may change from symptom elimination to protecting the client from further hazards of radiation, excessive medication, and surgery. Also, an additional outcome could be for the client to verbalize other factors that may be affecting the symptoms.

## THE FUTURE ARRIVES GRADUALLY

Health education involves an ongoing process of reducing common organizational barriers of language, oversimplified views of behavior change, educational fallacies, and interdisciplinary conflict. Many small changes can occur through the development of effective interpersonal relationships with clients and staff. It is useful to build an informal foundation of support before seeking large-scale organizational involvement. Annual health education performance evaluations and annual goal setting can be used to obtain staff input and formal organizational sanction for further work. Building educational assessment into interventions is a gradual process.

Opportunities for educational assessment to be fully integrated into medical care and educational services will expand in the future as the health care system adapts to the changing medical needs of the population and to new economic realities. Health education has the potential to play a major role in this change process, reorienting the medical care system from a traditional provider-centered model to a model based on a therapeutic partnership with the client. Such a reorientation allows the forces affecting health and behavior to be fully mobilized to improve health status and change health behaviors.

This process demands an expanded role for the health educator in clinical health education practice. Building on the existing roles of program administrator and coordinator, the new role would include health educators as behavior change specialists. This new role would also contribute to further effectiveness of staff education and consultation services. In order to gain skill and clinical credibility, health educators need to obtain additional training in psychosocial assessment, interviewing, and counseling techniques, as well as some content areas, such as disease entities, addiction treatment, or chronic disease management. As we recognize that simple paradigms do not work for us in the medical care system, we will become free to draw on a variety of professional traditions for approaches that integrate the whole person's well- and sick-care experiences.

Health educators in medical care face a challenge: instead of only offering classes, they can become integrated into the everyday provision of services. We must continue to demand a model of service involving the client in a self-assessment process that integrates an expanded view of the forces affecting health and behavior. This model of educational assessment takes health education interventions beyond the mere giving of information to the mobilizing of various influences on positive health action. This model will more effectively meet the health care needs of consumers.

# APPENDIX 8.1

## Health Improvement Questionnaire*

### Questionnaire: Evaluation of Health Status

This form is to help give you better health care. It is completely confidential and will be part of your medical record.

The _____ Clinic is pleased that you have made a health evaluation appointment. This evaluation is designed to review your health and to help you get to know yourself better.

Your feelings of health and well-being are affected by many aspects of your daily life. For this reason, we have included this questionnaire to find out about your interests, personal relationships, and work situation. Gathering this information will allow you and your health care provider to work more effectively together.

Please take time *before* your health-testing appointment to think about each question and fill out this questionnaire as openly and honestly as possible. *Bring the completed questionnaire with you at the time of your health-testing visit.*

---

### Section I: Health Promotion and Information

Consider each of the health actions listed below. We want to work with you to feel better now and reduce your risk of future health problems. Place a check next to the health actions that *you want to work on now.*

Check the health actions you want to work on now:

| | | | |
|---|---|---|---|
| Improve my diet: | | Reduce drinking | ( ) |
| Reduce salt | ( ) | Use or change birth control methods | ( ) |
| Reduce sugar | ( ) | Do breast self-exam monthly | ( ) |
| Reduce fat and cholesterol | ( ) | Do testicular self-exam monthly | ( ) |
| Increase fiber and whole grain | ( ) | Communicate better with medical providers | ( ) |
| Lose weight | ( ) | | |
| Reduce/quit smoking | ( ) | Care for home medical problems and emergencies | ( ) |
| Increase exercise/fitness | ( ) | | |
| Increase seat belt use | ( ) | Other _____ | ( ) |
| Manage stress more effectively | ( ) | Take no actions now | ( ) |
| Reduce drug use | ( ) | | |

*Reprinted with permission of the Total Health Care Program of Kaiser-Permanente Medical Care Program, Oakland, California.

Check the medical problems that you would like to learn more about:

| | | | |
|---|---|---|---|
| High blood pressure | ( ) | Heart disease | ( ) |
| Diabetes | ( ) | Arthritis | ( ) |
| Back pain | ( ) | Respiratory problems | ( ) |
| Venereal disease | ( ) | Cancer (What kind?) _____ | ( ) |
| Headaches | ( ) | Hemorrhoids | ( ) |
| Herpes | ( ) | Constipation | ( ) |
| Vaginitis | ( ) | Other _____ | ( ) |
| | | None | ( ) |

Some people with health problems have found it helpful to meet in a group to share information, discuss feelings, and solve problems. If you or a family member has one of the problems listed above, would you like to join such a group? Yes (  )  No (  )  Unsure (  )

---

### Section II: Important Life Areas

Important areas of your life are listed below. How well are your needs being met in each area? Check only *one* box for each question. If you have a particular concern, describe it as completely as you can in the space provided.

A. *Relationship with Family* (communicating, visiting, helping and being helped by your family)

My needs are being met:
    Very well (  )   Well (  )   Slightly (  )   Not well (  )

Specific concern: _____

_____

B. *Intimate Relationships* (close personal and/or sexual relationship with spouse or other loved one)

My needs are being met:
    Very well (  )   Well (  )   Slightly (  )   Not well (  )

Specific concern: _____

_____

C. *Children* (helping, teaching, giving and receiving love from your children) (answer if you are a parent)

My needs are being met:
    Very well (  )   Well (  )   Slightly (  )   Not well (  )

Specific concern: _____

_____

D. *Close Friends* (sharing activities and interests, being accepted, giving and receiving help, trust, and support)

My needs are being met:
Very well (  )   Well (  )   Slightly (  )   Not well (  )

Specific concern: _____

_____

E. *Work* (interesting, rewarding work at home or in a job outside the home, with an acceptable level of pressure and generally satisfying relationships)

My needs are being met:
Very well (  )   Well (  )   Slightly (  )   Not well (  )

Specific concern: _____

_____

F. *When You Are Troubled*, what is it usually about? Use the following space to describe your one most frequent concern (e.g., marriage, family, finances, work)

_____

_____

What do you do to deal with this concern? _____

_____

## Section III: Overall Health Review

A. What concerns you most about your health and well-being?

_____

_____

B. What in your daily activities, relationships, and surroundings is especially *good* for your health?

_____

_____

C. What in your daily activities, relationships, and surroundings is especially *harmful* to your health?

_____

_____

D.  What advice would you *give yourself* to improve your health and well-being?

_____

_____

E.  Use this space for any other comments you would like to make.

_____

_____

_____

_____

*Reminder:* Your health evaluation involves *two* visits.

*First Visit:* Health testing and questionnaires.
*Second Visit:* A follow-up visit a few weeks later with your personal health care provider for a physical exam, a review of your health questionnaires and test results, and to develop a health improvement program.

We are glad you are interested in your health and look forward to working with you. If you should have an urgent medical problem before the appointment with your health care provider, call the clinic for prompt assistance.

# APPENDIX 8.2

## Educational Assessment Review Form

### Influences on Client Behavior

Name: _____

Health condition/risks/habits: _____

_____

Presenting symptoms: _____

_____

| | Check appropriate space below: | | | | | Comments |
|---|---|---|---|---|---|---|
| | Poor Low 1 | 2 | 3 | 4 | 5 | |
| 1. Daily routine | | | | | | |
| 2. Support system | | | | | | |
| 3. Health belief system | | | | | | |
| 4. Experience with medical care system | | | | | | |
| 5. Environment | | | | | | |
| 6. Previous experience with change | | | | | | |
| 7. Self-management skills | | | | | | |
| 8. Stress coping skills | | | | | | |
| 9. Readiness to change | | | | | | |
| Total ratings | | | | | | |

Overall assessment: _____

Follow-up agreed on with client: _____

_____

_____

Date: _____ Staff: _____

# APPENDIX 8.3

Health Education Training Workshop, Pretraining
Assessment Questionnaire

### Pretraining Evaluation

1. What experience and/or training have you had in health education or patient teaching? (Include formal, informal, individual, and group situations.)

_____

_____

_____

2. How do you feel about your current health or patient education course? (Circle a number on each scale.)
   A. Very satisfying  1  2  3  4  5  Very unsatisfying
   B. Low frustration  1  2  3  4  5  Very high frustration

   Comments: _____

_____

_____

3. What teaching methods do you currently use? (Check your answer.)

| Teaching Methods | Use | Never Use | Interested in Trying |
|---|---|---|---|
| Lecture | _____ | _____ | _____ |
| Total group discussion | _____ | _____ | _____ |
| Small group exercises | _____ | _____ | _____ |
| Demonstration (e.g., instructor shows use of blood pressure cuff) | _____ | _____ | _____ |
| Practice of skills (e.g., patient practices using blood pressure cuff) | _____ | _____ | _____ |
| Role playing | _____ | _____ | _____ |

| Teaching Methods | Use | Never Use | Interested in Trying |
|---|---|---|---|
| Audiovisual aids | | | |
|   Films | —— | —— | —— |
|   Overhead transparencies | —— | —— | —— |
| Question and answer period | —— | —— | —— |
| Brainstorming | —— | —— | —— |
| Handouts | —— | —— | —— |
| Displays, exhibits | —— | —— | —— |
| Reading list | —— | —— | —— |
| Other: _____ | —— | —— | —— |

Comments: _____

_____

_____

4. Of the methods you currently use, which would you label *most* effective and appropriate? Why? (Choose one or two methods.)

_____

_____

_____

5. Of the following topics, which would you find useful if covered during the health education workshop? (Circle a number on each scale.)

|  | Not Very Useful | | | Very Useful |  |
|---|---|---|---|---|---|
| • Basic principles of health education | 1 | 2 | 3 | 4 | 5 |
| • How to | | | | | |
|   a. Adapt your class plan to meet the needs of each new group | 1 | 2 | 3 | 4 | 5 |
|   b. Revitalize your current class plan | 1 | 2 | 3 | 4 | 5 |
|   c. Keep class participants on the topic | 1 | 2 | 3 | 4 | 5 |
|   d. Involve participants effectively in the lesson | 1 | 2 | 3 | 4 | 5 |
|   e. Find and select effective instructional materials | 1 | 2 | 3 | 4 | 5 |
|   f. Best use instructional and informational handouts | 1 | 2 | 3 | 4 | 5 |
|   g. Use participant evaluations to improve your classes | 1 | 2 | 3 | 4 | 5 |
|   h. Assess the effectiveness of your presentation | 1 | 2 | 3 | 4 | 5 |
|   i. Increase hospital staff support and referral | 1 | 2 | 3 | 4 | 5 |

6. Can you suggest another topic(s) that would be useful to you if covered?

_____

_____

_____

7. Would you find it helpful to share success stories, problem-solving strategies, and materials with other workshop participants?

   Yes _____   No _____

   Would you like to contribute stories, strategies, or materials to the workshop? Yes _____   No _____ (If yes, please explain.)

   _____

   _____

   _____

8. What concerns, questions, doubts, problems, or comments do you have related to the proposed workshop on health education? (Please discuss below.)

   _____

   _____

   _____

9. Which day of the week would be most convenient for you to attend the proposed workshop? (Please circle.)   M   Tu   W   Th   F   No preference

10. Additional comments:

   _____

   _____

   _____

   _____

   _____

Thank you once again for your assistance in the planning of this project. We hope your efforts will be rewarded by a meaningful training workshop experience.

# APPENDIX 8.4

## Instructor Self-Assessment Form

### Self-Evaluation for Instructors

Course: _____    Date: _____

Instructor: _____

| Introduction | EXC | SAT | N.I. | Comments |
|---|---|---|---|---|
| 1. Introduced content area | | | | |
| 2. Established mood and climate | | | | |
| 3. Motivated students to learn | | | | |
| 4. Related utility of the skill | | | | |
| 5. Established a knowledge base | | | | |
| 6. Stated objectives clearly | | | | |
| **Presentation (Lecture) Techniques** | | | | |
| 1. Organized content | | | | |
| 2. Made transitions | | | | |
| 3. Changed pace | | | | |
| 4. Clarified technical terminology | | | | |
| 5. Used visuals and examples | | | | |
| 6. Introduced resource material | | | | |
| 7. Responded to student feedback | | | | |
| **Closure** | | | | |
| 1. Introduced no new materials | | | | |
| 2. Summarized major points | | | | |
| 3. Provided sense of achievement | | | | |
| 4. Related to introduction | | | | |

| Teacher Tactics | EXC | SAT | N.I. | Comments |
|---|---|---|---|---|
| 1. Involved students in the lesson | | | | |
| 2. Provided reinforcement and feedback | | | | |
| 3. Used questioning techniques | | | | |
| 4. Exhibited enthusiasm for lesson | | | | |
| Verbal and Nonverbal Behaviors | | | | |
| 1. Voice | | | | |
| 2. Eye contact | | | | |
| 3. Gestures | | | | |
| 4. Movement | | | | |
| 5. Use of silence | | | | |
| 6. Facial expression | | | | |

KEY: EXC = Excellent    SAT = Satisfactory    N.I. = Needs Improvement

# EXERCISES

1. Give at least five reasons why educational assessment should be integrated, as a behavior change intervention, into the educational process and medical care system.

2. Imagine that you have been asked to conduct a series of three inservice programs on educational assessment for the physicians in the obstetrics-gynecology department. You have had the first session, which identified physicians' needs and concerns. The following questions were raised and will be discussed in the second session. As you sit down to prepare for the session, start by answering the questions yourself first. Write your answers on a separate sheet of paper.
   a. What behaviors by the health practitioner are most critical in establishing a new helping relationship?
   b. Describe the most effective questions to determine the client's view of the situation. Support your answer and give examples.
   c. Describe the most effective types of questions to obtain specific information from the client. Support your answer and give examples.
   d. How can you let your client know you understand his or her feelings and situation? Support your answer and give examples.
   e. What is the most effective way to end an educational session or client interview? Support your answer and give examples.

3. Imagine that you are a health educator and are now preparing for an appointment with a client who has been referred to you by an internal medicine physician. Your client is a fifty-two-year-old divorced white male with a nine-month history of tension headaches. In reviewing his medical record prior to the visit, you obtain the following information:

   • Patient-identified concerns are diet, lack of exercise, difficulty sleeping, constipation, and work-related concerns.
   • Family history: diabetic mother.
   • Two previous physician appointments: one a complete health evaluation with no identified medical problems three months ago, the second two weeks ago with continued concern about frequent headaches.

   How would you begin the interview? What questions would you use during your initial appointment with this client? Pair up with another person and role play the educational assessment interview.

**4.** A large hospital has had many requests from clients for information regarding detection of breast cancer. A physician and nurse practitioner in the obstetrics-gynecology department have approached you for help in organizing an educational program on breast self-exam to meet these needs. You are preparing for a meeting with them by organizing your thoughts on educational assessment, opportunities, issues, and tasks to be done. In developing your ideas on the breast self-exam program, you look at the situation on three levels.

a. *Organizational:* policy, financial, administrative, and medical support

b. *Programmatic:* goals and opportunities for educational assessment, staffing needs, and coordination of educational activities

c. *Individual:* Client influences on behavior and types of needs

Prepare a two-page outline summarizing your view of this situation. List the issues, and specify your approach.

# RESOURCES

American Hospital Association, Center for Health Promotion. *Strategies to Promote Self-Management of Chronic Disease.* Chicago: American Hospital Association, 1982.

This book is a helpful compilation of literature on adherence, interviews with clients themselves, and the experiences and suggestions of providers. It suggests a step-by-step approach to self-management educational strategies, similar to the same type of step approach used in drug treatment. The book identifies a variety of initial strategies and then more costly interventions for clients who are having trouble managing their condition. The annotated bibliography reviews studies regarding outpatient chronic disease self-management that meet acceptable research standards or provide interesting qualitative information about client-provider experience.

Cormier, L. S., and Cormier, W. H. *Interviewing Strategies for Helpers: A Guide to Assessment, Treatment and Evaluation.* Monterey, Calif.: Brooks/Cole, 1979.

This book is a good introduction to helping skills. It can be used on a self-instructional basis or within an organized course. The first part of the book describes verbal and nonverbal behaviors that can be used during the assessment phase of helping. The second part presents additional techniques that can be used to facilitate client action and behavior change. Some of the techniques include setting goals, cognitive modeling and thought stopping, meditation and muscle relaxation, systematic desensitization, and self-management.

Jenkins, C. D. An Approach to the Diagnosis and Treatment of Problems of Health Behavior. *International Journal of Health Education*, 2 (April/June 1979): 1–24.

This article provides a good framework for examining problems of individuals and groups in adopting and maintaining health-related behaviors, both preventive and therapeutic. Jenkins presents techniques for making a behavioral diagnosis, improving the delivery of health services, and improving the effectiveness of self-directed behavior change. He also offers literature references to practice-oriented guidebooks.

*Journal of Nursing Research*
555 West 57th St.
New York, NY 10019

*Journal of the American Medical Association (JAMA)*
535 N. Dearborn St.
Chicago, IL 60610

Lefrancois, G. R. *Psychological Theories and Human Learning: Kongor's Report*. Monterey, Calif.: Brooks/Cole, 1972.

Lefrancois gives an overview and interpretation of the major theories of human learning. His use of humor is an enjoyable addition to the theoretical text. Lefrancois begins by discussing memory, attention, and motivation and then reviews the major theorists of behaviorism, neobehaviorism, and cognitionism. Finally, he integrates and evaluates, providing a succinct summary of learning theory.

*Medical Self-Care*
P.O. Box 717
Inverness, CA 94937

This magazine is a useful source of current skill-oriented self-care educational materials. You can write to the editors for reprint permission for in-clinic distribution.

Melamed, B., and Siegel, L. *Behavioral Medicine: Practical Applications in Health Care*. New York: Springer, 1980.

This book is an excellent introduction to the field of behavioral medicine, which represents an intersection of behavioral science and the practice of medicine. The field involves the disciplines of sociology, education, psychology, and medicine. The book's main goal is to give providers additional techniques to help patients cope with stress as a reaction to illness or an overwhelming life circumstance such as job loss or divorce. The authors review the theoretical foundations of behavioral medicine and discuss program design as well as applications of behavior therapy to specific health care problems such as health risk reduction, pain, and eating disorders.

*New England Journal of Medicine*
P.O. Box 4772
Boston, MA 02212

Peters, K. Headaches: They Are Not All in Your Head. *Medical Self-Care*, 18 (Fall 1982): 10–15.

Peters's article is a good example of a broad-based approach to the diagnosis and treatment of headaches. He includes a summary of types of headaches and suggests self-observation and diary keeping as a means to assess the environmental, nutritional, physical, and psychological factors that are considered related to headaches. Treatments suggested include nutritional and environmental changes, increased aerobic exercise, stress management techniques, and judicious use of medication to break pain cycles.

Stone, G. C., Cohen, F., and Adler, N. E. *Health Psychology, Theories, Applications and Challenges of a Psychological Approach to the Health Care System*. San Francisco, Calif.: Jossey-Bass, 1979.

This handbook is a collection of writings from a number of fields and their application to improving the health care system. Chapters of most interest to health educators include those on changing self-destructive behaviors, patients' problems in following recommendations, coping with the stresses of illness, interpersonal skills, and the social-ecological perspective.

U.S. Department of Health and Human Services. *Report of the Working Group on Critical Behaviors in the Dietary Management of High Blood Pressure*. NIH [National Institute of Health] Publication no. 71-2269. Washington, D.C.: U.S. Government Printing Office, 1981.

An interdisciplinary group developed this report as an aid to those who counsel on the dietary management of hypertension through controlling sodium and weight. The protocol integrates content with the identification of patient and professional behaviors for a successful outcome. It identifies a series of ten steps to achieve the goal of blood pressure control; the steps are generalizable to other health behavior changes.

# 9

# Risk assessment and health improvement

RISK ASSESSMENT IS receiving increased attention and use as a motivational tool for health improvement. One of the most popular approaches, called *health risk appraisal* (HRA), is the major focus of this chapter, because it has received the widest application thus far. We review the current state of the HRA process, using two settings to illustrate its application.

Problem-oriented health education programs—the most common in medical care practice—often have a major weakness: their overemphasis on content. HRA's problem-oriented approach to assessment helps reduce this weakness. This chapter illustrates how the generic process of assessment as intervention (as discussed in Chapter 8) can be integrated with HRA to increase the educational impact of the process. And, finally, we suggest resources for exploring other risk assessment approaches, such as lifetime health monitoring. This chapter is one of four (8, 9, 10, 11) that emphasize contemporary strategies and interventions for health educators who practice in medical care settings.

## OVERVIEW OF HEALTH RISK APPRAISAL (HRA)

Health risk appraisal (HRA) is based on the principles of prospective medicine, which use client risk factors to quantify the risk of client death in the next ten years (Berry et al., 1981). Then, as a technique to stimulate health behavior change, the client is given feedback regarding the prediction. The popularity of HRA reflects the major shift in causes of mortality from infectious disease to chronic disease, with the resulting recognition that the risk factors associated with these chronic problems are primarily linked to health behaviors.

At this time, the scientific basis for HRA risk prediction is weak and changing. Epidemiological data, which constitute the foundation for HRA's ability to predict risk, are debated regularly in scientific journals and public newspapers (epidemiology is the study of the occurrence of disease in human populations). Belief in HRA's efficacy is not substantiated, yet HRA has been widely accepted and has been promoted extensively.

The technique holds promise as a motivational tool if integrated into the context of an educational program. A description and analysis of HRA programs prepared for the National Center of Health Services Research by North Carolina University at Chapel Hill identified the major factors contributing to the recent attention paid to HRA.

First, HRA relates well to current health education theories about motivation as exemplified by the health belief model. The health belief model identifies relevant health beliefs that are presumed to influence the decision-making process to adopt a health behavior. HRA is designed to activate the following factors to increase client motivation: susceptibility to a condition, severity of a condition, and benefits of preventive action in comparison with barriers to taking action (Rosenstock, 1974).

Second, HRA relies on self-administered questionnaires, simple physiologic measures, and computer-assisted or hand-done calculations, making applications to large groups feasible, efficient, and relatively inexpensive. Third, the report notes that HRA has the appearance of a scientific approach to health promotion and is therefore consistent with the established values of many segments of American society. Fourth, it is consonant with current thinking and publicity about the role of lifestyle in disease etiology. And, fifth, the data-gathering instruments, computer software, and other aspects of the program can be marketed as a package (Berry et al., 1981).

Given these attractive factors, it might be easy to overlook a number of problematic issues. These include the actual utility of HRA as a motivational tool, potential adverse effects, the lack of attention to environmental factors, and the unreliability of the epidemiological and statistical data on which the program is based.

Two physicians, Lewis Robbins and Jack Hall, originated HRA in the 1960s, at Methodist Hospital in Indiana. They describe their technique in detail in their book *How to Practice Prospective Medicine* (1970). The intended audience was practicing physicians who would use it as a tool to highlight risks and emphasize preventive medicine. Initially physicians had little enthusiasm for this approach, and over time the audience expanded to industrial settings and fitness groups. Recent concerns with rising costs for medical care and recognition of the role of lifestyle have now increased medical attention given to HRA.

The HRA predictions are based on the available epidemiological data that relate the presence of particular risk factors to mortality from a specific disease. In theory, by modifying risk factors people can reduce the probability that they will die of a particular disease. A series of questions are used to collect data that are then compared with epidemiological data and national mortality statistics of the client's age, sex, and racial group. Data are gathered on past family and medical history, simple physiological measures of blood pressure, height, weight, and cholesterol level, and lifestyle patterns such as smoking, drinking, and support systems. A sample HRA questionnaire in a computer printout form is shown in Appendix 9.1. It is part of an HRA program available from the U.S. Centers for Disease Control (CDC) in Atlanta, Georgia. The data obtained from an HRA questionnaire are then translated into statistical predictions of life expectancy, likelihood of death in the next ten years, or level of risk in relationship to age, sex, or racial group. Usually a computer prints this information on a report; this report also makes recommendations to the user to reduce risks.

Many adaptations can and have been made to the basic questions needed for statistical analysis. Questionnaires range in length from 20 to 300 questions. Simplified, low-cost, self-scoring questionnaires can categorize the risk level without the detailed quantification the computerized version offers. See Appendix 9.2 for the Healthstyle Test, an example of this type of assessment that was distributed by a large hospital through its community newsletter as part of a national media campaign sponsored by the U.S. Department of Health and Human Services. At the other end of the spectrum of complexity are computerized versions of HRA that provide a forty-eight-page report with personalized health analysis as well as detailed information on the particular health risk area.

## A STATE-OF-THE-ART REVIEW OF HRA

The study we referred to earlier, by the University of North Carolina's Health Services Center (Berry et al., 1981), presents the results of a state-of-the-art review of HRA. It is an excellent discussion of the major issues. The purpose of the study was to document the extent and manner in which HRA is being applied and to review its scientific basis and effectiveness. A literature review, consultation with experts, and site visits of fifteen operational programs provided the basis for the analysis. Resources such as this study are very useful when developing a new program. The following sections summarize the major areas of inquiry and findings.

## Controversial risk factors

After an extensive review of each computational step of HRA, Berry and his associates (1981) concluded that the current technique for risk assessment is reasonably accurate, but several areas of concern were raised. First, some of the risk factors measured are plagued by controversy regarding how well they predict health problems as well as regarding the impact that behavior change has on reducing risk. For example, increased exercise does not completely predict decreased coronary heart disease; cholesterol level may not respond to changes in food intake. The lack of agreement in these areas makes it difficult to select the best direction for health promotion efforts.

## Data limitations

Second, the data used are derived from the Framingham Heart Disease and American Cancer Society studies, which are conducted primarily with middle-aged white subjects. The data are subsequently generalized to blacks, hispanics, teenagers, and other dissimilar groups. Particular questions are raised regarding the usefulness of the HRA with individuals under age thirty-five because the ten-year-risk-of-death reports and extrapolations from older individuals are limited. For example, at age twenty-two there is only a minute risk of dying of cancer or heart disease in the next ten years. Therefore, the ten-year risk-of-death prediction for a twenty-two-year-old individual will not reflect the impact of risk factors related to cancer or heart disease, which are the two major causes of mortality in this country.

Another key concern raised is the reliability of client data, particularly since it is self-reported. Questionnaire construction and physiologic measures need more attention and refinement for accuracy and reliability. Although many clinical programs that use the HRA do not view arithmetic precision as important, the University of North Carolina report made an issue of this perception. Client variability in answers has been shown in time spans as little as three to four weeks apart, which could completely invalidate the feedback aspects of HRA (Berry et al., 1981, pp. 75–76).

## HRA expectations

The study also listed the many expectations that users have of HRA. They ranged from (1) using HRA as a tool to organize client data or to grab client attention, to (2) a motivational technique to stimulate behavior change and reduce health care costs. Evidence supporting HRA's success in influencing behavior is not available at this time. Methodological problems have continued to weaken the validity of many studies that have been done. However, several of the programs visited as part of the study were engaged in sophisticated evaluation research, which will soon provide more reliable evidence (Berry et al., 1981, pp. 87, 113). Also, programs that were made part of the client's social environment, such as the workplace or doctor's office, had higher participation rates and effectiveness.

The University of North Carolina report suggested more study on the measurement of physical or psychological risk. Two major areas of negative effects should be examined: first, depressive client responses on the HRA questionnaire could result in increased anxiety, depression, and hypochondriasis. These symptoms would eventually lead to somatic complaints and unnecessary health care expenses for assessment and diagnosis of these symptoms and for follow-up on false positive test results. Second, HRA may overemphasize the individual's lifestyle and personal responsibility for change. Thus it may promote excessive client guilt and frustration; in reality, economic and environmental factors may play an equally important role in the incidence of disease.

**Overemphasis on lifestyle**

An overemphasis on lifestyle may contribute to the fact that most programs using HRA continue to find low participation by disadvantaged social groups. Other life necessities often have greater priority in the lives of the disadvantaged. Since poverty, inadequate housing, hunger, and political impotency have tremendous effects on health risks, the effect of lifestyle on health risk reduction offers less promise for this population. The emphasis of HRA on individual solutions could detract attention from important policy and societal issues that may yield greater health promotion and risk reduction outcomes.

**Recommendations and summary**

The investigators (Berry et al., 1981) recommend that the federal government continue involvement with HRA; however, they caution that the government runs the risk of being perceived as endorsing the HRA technique, whose efficacy has not yet been established. Increased use of a peer-reviewed granting mechanism to answer specific questions raised by this study may offset a misperception of government support for HRA. Further funding for refinement and distribution of HRA for implementation is not recommended at this time. The following summary lists recommendations for future research (Berry et al., 1981, pp. 118–122):

- Factors determining the adoption and maintenance of health-related behaviors
- Positive strategies for motivating and supporting health-related behavior change (such as an orientation toward benefits over losses or death)
- The attitudes and beliefs of minority groups toward health promotion and disease prevention and the barriers to their participation
- The role and impact of the medical practitioner in health promotion and disease prevention
- The possible harmful effects of health promotion and disease prevention interventions
- The source of errors in data collection and their impact on the feedback given to clients in HRA programs
- The perceptions of HRA clients regarding the importance and meaning of the data collected from them and returned to them
- The effectiveness of HRA as compared to other educational approaches in stimulating participation in risk-reduction activities and producing health-related behavior change

The University of North Carolina report (1981, p. 9) summarizes itself as follows:

> Health risk appraisal is an appealing technique which may have potential as a tool in health promotion/disease prevention efforts. Its attraction derives probably as much from the lack of packaged options for individuals working in health promotion and disease prevention as from demonstrable effects of the health risk assessment process. The current degree of attention given specifically to health risk assessment may be excessive, and such a concentration of interest risks missing the forest of health promotion for the tree of the health risk appraisal.
>
> Health promotion and disease prevention is an area which requires innovative programming and careful evaluation of results. Health risk appraisal is but one approach and should be viewed with care and circumspection—care to ensure that assumptions are tested in view of the paucity of current evidence regarding its effectiveness. Caution is also indicated since HRA programs, like other health promotion efforts aimed at modifying personal behaviors, have the potential for the promulgation of lifestyles possibly inadequately supported by existing scientific evidence and/or inconsistent with values and traditions of specific

population groups. There are also concerns that such programs may constitute "blaming the victim" or may pay insufficient regard to the influence of environmental and social factors on health and health-related behaviors.

Programs attempting to change behaviors and improve health have been searching for effective tools. Our evaluation of the current state of the art in HRA suggests that there is no reason to abandon that search. [Berry et al., 1981, p. 124]

Since the promise of health hazard appraisal and the limitations of its current scientific and methodological base are both so great, we dedicate the rest of this chapter to examples that demonstrate that it is possible, without succumbing to the problems of one finite approach, to conduct risk assessment as an educational strategy.

## ADAPTING HRA TO ORGANIZATIONS: TWO EXAMPLES

The following examples show how risk assessment can be built into existing services. Two medical care settings, a health maintenance organization (HMO) and a university student health service, have developed risk assessment programs by adapting existing programs for their particular target groups. Each shows the importance of considering the needs of both the target population and the institution staff as well as the consistency of the approach and health information given. As you read these profiles, look for the tradeoffs that each health educator made in designing the program, managing the institutional issues, and increasing the educational effectiveness of the risk assessment intervention.

### HRA in a primary care clinic

In the first profile, a primary care clinic serving 12,000 members of a large HMO (150,000 total membership) in an urban setting has been using HRA as part of complete health evaluations for the past year. The administration introduced it as a strategy to meet the overall goal of the clinic: to maintain and improve the health of the membership. In addition, the administration viewed it as a low-cost mechanism to maintain contact with well members who often receive little attention and service yet provide major financial support for the HMO. Such contact would increase member satisfaction and member retention. Initially, the clinic operations staff and administration disagreed regarding the implementation of a computerized HRA program. The staff felt it was a costly investment with unproven outcomes. The administration made the firm decision to implement a computerized HRA program and assigned to the health education staff responsibility for developing and implementing the program. Reservations about its use were channeled into identifying strategies to increase its educational potential.

The primary target group of the HRA program is new members receiving complete health evaluations. An invitation to obtain a complete health evaluation is included in the mailing of new membership materials. Referrals to HRA derive from a second mailing. Spot phone calling as time permits and referral by medical staff are used as additional outreach mechanisms.

HRA complements the usual aspects of a health evaluation, which focus on laboratory testing, physical examination, psychosocial assessment, and medical history. Two visits are scheduled, resulting in the development of a health improvement program with the member. The first visit is devoted to multiphasic testing, which includes a series of laboratory screening tests and HRA. The second visit takes place between the client and a medical provider (nurse practitioner or physician) to review the test results, health risks, perform a physical examination, review other assessment questionnaires, deal with individual concerns, and formulate a health improvement program. See Figure 9.1 for an example of documentation of a client's health improvement program.

In order to integrate HRA into the complete health evaluation, the clinic added one more testing station in the primary care clinic's health education resource center. The station involves a three-minute physical fitness step test and a computerized HRA program. Members receive a handout that lists the physiologic measurements gathered during the multiphasic testing process. A screening questionnaire is administered to identify any preexisting conditions that would preclude clients from undergoing the fitness test.

The clinic obtained an HRA computer program at a low cost from the U.S. Centers for Disease Control (CDC). It was a standard program to be operated on a large computer (see Appendix 9.1 for the CDC questionnaire and printout). In reviewing and pretesting the program, staff mentioned a number of concerns:

**1.** The language of the questions and printout was confusing and difficult to understand.

**2.** The report produced by the computer strongly emphasized fear of death (manipulative approach).

**3.** The design required a lapse of one to two weeks between the time the questionnaire was completed and when the report was available.

**4.** Some risk levels and some advice were unacceptable to clients as well as inconsistent with the clinic's medical recommendations. For example: standards for alcohol consumption were set at less than six

## Figure 9.1 A client's health improvement plan

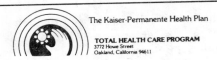

The Kaiser-Permanente Health Plan

**TOTAL HEALTH CARE PROGRAM**
3772 Howe Street
Oakland, California 94611

### PERSONAL HEALTH RECORD AND HEALTH IMPROVEMENT PROGRAM

(Imprint Area)

| DIAGNOSES OR OPERATIONS | Date | DRUG SENSITIVITIES |
|---|---|---|
| ☐ Cystic Breast Disease-OP 59 | | ☐ None |
| ☐ | | ☐ |
| ☐ | | ☐ |
| ☐ | | ☐ |

IMMUNIZATIONS: Date last done / Date last done

| | Date last done | | Date last done |
|---|---|---|---|
| ☐ RUBELLA TITER | due now | ☐ RUBELLA IMM. | |
| ☐ INFLUENZA | | ☐ PNEUMOVAX | |
| ☐ DIP-TETANUS | 79 | ☐ PPD | |

| CURRENT PROBLEMS AND HEALTH RISKS | TREATMENT PLAN |
|---|---|
| ☐ Elevated Blood Pressure | ☐ Return for BP Check in 2 weeks |
| ☐ | ☐ Reduce salty foods and table salt use |
| ☐ | ☐ |
| ☐ Smoker | ☐ Switch to low tar brand |
| ☐ | ☐ Contact health ed in next month |
| ☐ | ☐ |
| ☐ Marital Concerns | ☐ Read Couples Self Care with Spouse |
| ☐ | ☐ Consider contacting mental health |
| ☐ | ☐ |
| ☐ Health Promotion | ☐ Do Breast Self Exam monthly |
| ☐ | ☐ Decrease fat in diet |
| ☐ | ☐ Obtain Rubella Titer |
| ☐ | ☐ |
| ☐ Contraception - CU7-IUD | ☐ Check IUD string monthly |
| ☐ | ☐ Remove/change next year |
| ☐ | ☐ |
| ☐ | ☐ |
| ☐ | ☐ |
| ☐ | ☐ |
| ☐ | ☐ |
| ☐ | ☐ |
| ☐ | ☐ |
| ☐ | ☐ |

NEXT HEALTH VISIT CHECKUP ___1986___ NEXT PAP SMEAR ___1983-Oct___

NEXT FITNESS EVALUATION ___1983-Oct___

WHEN YOU HAVE HEALTH CONCERNS, CALL TOTAL HEALTH CARE TEAM ADVICE NURSE (428-7444).

_____ (MD/MNP)

THC 10/82-1

SOURCE: Reprinted with permission of the Total Health Care Program of Kaiser-Permanente Medical Care Program, Oakland, California.

drinks per week, whereas the clinic's medical recommendations were not to exceed two drinks per day or fourteen per week.

**5.** Certain factors that influence health were not included in the questionnaire; for example, health hazards in the environment and testicular self-examination.

Then the clinic made and pretested a series of adaptations to the basic program. The staff simplified the questions and report, softened the emphasis on death, and added reinforcement for positive health habits. An interactive computer program was designed, with the computer asking questions to which the client responds (this approach reduces the time required to process the HRA reports, while capitalizing on the fact that clients like using an interactive computer). The staff also raised risk levels for alcohol and weight to conform to the clinic's medical recommendations, and added a few questions that are not used in the computations but that do generate advice on the member's report. And staff prepared a member handout that addressed some of these concerns. Finally, the clinic allocated time for personalized discussion after receiving the report. See Figure 9.2 for an example of the HRA report, done on an Apple II microcomputer. A double copy of the HRA report is made; one copy goes to the member, and an additional copy documents the visit in the medical record. Appendix 9.3 includes the HRA informational handout that clients read after completing the interactive HRA program and while waiting one to two minutes for their computerized HRA report to be printed. Table 9.1 specifies the start-up costs of the HRA program.

**Table 9.1  HRA program start-up costs**

| | |
|---|---:|
| Total HRA program start-up costs | $11,000 |
| 1. Apple II microcomputer with printer | 5,000 |
| 2. Computer specialist time to translate Centers for Disease Control computer software to Apple computer | 6,000 |
| 3. Health educator planning and development time | Unknown |
| Total ongoing costs (volume 2,200 per year) | $9,400 |
| 1. Two-part report forms ($.40 ea.) | 900 |
| 2. Health education assistant, half-time | 8,500 |
| 3. Health education supervision | Unknown |
| Cost per participant | $4.27/HRA |

SOURCE: Data from Total Health Care Project, Kaiser-Permanente Medical Center, Oakland, California.

**Figure 9.2   Computer-produced HRA report**

```
        TOTAL HEALTH CARE PROGRAM
             PERSONAL HEALTH RISK REPORT

        FOR:                     MR#              DATE      4/12/8

──────────────────── AGE APPRAISAL ────────────────────
  ACTUAL AGE:    36      HEALTH AGE:    38.5   ACHIEVABLE AGE:   33.7

──────────── HIGHER THAN AVERAGE HEALTH RISKS ────────────
   REASON FOR HEALTH RISK            HEALTH PROBLEM           DEGREE OF RISK**
 HIGH STRESS FACTORS       :              SUICIDE:       3 TIMES AVERAGE

 ***-ADVICE---REACH OUT TO OTHERS TO TALK ABOUT YOUR CONCERNS.
 ----------------------------------------------------------------------
 HIGH DIA. BLOOD PRESSURE:       HEART DISEASE:      2 TIMES AVERAGE
                          :              STROKE:      2 TIMES AVERAGE

 ***-ADVICE---SEEK MEDICAL ADVICE AND REDUCE SALT IN YOUR MEALS.
 ----------------------------------------------------------------------
 FREQUENT DRUG USE        : AUTOMOBILE ACCIDENTS:      3 TIMES AVERAGE

 ***-ADVICE---ASK US ABOUT OTHER WAYS TO RELAX AND SLEEP BETTER.
 ----------------------------------------------------------------------
 INADEQUATE EXERCISE      :       HEART DISEASE:      2 TIMES AVERAGE

 ***-ADVICE---START EXERCISING. BRISK WALKING FOR 15 MIN/DAY IS A GOOD START
 ----------------------------------------------------------------------
 SMOKING                  :       HEART DISEASE:      3 TIMES AVERAGE
                          :              STROKE:      2 TIMES AVERAGE
                          :         LUNG CANCER:      3 TIMES AVERAGE

 ***-ADVICE---STOP SMOKING NOW.
 ----------------------------------------------------------------------


 CONTACT THE TOTAL HEALTH CARE STAFF FOR THE MANY SERVICES OFFERED TO HELP YOU IMPROVE YOUR HEALTH
 ** = ESTIMATE OF YOUR RISK COMPARED TO THE AVERAGE PERSON OF YOUR AGE AND SEX.

──────────── OTHER WAYS TO IMPROVE YOUR HEALTH ────────────
   -YOU FEELINGS OF DISSATISFACTION AND ALONENESS ARE HIGH.
    TALK TO YOUR MEDICAL PROVIDER.
   -ALWAYS USE A SEATBELT TO LOWER YOUR RISK OF INJURY/DEATH.
   -EXAMINE YOUR BREASTS MONTHLY FOR  CHANGES.




──────────── YOUR POSITIVE HEALTH HABITS ────────────
 BY CHOOSING THESE HABITS, YOU REDUCE YOUR RISK OF FUTURE HEALTH PROBLEMS. WE URGE YOU TO CONTINUE TO:

 -DRINK IN MODERATION      -MAINTAIN GOOD WEIGHT      -GIVE&RECEIVE SUPPORT
 -GET ANNUAL PAP SMEAR


 ALERT:  IF YOU SMOKE, OVEREAT OR DO NOT EXERCISE REGULARLY THESE HABITS WILL HAVE A MORE SEVERE EFFECT WHEN YOU ARE
 OLDER. THESE LONG TERM EFFECTS OFTEN DO NOT SHOW UP IN THIS REPORT IF YOU ARE UNDER AGE 40, BUT THEIR HARMFUL EFFECTS ARE
 TAKING THEIR TOLL. REMEMBER, THE YOUNGER YOU ARE, THE EASIER IT IS TO CHANGE, OR, IF YOU ARE OLDER, IT IS NEVER TOO LATE.
```

SOURCE: Reprinted with permission of the Total Health Care Program of
Kaiser-Permanente Medical Care Program, Oakland, California.

After the HRA report is made, an individualized ten-minute discussion takes place between the client and a health education assistant. The health education assistant has two years of post–high school education, special courses, and on-the-job training in the basis of HRA and educational techniques, plus three years' experience working in a health education program in a medical care setting. During the post-HRA discussion, the following minimum activities occur. These are called the "client behavior change steps." The health education assistant uses open-ended questioning and active listening skills to facilitate this discussion. The following list describes the client behavior change steps:

1. Client makes self-assessment of health risks.

2. Staff supports and supplements client self-assessment using health risk appraisal, medical testing, and history.

3. Client accepts health risks.

4. Client states willingness to accept recommendation, make changes, and identify benefits.

5. Health educator and client identify risk reduction area to start with.

6. Health educator and client identify first specific health action to take.

7. Client and health educator review appropriate health information referral resources; health educator schedules follow-up if applicable.

During this interview, the health education assistant classifies the client as low, medium, or high cardiovascular risk. The major goals of this first interaction are (1) to establish two-way communication, (2) to get the client to agree (or disagree) to the cardiovascular risk status classification, (3) to estimate the client's willingness to explore health behavior change, and (4) to identify the first step toward this change. The assistant also offers health information materials, along with referrals to educational programs for weight management, increased exercise, smoking cessation, and stress reduction.

Between the two visits of the complete health evaluation, most clients identify a health behavior change to make. The assistant notes the change goal on the copy of the HRA report that goes in the client's medical record. Occasionally, additional client medical and mental health needs surface during this visit. The health education coordinator, a psychologist, and medical staff are available for on-the-spot consultation if necessary.

When clients return three weeks later for the second visit, they discuss health promotion with their medical provider. The provider then enters the clients' health risks into their overall problem list kept in the medical record. The provider summarizes clients' current health problems, risks, and treatment plans, and gives them a copy of the report. Clients who are at high risk for health problems receive more frequent and individualized follow-ups, usually with the health education staff. The medical provider follows medical needs, also paying attention to health promotion, psychosocial, and behavioral issues.

In this HMO, routine follow-up of the initial HRA will soon be added. Clients will be invited back for annual health improvement visits. The clinic has designed these visits to complement the periodic health evaluations. The health improvement visits, conducted by the health education staff, will include a blood pressure check, fitness test, and a repeat HRA computer report with personalized discussion regarding health improvement.

Members have responded positively to the health appraisal component of the complete health evaluation. The program has generated approximately 1,650 such HRA reports, or 45 per week, in nine months of operation. Outreach efforts have yielded a 45 percent response (of total). This does not include the 36 percent of clients (of total) who schedule an appointment but fail to keep it.

Clients have accepted the additional thirty to forty-five minutes that were added to the complete health evaluation visit. Staff find that members comment about the experience and cite health behavior changes made between the first and second visit. Also, during informal discussions with the clinic staff, both clients and staff report satisfaction with the increased recognition of health promotion as an element of medical care practice. The risk classification notation on the medical chart problem list allows for follow-up and discussion during future medical encounters.

On the other hand, problems have also surfaced as the program goes on. For example, clients with preexisting conditions (such as cancer or kidney disease) that health education staff did not know about may receive inaccurate HRA reports. Staff resistance to the computerized aspect of the HRA has decreased, but still remains to some measure. Another concern expressed by staff and clients is that the program does not recognize environmental health risks, such as exposure to chemical hazards. Reports for clients in their late fifties and sixties and who have a high number of risk factors are sometimes incomplete because such clients may have exceeded the average life expectancy for someone of their age and risk status. For example, a sixty-year-old man with elevated blood pressure, a twenty-year history of smoking, and poor physical fitness has already exceeded his life expectancy. The computer therefore leaves part of the report blank, because it cannot quantify his health age. Moreover, young people who are at high cardiovascular risk may receive false reassurance because their risk of dying of heart disease in the next ten years is extremely low.

Such problems are discussed during the individualized discussion with the health education assistant and with the medical staff. Thus far it seems that personalized discussion is an effective way to deal with these limitations.

## HRA in a student health service

In the second example, a university student health service serving 30,000 students is developing a personal health assessment program (PHA).* The new program incorporates a disease prevention and health promotion perspective into outpatient clinical services. Recently the outpatient services were reorganized into clinical groups; two primary care clinical groups were given part-time health educators. This is a new role for health educators in the student health service. At this time the role calls for the health educator to plan patient education and self-care programs, provide staff consultations, and give individual lifestyle education to students. This new role for health educators has increased collaboration with clinical staff and given health educators in the student health service a better understanding of the medical care process than before.

The need for the personal health assessment program was indicated by a combination of factors:

- Positive feedback from health promotion programs
- Favorable student environment
- Research findings and experience of other health centers
- Commitment of student health service administration to health promotion
- Requests from some student health service physicians and nurse practitioners for help in dealing with health and medical history

The student health service staff—particularly the health educators—had developed their experience with a self-assessment program that included a workbook, *Picture of Health* (Health Education, Student Health Services, University of California at Berkeley, 1979). The staff found, however, that students often could not understand the connection between their lifestyle and their health. Although many students found the workbook valuable and identified the need to do periodic

*This example is derived from a series of interviews with Eileen Babitt, M.P.H., Coordinator, Health Promotion and Clinical Health Education, and Cathy Tassan, M.P.H., Director of Health Education, Student Health Services, University of California at Berkeley, in January 1983.

health self-assessment when they were well, they had some problems using the workbook. Some students felt that the workbook was too long (120 pages), and that they did not receive enough personal help in interpreting the results of the exercises. They also said they needed more specific health information.

Debates among professionals over the usefulness of many health-screening tests made it particularly difficult to design a health assessment tool. The general physical exam had not proven cost effective in this age group in uncovering disease that could be prevented with early detection. And the American Cancer Society (1980), the Canadian Task Force on Periodic Health Examinations (1979), and many other medical publications were making new and sometimes conflicting recommendations about what should be included in risk assessment (Frame and Calson, 1975; American College of Physicians, 1981). In all this confusion, one thing was clear: health promotion and risk reduction were receiving greater attention than traditional health-screening tests.

The health educators interviewed the clinical staff and found that many students had numerous questions and concerns that went beyond their presenting medical problem, yet the routine medical appointment was not long enough to address these concerns. For example, a student might come in showing symptoms of a urinary tract infection and also raise concerns regarding her diet, intimate relationship, and sleep habits. In addition, the clinical staff felt that more education should be offered about personal health history and health behavior as it relates to the risk of specific illness. Efforts were begun to create a clinical health assessment for well students. This assessment was field tested with students.

A nurse practitioner and health educator developed a personal health assessment questionnaire, using input from the student health service administration, clinicians, and support staff. The two undertook a number of critical developmental tasks while they continued to seek further clinical administrative support, in preparation for a pilot program. A core group of involved clinicians and support staff drafted and reviewed materials, interventions, and protocols to be used in conjunction with the questionnaire. This first phase of the PHA program development took one year. The health educator and the nurse practitioner are now working with other student health service staff, students, and community experts to improve their prototype questionnaire.

The following categories of referrals guided intake during the preliminary testing:

1. *Referrals by clinicians*
   a. Students with multiple risk factors requiring more time for education than available during a medical visit

   b. Students motivated to improve their health or reduce their risks for disease

   c. Worried but well students who could benefit from a complete assessment

   d. Students referred for help in managing stress

   **2.** *Referrals by support staff:* Students with no particular health problem seeking a general assessment of health or a general physical exam

   **3.** *Student self-referrals:* Any student who sees the handout sheets in the student health service and wants to participate

Before drafting the questionnaire and appointment format, the developers reviewed a number of packaged, computerized health risk assessment programs, a lifetime health-monitoring approach, and many publications. They used the following criteria to identify the appropriate personal assessment areas and techniques:

   **1.** The benefit of early detection

   **2.** The costs

   **3.** The benefit of disease prevention and health promotion

   **4.** The comprehensive health needs of an eighteen- to thirty-year-old population

   **5.** The availability of known strategies that reduce students' risks of heart disease, cancer, and premature death

The reviewers felt that a prepackaged, computerized health risk appraisal approach that quantified risks of disease and premature death was ineffective, because that approach minimizes personal interaction and uses the goal of extending life span, which is of little interest to a younger population. The lifetime health-monitoring approach was useful as a beginning point, even though the staff considered it to be an incomplete review of health influences (Breslow and Somers, 1979). The staff have not ruled out other adaptations of a computerized approach for the duration of the program.

The initial pretest consisted of a handscored assessment questionnaire in combination with two individualized appointments with a nurse practitioner or health educator. This format worked well for the students and for the staff, but did represent a substantial time commitment for both students and staff. The following list shows the topics that were included on the written assessment questionnaire (see Appendix 9.4 for the questionnaire itself):

   • Demographic data to examine the characteristics of the students who use the services

- Review of health habits such as smoking, drinking, exercise, sleep, diet, and contraceptive use
- Incidence of acute and chronic health problems such as accidents, respiratory infections, low back pain, and headaches
- Psychosocial issues such as stress level, support system, and sexuality
- Family and personal medical history
- Review of environment, including noise, living situation, and exposure to hazardous substances
- Open-ended questions that leave room for students to identify additional health beliefs and concerns

The nurse practitioner or health educator reviewed the student's questionnaire and completed a health assessment summary sheet. The following list shows the sections of the summary sheet (the whole sheet is shown in Appendix 9.5).

- Health behaviors
- Psychosocial factors
- School environment
- Risk factors from personal or family health history
- Recurrent health problems that may benefit from intervention
- Self-assessment
- Health professional assessment and recommendations
- Referrals

The summary sheet was reviewed with the student during the 50-minute initial assessment appointment, and options discussed for improvement or changes in individual lifestyle. Students were asked to think about their priorities. At the second visit (20–30 minutes long), these priorities provided direction for the educational efforts for students needing help with a health problem or interested in health promotion. The goal is to match the student with the most appropriate service.

The services available to students are extensive and include health information handouts, referrals to medical staff, individual follow-up on behavioral change with the health educator or nurse practitioner, health education group programs on a variety of illness and health promotion topics, referral to the university counseling center, and in-depth self-assessment workbooks for home study.

Discussion is underway at the student health service to determine the need for adding personal health assessment data to the students' medical records. The health educators are also working on a mechanism to get student feedback to each student's medical provider. Participants in the pretesting filled out an evaluation questionnaire, which has provided the clinic staff with student feedback (see Appendix 9.6). Table 9.2 summarizes the program's costs.

Thus far, administration and the medical staff in the clinic where the program has been initiated support further development of the assessment process and integration of health promotion in a clinical setting. The preliminary pretesting efforts have helped identify ways to improve the questionnaire, the information given to students, and the protocols used by staff in their appointments with students. And the student response has been favorable. Participants perceive the service as more comprehensive than the usual medical appointments in meeting their health needs. Strategies to gain further clinical and administrative support are necessary before a formalized pilot program is initiated.

Based on the first year of pretesting and developmental work, the following recommendations were made to the director of the student health services:

**1.** Involve more clinicians in the development of the personal health assessment program, with the recognition that their disease-oriented training may contribute to a resistance to focus on health as well as a lack of understanding of how to change to a health focus.

**2.** Refine and simplify the questionnaire, using the help of research consultants.

**3.** Continue the initial assessment appointments.

**Table 9.2   Developmental costs of personal health assessment program start-up**

| | |
|---|---|
| Total clinical health educator and nurse practitioner time for start-up (1 year planning) | $4,000 |
| Proposal packets for marketing | $200 |
| Administrative supervision | Unknown |
| Per participant costs | |
| Materials | $4 |
| Individual appointment with health educator or nurse practitioner | $12 |
| Pretesting per participant cost | $16 |
| Continued planning costs for next year | $4,000 |

**4.** Identify a mechanism for medical record documentation and medical staff feedback.

**5.** Continue to offer the *Picture of Health* self-assessment workbook as a self-directed program in the self-care center (it seems to attract a different group of students than does the personal health assessment program).

**6.** Broaden the focus of the clinical care setting to incorporate routine attention to health and health promotion; develop protocols to integrate health promotion into illness care.

This example describes the efforts of a student health service to adapt the health risk assessment process to a younger population and to deal with some of the problems of targeting this age group in the context of a student health services setting. The coordination between health education and clinic staff allowed for a more comprehensive student needs assessment and intervention than is usually available in university student health services.

## HRA: IMPLICATIONS FOR HEALTH EDUCATION

Inevitably health educators will be involved with various forms of risk assessment when working in a medical care setting. We should be conversant with the HRA process and be assertive in order to tap its educational potential. This section of the chapter highlights some of the major issues we face in doing so.

Realizing the full educational potential of HRA remains a challenge. HRA can be a meaningful aspect of the expanded educational assessment process described in Chapter 8. If health educators capitalize on its problem orientation, HRA can become an effective way to gain further recognition of the preventive medicine and health promotion aspects of medical care. In addition, medical staff can actively involve the client in the collection and assessment of physiologic data for HRA use. For example, the client can learn how blood pressure is measured and what the readings mean while the blood pressure is being taken. During a physical fitness step test, the client can learn how to take his or her pulse and interpret the results. By setting up interactions between the medical staff and clients, we can transform the collection of simple physiologic data into an educational experience, inviting the client to become more actively involved in the medical care process.

Epidemiological evidence forms an important basis for health promotion and disease prevention efforts. Since the scientific basis of health risk appraisal is the relationship between risk and disease, proven epidemiological relationships between these two need to be the starting point for educational intervention. Although health educators are not epidemiologists, we need skills to be wise consumers of the literature and to interpret epidemiological data. It is essential for the health educator to remain abreast of current epidemiological developments that influence program directions. The Centers for Disease Control run by the federal government maintain a clearinghouse for risk assessment information. Medical staff, journals, and professional organizations also can offer updated information. Periodic review of program content by medical staff further assures a direction for programs that is current and consistent with medical center recommendations.

Personalized discussion and educational materials on psychosocial, occupational, and community health needs can supplement the emphasis on traditional lifestyle risks in the HRA program. For example, health educators and clients can work with employers and community groups to create exercise periods and safe facilities; to increase the availability of nutritious, low-cost foods in the cafeteria and vending machines; to pressure local government for safer sidewalks and opportunities for low-cost adult education programs. These examples are health-promoting changes, made at the community level, that can complement HRA's individual lifestyle orientation.

Many variations of HRA programs exist, ranging from sophisticated computer programs to simple pencil-and-paper scored scales. Although the computerized versions exert an attention-grabbing, science-oriented attraction, a self-scoring questionnaire can also provide a useful basis for discussion between staff and client. An additional variation, called a "lifetime health-monitoring program" (Breslow and Somers, 1979), was discussed in the example of the university health services. The lifetime health-monitoring program divides the adult life span into ten stages and identifies psychosocial, medical testing, and health promotion needs for each stage. Lester Breslow and Anne Somers developed the program, to be used by physicians to promote a systematic, age-adjusted approach to meeting health needs and replace the annual checkup concept. When developing risk assessment programs, health educators may find a review of this existing program to be a useful beginning point. Table 9.3 shows the preventive procedures recommended for one stage of the adult life span. The table summarizes the recommendations for preventive health care for the young adult. The column on the left lists the condition to be prevented or detected; the middle column lists the procedure to be used; and the column on the right lists how frequently the procedure should be repeated between ages 25 and 39.

Whatever the variation, integrating a risk assessment process into a primary care clinic, preventive medicine department, or health evaluation process is preferable to developing services isolated in the health

**Table 9.3   Lifetime health-monitoring program, recommended preventive procedures for adults of age 25–39**

| Condition | Procedure | Frequency |
|---|---|---|
| Smoking | History and counseling | Every 2 years |
| Obesity or poor eating habits | History and counseling; weight [measurement] | Every 2 years Every 2–4 years |
| Lack of exercise | History and counseling | Every 2 years |
| Accidental injury or death | History and counseling | Every 2 years |
| Problem drinking, alcoholism | History and counseling | Every 2–4 years |
| Drug abuse | History and counseling | Every 2–4 years |
| Unwanted pregnancy | History and counseling | Every 2 years |
| Hypertension | Blood pressure measurement | Every 2 years |
| Breast cancer | Breast examination; counseling about self-examination | Every 1–2 years |
| Tetanus and diphtheria | Immunization | Every 10 years |
| Cervical cancer | Pap smear | Every 2–3 years |
| Tuberculosis | Skin test | |
| Diabetes | Urinalysis[a] | Every 4 years |
| Bacteriuria | Urinalysis[a] | Every 4 years |
| Proteinuria | Urinalysis[a] | Every 4 years |
| Coronary artery disease | Serum cholesterol determination[a] | Every 4 years |
| Vision defects | Examination[a] | Every 4 years |
| Anemia | Hematocrit or hemoglobin[a] | Every 4 years |
| Syphilis | Blood test[a] | Every 4 years |
| Dental caries and periodontal disease | Dental examination and cleaning | Every 1–2 years |

[a]There is a debate on whether this procedure should be included.

SOURCE: Breslow and Somers, 1979, p. 99. Reprinted with permission from *Patient Care* ® magazine. Copyright © 1979, Patient Care Communications, Inc., Darien, CT. All rights reserved.

education department. HRA programs that are integrated into the day-to-day experience of medical and nursing staff and clients have a higher participation rate because the HRA requirement of interactions lends credibility to both patient and provider. Health education staff can still be responsible for education and follow-up activities in this integrated context.

## High-risk clients

A system of health risk classification is useful to identify high-risk clients. Intensive educational activities can then be directed at this high-risk group. Three major elements support the process: linkages between programs, medical record documentation, and a follow-up system.

For example, Joe, a thirty-seven-year-old man involved in the risk assessment program, is found to have elevated blood pressure and to smoke one pack of cigarettes per day. In addition, a family history of cardiovascular disease places Joe in a high-risk category with three risk factors (elevated blood pressure, smoking, and family history of cardio-vascular disease). During the risk assessment program, Joe repeatedly says that he feels the blood pressure elevation is a fluke and that it only goes up when he comes in for a visit.

During the discussion with the health educator after the HRA, Joe recalls a prior experience with the medical care system during his father's hospitalization for congestive heart failure. Although this experience was three years ago, Joe is still quite angry about the medical staff's lack of understanding and poor explanation of the condition. A discussion ensues regarding Joe's views on effective medical care relationships, his need for assertiveness with medical staff, and his interpretation of his risk status.

No specific plans were made for risk factor reduction, but Joe did agree to observe his stress response and smoking patterns for two to three weeks and to consider the benefits and costs of behavior change. The health educator taught Joe a simple deep breathing, relaxation exercise, and discussed the availability of behavior change resources. A referral was made to Joe's medical provider for follow-up of elevated blood pressure; the appointment was scheduled before Joe left the clinic. Since Joe was classified as high risk, the health education staff suggested a follow-up appointment in one month, which Joe agreed to. The health educator made note of the discussion on the HRA report, and made a brief phone call to Joe's medical provider to alert her to his concerns. A follow-up system (on card file) will alert health education staff to follow up Joe's case in one month. This example illustrates an educational system that integrates the HRA with an expanded educational assessment process and with ongoing medical care while targeting high-risk individuals for more indepth follow-up.

### Conclusions

HRA is an educational tool that promises to increase client motivation for health behavior change. Although still in its developmental stage, it is gaining widespread acceptance. The appeal of HRA to consumers and medical care providers can be used by health educators to gain recognition of the need for health promotion services and to integrate specific activities for disease prevention into the provision of medical care. The principles and process of educational assessment outlined in Chapter 8 can be used to realize the full educational effect of HRA on client behavior change.

Further work is needed to refine this technique and reduce its limitations. In addition, a more accurate HRA process for people with chronic problems such as diabetes or hypertension would be useful. On the other hand, HRA continues to present problems, because it could perpetuate our societal orientation toward youth, on which advertising continues to capitalize. We must acknowledge that health education serves to fuel this dilemma even further. Health education needs to avoid the temptation to support the drive to beat death, over the goal of enhancing the quality of life.

We need health risk assessment programs that are based on educational principles and on a view of health that integrates physical, psychosocial, behavioral, and environmental influences. And we are in a position to demand such adaptations of current risk assessment programs—but we are also challenged to help develop them.

The key element of the strategies and interventions mentioned in this part of the book is client participation. The following two chapters, on decision making and self-care, are designed to augment educational approaches that begin with educational assessment and risk assessment. Once the client understands the behaviors that could be added or modified in order to reach his or her health goal, the educator could support the client by following up the interest with the interventions mentioned in Chapters 10 and 11.

# APPENDIX 9.1

## Health Risk Appraisal Form*

Ⓑ **HEALTH RISK APPRAISAL**

Health Risk Appraisal is a promising health education tool that is still in the early stages of development. It is designed to show how your individual lifestyle affects your chances of avoiding the most common causes of death for a person of your age, race and sex. It also shows how much you can improve your chances by changing your harmful habits. (This particular version is not very useful for persons under 25 or over 60 years old and for persons who have had a heart attack or other serious medical problem.)

**IMPORTANT:** To assure protection of your privacy, do NOT put your name on this form. Make sure that you put your Health Risk Appraisal "claim check" in your wallet or other safe place and insure that the number matches the number on this form. You must present your claim check to get your computer results.

PARTICIPANT NUMBER ⌊＿＿＿＿＿＿＿＿＿⌋ 1-6

PLEASE ENTER YOUR ANSWERS IN THE EMPTY BOXES ( use numbers only )

1. SEX  ☐1 Male  ☐2 Female  ☐ 7

2. RACE/ORIGIN  ☐1 White (non-Hispanic origin)  ☐2 Black (non-Hispanic origin)  ☐3 Hispanic  ☐4 Asian or Pacific Islander  ☐5 American Indian or Alaskan Native  ☐6 Not sure  ☐ 8

3. AGE (At Last Birthday)  Years Old  ☐☐ 9-10

4. HEIGHT (Without Shoes)  Example: 5 foot, 7½ inches = ☐5 ' ☐0 ☐8 "  (No Fractions)  ☐ ' ☐☐ 11-13

5. WEIGHT (Without Shoes)  Pounds  ☐☐☐ 14-16

6. TOBACCO  ☐1 Smoker  ☐2 Ex-Smoker  ☐3 Never Smoked  ☐ 17

(Smokers and Ex-smokers) — Enter average number smoked per day in the last five years (ex-smokers should use the last five years before quitting.)

Cigarettes Per Day  ☐☐ 18-19
Pipes/Cigars Per Day (Smoke Inhaled)  ☐☐ 20-21
Pipes/Cigars Per Day (Smoke Not Inhaled)  ☐☐ 22-23

(Ex-smokers only)  Enter Number of Years Stopped Smoking (Note: Enter 1 for less than one year)  ☐☐ 24-25

7. ALCOHOL  ☐1 Drinker  ☐2 Ex-Drinker (Stopped)  ☐3 Non-Drinker (or drinks less than one drink per week)  ☐ 26

If you drink alcohol, enter the average number of drinks per week:

Bottles of beer per week  ☐☐ 27-28
Glasses of wine per week  ☐☐ 29-30
Mixed drinks or shots of liquor per week  ☐☐ 31-32

8. DRUGS/MEDICATION  How often do you use drugs or medication which affect your mood or help you to relax?
☐1 Almost every day  ☐2 Sometimes  ☐3 Rarely or Never  ☐ 33

9. MILES Per Year as a driver of a motor vehicle and/or passenger of an automobile (10,000 = average)  Thousands of miles  ☐☐ 0 0 0 34-38

10. SEAT BELT USE (percent of time used)  Example: about half the time = ☐5 ☐0  ☐☐☐ % 39-41

11. PHYSICAL ACTIVITY LEVEL
☐1 Level 1 - little or no physical activity
☐2 Level 2 - occasional physical activity
☐3 Level 3 - regular physical activity at least 3 times per week
☐ 42

NOTE: Physical activity includes work and leisure activities that require sustained physical exertion such as walking briskly, running, lifting and carrying.

12. Did either of your parents die of a heart attack before age 60?
☐1 Yes, One of them  ☐2 Yes, Both of them  ☐3 No  ☐4 Not sure  ☐ 43

13. Did your mother, father, sister or brother have diabetes?  ☐1 Yes  ☐2 No  ☐3 Not sure  ☐ 44

14. Do YOU have diabetes?  ☐1 Yes, not controlled  ☐2 Yes, controlled  ☐3 No  ☐4 Not sure  ☐ 45

15. Rectal problems (other than piles or hemorrhoids).  Have you had:
Rectal Growth?  ☐1 Yes  ☐2 No  ☐3 Not sure  ☐ 46
Rectal Bleeding?  ☐1 Yes  ☐2 No  ☐3 Not sure  ☐ 47
Annual Rectal Exam?  ☐1 Yes  ☐2 No  ☐3 Not sure  ☐ 48

(Continued on Other Side)

*SOURCE: Reprinted with permission of the Total Health Care Program of Kaiser-Permanente Medical Care Program, Oakland, California.

16. Has your physician ever said you have Chronic Bronchitis or Emphysema?   [1] Yes    [2] No    [3] Not sure      □ 49

17. Blood Pressure (If known — otherwise leave blank)       Systolic (High Number)    50-52

                                         Diastolic (Low Number)    53-55

18. Fasting Cholesterol Level (If known — otherwise leave blank)                  MG/DL    56-58

19. Considering your age, how would you describe your overall physical health?
     [1] Excellent    [2] Good    [3] Fair    [4] Poor      □ 59

20. In general how satisfied are you with your life?
     [1] Mostly Satisfied    [2] Partly Satisfied    [3] Mostly Disappointed    [4] Not Sure      □ 60

21. In general how strong are your social ties with your family and friends?
     [1] Very strong    [2] About Average    [3] Weaker than average    [4] Not sure      □ 61

22. How many hours of sleep do you usually get at night?
     [1] 6 hours or less    [2] 7 hours    [3] 8 hours    [4] 9 hours or more      □ 62

23. Have you suffered a serious personal loss or misfortune in the Past Year? (For example, a job loss, disability, divorce, separation, jail term, or the death of a close person)
     [1] Yes, one serious loss    [2] Yes, Two or More serious losses    [3] No      □ 63

24. How often in the Past Year did you witness or become involved in a violent or potentially violent argument?
     [1] 4 or more times    [2] 2 or 3 times    [3] Once or never    [4] Not sure      □ 64

25. How many of the following things do you usually do?

     ● Hitch-hike or pick up hitch-hikers    ● Criticize or argue with strangers
     ● Carry a gun or knife for protection    ● Live or work at night in a high-crime area
     ● Keep a gun at home for protection    ● Seek entertainment at night in high-crime areas or bars

     [1] 3 or more    [2] 1 or 2    [3] None    [4] Not sure      □ 65

26. Have you had a hysterectomy? (Women only)      [1] Yes    [2] No    [3] Not sure      □ 66

27. How often do you have Pap Smear? (Women only)
     [1] At least once per year    [2] At least once every 3 years    [3] More than 3 years apart
     [4] Have never had one    [5] Not sure    [6] Not applicable      □ 67

28. Was your last Pap Smear Normal? (Women only)    [1] Yes    [2] No    [3] Not sure    [4] Not applicable      □ 68

29. Did your mother, sister or daughter have breast cancer? (Women only)    [1] Yes    [2] No    [3] Not sure      □ 69

30. How often do you examine your breasts for lumps? (Women only)
     [1] Monthly    [2] Once every few months    [3] Rarely or never      □ 70

31. Have you ever completed a computerized Health Risk Appraisal Questionnaire like this one?
     [1] Yes    [2] No    [3] Not sure      □ 71

32. Current Marital Status
     [1] Single (Never married)    [2] Married    [3] Separated
     [4] Widowed    [5] Divorced    [6] Other      □ 72

33. Schooling completed (One choice only)
     [1] Did Not graduate from high school    [2] High School
     [3] Some College    [4] College or Professional Degree      □ 73

34. Employment Status
     [1] Employed    [2] Unemployed
     [3] Homemaker, Volunteer, or Student    [4] Retired, Other      □ 74

35. Type of occupation (SKIP IF NOT APPLICABLE)
     [1] Professional, Technical, Manager, Official or Proprietor    [2] Clerical or Sales
     [3] Craftsman, Foreman or Operative    [4] Service or Laborer      □ 75

36. County of Current Residence (SKIP IF NOT KNOWN)

                                                   [9][9][9] Other    76-78

37. State of Current Residence                           [9][9] Other    79-80)

# APPENDIX 9.2

## The Healthstyle Self-Test*

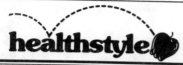

### Your lifestyle can make a difference...

No one can control all the factors that contribute to good health. Some risks are beyond the control of the individual — environmental pollution and unsafe highways, for example. However, you do have control over your behavior and habits. Improving those aspects of your lifestyle can make a difference in both the quality and quantity of your life.

Health experts now consider lifestyle to be one of the most important factors affecting health. It is estimated that as many as seven of the 10 leading causes of death in the United States could be reduced through common sense changes in lifestyle.

What type of changes should you make? The most important are: stopping smoking, moderation in drinking, developing good eating habits, proper handling of stress, regular exercising, and using safety measures in your car and around work and home.

Unfortunately, too few of us make the effort. Maybe you will after considering the following:

### Smoking

Cigarette smoking is the single most important preventable cause of illness and early death. It is especially risky for pregnant women and their unborn babies. Persons who stop smoking reduce their risk of getting heart disease and cancer.

So if you're a smoker, think twice about lighting up that next cigarette. But if you choose to continue smoking, at least try decreasing the number of cigarettes you smoke and switch to a low tar and nicotine brand.

### Drinking

Alcohol produces changes in mood and behavior. Most people who drink are able to control their intake of alcohol and to avoid undesired and often harmful effects. Heavy, regular use of alcohol can lead to cirrhosis of the liver — a leading cause of death.

If you do drink, do it wisely and in moderation. Statistics clearly show that mixing drinking and driving is often the cause of fatal or crippling accidents.

Use care in taking drugs too. Today's greater use of drugs — both legal and illegal — is one of our serious health risks. Even some of the drugs prescribed by your doctor can be dangerous if taken when drinking alcohol or before driving.

Using or experimenting with illicit drugs can lead to a number of damaging effects and even death. Physical and mental problems can develop from the excessive continued use of tranquilizers (or "pep pills").

### Overeating

Overweight individuals stand a greater risk of developing diabetes, gall bladder disease, and high blood pressure.

It makes good sense to maintain your proper weight. Good eating habits also include holding down the amount of fat (especially saturated fats), cholesterol, sugar, and salt in your diet. If you must snack, try nibbling on fresh fruits and vegetables.

### Regular Exercise

As little as 15 to 30 minutes of vigorous exercise three times a week will help you to have a healthier heart, eliminate excess weight, tone up sagging muscles, and sleep better.

Almost everyone can adopt some form of exercise program which will meet both his or her needs and ability. (If you have any doubt, check with your doctor first.)

### Handling Stress

Stress is a normal part of living. Everyone faces it to some degree. The causes of stress can be good or bad — a promotion on the job or the loss of a spouse.

Properly handled, stress need not be a problem. But unhealthy responses to stress — such as driving too fast or erratically, drinking too much, or prolonged anger or grief — can cause a variety of physical and mental problems.

Even on a very busy day, find a few minutes to slow down and relax. Talking over a problem with someone you trust can often help you find a satisfactory solution. Learn how to distinguish between things that are "worth fighting about" and things that are less important.

### Safety

Think "safety first" at home, at work, at school, at play, and on the highway. Buckle seat belts and obey traffic rules. Keep poisons and weapons out of the reach of children, and keep emergency telephone numbers handy. When the unexpected happens, you'll be prepared.

Now that you know why you should improve your lifestyle, find out what areas you should start to work on. Take a few minutes to complete the following test. Its purpose is simply to tell you how well you are doing in staying healthy.

The behaviors covered in the test are recommended for most Americans. However, persons with certain chronic diseases, handicapped individuals, or pregnant women may require special instructions from a physician or other health professional.

After you have taken the test, add up the score. Based on the results, you will know how much you will have to work on improving your lifestyle.

If you have already tried to change your health habits and haven't succeeded, don't be discouraged. The difficulty you have encountered may be due to influences you never really have thought about or to a lack of support and encouragement. Understanding those influences is an important step toward changing the way they affect you.

And, you don't have to do it by yourself. We can help. For more information, read the section, "Where Do You Go From Here," which follows the test.

The health suggestions and the following test were adapted from an article from the Department of Health and Human Services.

*SOURCE: U.S. Office of Health Information and Health Promotion, Department of Health and Human Services (Washington, D.C.: U.S. Government Printing Office, 1981).

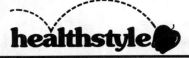

# healthstyle  A self-test

You will find that the test has six sections: smoking, alcohol and drugs, nutrition, exercise and fitness, stress control, and safety. Complete one section at a time by circling the number corresponding to the answer that best describes your behavior (2 for "Almost Always", 1 for "Sometimes", and 0 for "Almost Never"). Then add the numbers you have circled to determine your score for that section. Write the score on the line provided at the end of each section. The highest score you can get for each section is 10.

*Almost Always / Sometimes / Almost Never*

### Cigarette Smoking

If you never smoke, enter a score of 10 for this section and go to the next section on *Alcohol and Drugs.*

1. I avoid smoking cigarettes.  2 1 0
2. I smoke only low tar and nicotine cigarettes *or* I smoke a pipe or cigars.  2 1 0

**Smoking Score:**_____

### Alcohol and Drugs

1. I avoid drinking alcoholic beverages *or* I drink no more than 1 or 2 drinks a day.  4 1 0
2. I avoid using alcohol or other drugs (especially illegal drugs) as a way of handling stressful situations or the problems in my life.  2 1 0
3. I am careful not to drink alcohol when taking certain medicines (for example, medicine for sleeping, pain, colds, and allergies), or when pregnant.  2 1 0
4. I read and follow the label directions when using prescribed and over-the-counter drugs.  2 1 0

**Alcohol and Drugs Score:**_____

### Eating Habits

1. I eat a variety of foods each day, such as fruits and vegetables, whole grain breads and cereals, lean meats, dairy products, dry peas and beans, and nuts and seeds.  4 1 0
2. I limit the amount of fat, saturated fat, and cholesterol I eat (including fat on meats, eggs, butter, cream, shortenings, and organ meats such as liver).  2 1 0
3. I limit the amount of salt I eat by cooking with only small amounts, not adding salt at the table, and avoiding salty snacks.  2 1 0
4. I avoid eating too much sugar (especially frequent snacks of sticky candy or soft drinks).  2 1 0

**Eating Habits Score:**_____

### Exercise/Fitness

1. I maintain a desired weight, avoiding overweight and underweight.  3 1 0
2. I do vigorous exercises for 15-30 minutes at least 3 times a week (examples include running, swimming, brisk walking).  3 1 0
3. I do exercises that enhance my muscle tone for 15-30 minutes at least 3 times a week (examples include yoga and calisthenics).  2 1 0
4. I use part of my leisure time participating in individual, family, or team activities that increase my level of fitness (such as gardening, bowling, golf, and baseball).  2 1 0

**Exercise/Fitness Score:**_____

### Stress Control

1. I have a job or do other work that I enjoy.  2 1 0
2. I find it easy to relax and express my feelings freely.  2 1 0
3. I recognize early, and prepare for, events or situations likely to be stressful for me.  2 1 0
4. I have close friends, relatives, or others whom I can talk to about personal matters and call on for help when needed.  2 1 0
5. I participate in group activities (such as church and community organizations) or hobbies that I enjoy.  2 1 0

**Stress Control Score:**_____

### Safety

1. I wear a seat belt while riding in a car.  2 1 0
2. I avoid driving while under the influence of alcohol and other drugs.  2 1 0
3. I obey traffic rules and the speed limit when driving.  2 1 0
4. I am careful when using potentially harmful products or substances (such as household cleaners, poisons, and electrical devices).  2 1 0
5. I avoid smoking in bed.  2 1 0

**Safety Score:**_____

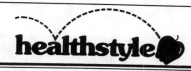

# What your scores mean to YOU

Remember, there is no total score for this test. Consider each section separately. You are trying to identify aspects of your lifestyle that you can improve in order to be healthier and to reduce the risk of illness. So let's see what your scores reveal:

**Scores of 9 and 10**

Excellent! Your answers show that you are aware of the importance of this area to your health. More important, you are putting your knowledge to work for you by practicing good health habits. As long as you continue to do so, this area should not pose a serious health risk. It's likely that you are setting an example for your family and friends to follow. Since you got a very high test score on this part of the test, you may want to consider other areas where your scores indicate room for improvement.

**Scores of 6 to 8**

Your health practices are good, but there is room for improvement. Look again at the items you answered with a "Sometimes" or "Almost Never." What changes can you make to improve your score? Even a small change can often help you achieve better health.

**Scores of 3 to 5**

Your health risks are showing! Would you like more information about the risks you are facing and why it is important for you to change these behaviors? Perhaps you need help in deciding how to successfully make the changes you desire. In either case, help is available.

**Scores of 0 to 2**

Obviously, you were concerned enough about your health to take the test, but your answers show that you may be taking serious and unnecessary risks with your health. Perhaps you are not aware of the risks and what to do about them. You can easily get the information and help you need to improve, if you wish. The next step is up to you.

# Where do you go from here?

Many health education programs are offered at our facilities which can help you identify and deal with lifestyle problems. If you want to make a change in any of the areas listed below, call the appropriate number for more information. Richmond Medical Center patients are encouraged to participate in the programs sponsored at our Oakland Medical Center.

**Stop Smoking Clinic:** Stopping smoking would be the best present you could give yourself in 1981. Our clinic calls for an evaluation meeting with a counselor during regular office hours to determine what would work best for you. Group classes, held in the evening at the Oakland Medical Center, provide the structure and group support necessary for changing smoking behavior and attitudes. The program has been successful in maintaining smoking abstinence and preventing relapse. For information call 428-6561.

**Weight Control:** Group meetings provide peer support and an opportunity to join with others in discussing behavior modification techniques, nutrition, and exercises. Meetings are held in the evenings at the Oakland Medical Center. For information, call 428-6552.

**Alcoholism and Drug Abuse:** Richmond Medical Center patients who want help should consult with their personal physician. Oakland Medical Center patients can make an appointment with the alcoholism and drug abuse clinic. There you can get a professional assessment of your problem. Support and education programs are available three days a week at the center. For information call 428-6984.

**Stress:** Help in identifying and managing the stress in your life is available through a series of popular evening classes held at the Oakland Medical Center. For information call 428-6552.

In addition to the above health education programs, packets of information on each of the topics are available at the Oakland Health Library. The packets include directories with referrals to educational programs, pamphlets, and lists of books and films available. The library is located on the 12th floor of the Oakland Medical Center, 280 West MacArthur Blvd. The hours are 9 a.m. to 5 p.m., weekdays. On Tuesdays, the library remains open until 8 p.m. The phone number is 428-6569.

# APPENDIX 9.3

## General Information for Your Personal Health Risk Report*

Working with you to improve your health is what the Total Health Care Program is all about. This Health Risk Report gives you important information about doing just that. It predicts your potential health problems, then gives you advice on how to reduce your risks and feel better every day.

A high-quality life is as important as how many years you live. Self-care is how you can make a difference. This means taking responsibility and action to improve your health. Caring for others and your environment is also necessary to really care for yourself.

So . . . what can you get for being more involved with self-care?

- A greater feeling of self-control and confidence
- More energy, vitality, and enthusiasm
- New interests in yourself, others, and your community
- A greater resistance to illness and health problems

We hope you will use your Personal Health Risk Report to take some new action for your health.

### PERSONAL HEALTH RISK REPORT

Your report is based on the answers you gave to the computer's questions. These are analyzed by the computer and compared to statistics given us by the U.S. Centers for Disease Control. Your report is divided into *four* sections.

1. "Age Appraisal"
2. "Higher Than Average Health Risks and Advice for Risk Reduction"
3. "Other Ways to Improve Your Health"
4. "Your Positive Health Habits"

*SOURCE: Reprinted with permission of the Total Health Care Program of Kaiser-Permanente Medical Care Program, Oakland, California.

Here is a brief description of each:

**1.** *Age Appraisal:* In this section, your actual age is compared with your

    a. Health age: This is an estimate of your *total* health risk based on the health problems listed for you. It tells you whether you have the health risks of someone older or younger than yourself.

      Example: Actual age 32. Health age 35.

      This means that even though you are only 32 years old, you have the health risks of someone who is 35 years old.

    b. Achievable age: This is an estimate of your possible health age if you follow the advice on your report.

      Example: Actual age 32. Health age 35. Achievable age 28.

**2.** *Higher Than Average Health Risks:* This section predicts your potential health problems. Your risk is greater than average for those listed.

With no habit changes on your part, the same possible problems will remain with you throughout your life. However, your highest risk area will change as you get older. For example, in your 20's, automobile accidents cause the greatest amount of death and disability. Later in life, your highest risk area will change to chronic problems like heart disease.

Take note of the advice listed. It can allow you to feel better now—and in the future.

**3.** *Other Ways to Improve Your Health:* Here you will find other important suggestions for how to improve the quality of your life, based on your answers.

**4.** *Your Positive Health Habits:* These are worthy of congratulations. Keep it up. Taking care of yourself enriches your life, increases your enjoyment, and assists you in reaching your goals.

## MAJOR INFLUENCES ON YOUR HEALTH

The Total Health Care Program's philosophy recognizes that the mind, body, environment, and personal relationships need to be considered when providing your medical care. When you read your Health Profile, consider these major influences on your health.

- *Self-care* includes the choices you make about your daily habits and lifestyle. This includes things like nutrition, exercise, stress management, communication skills, and using medication effectively. This area has the greatest potential for positive influence on your health. Even with small changes, you can feel better and reduce your health risks.

- *Environment* includes your home, work, and community surroundings. Exposure to dangerous materials and chronic high-stress jobs are examples. Although this area is difficult to change, it's easier if you join with others. (*Note:* Your report does not include the influence of your environment. It is very difficult to calculate in this manner. Nevertheless, this area remains very important.)

- *Health care practices* include periodic health testing and self-examination to identify problems early. If you have a health problem (such as high blood pressure), work with your health care provider to develop a treatment plan. Then, stick to it. *Note:* If you do have an existing health problem, this Health Risk Appraisal will underestimate your risk. Therefore, taking action is very important to keep the quality of your life high.

- *Heredity* is an area to be aware of even though it cannot be changed. You may be able to reduce your risk by choosing positive health habits. For example, if you have a family history of heart disease, stopping smoking, increasing exercise, and good nutrition will reduce your risk.

# APPENDIX 9.4

## Personal Health Assessment Questionnaire*

### Personal Health Assessment Questionnaire

Congratulations! You've decided to take an active role in assessing your health status and in doing what you can to stay healthy.

Please take the time to answer the assessment questions carefully. The benefits to you will be enhanced if you are honest and complete in your answers. The questionnaire will be kept confidential. When you return for your assessment appointment, a health educator or nurse practitioner will go over your questionnaire with you and fill out a summary sheet. You will get a copy of this summary sheet, and one copy will go into your medical record.

This assessment process is for you. We hope you enjoy getting to know yourself and your health profile and will use the information to make your time at the university more healthful and satisfying.

Name _____ Age _____

Campus Address _____

Campus Phone _____ Student Health ID No. _____

Permanent Address _____

Department/Academic Major _____

Check one:  _____ Freshman
            _____ Sophomore
            _____ Junior
            _____ Senior
            _____ Graduate

Number of years enrolled at college: _____

Living arrangements—check one:  _____ Dorm
                                _____ Fraternity
                                _____ Sorority
                                _____ Co-op
                                _____ Off-campus—live alone
                                _____ Off-campus—live with family
                                _____ Off-campus—live with friends

*SOURCE: Reprinted with the permission of Student Health Services, Health Education Department, University of California, Berkeley.

I. *Recurrent Health Problems:* In the last three years have you ever missed school or work for any of the following health problems?

|  | Yes | No. of Days per Quarter |
|---|---|---|
| Menstrual cramps | _____ | _____ |
| Headaches | _____ | _____ |
| Low back pain | _____ | _____ |
| Neck pain | _____ | _____ |
| Cold or sore throat | _____ | _____ |
| Urinary infection | _____ | _____ |
| Stress or anxiety | _____ | _____ |
| Insomnia | _____ | _____ |
| Asthma | _____ | _____ |
| Bronchitis | _____ | _____ |
| Depression | _____ | _____ |
| Stomach problem or ulcer | _____ | _____ |
| Fatigue | _____ | _____ |
| Injuries or accidents | _____ | _____ |

Other—*Please list* any other recurrent health problem that you feel adversely affects your health now:

_____

_____

II. *Family Medical History* (parents, grandparents, etc.)

|  | Yes | Who? (Relationship) |
|---|---|---|
| Diabetes | _____ | _____ |
| High blood pressure | _____ | _____ |
| Mental depression | _____ | _____ |
| Suicide | _____ | _____ |
| Drinking problem | _____ | _____ |
| Breast cancer (include aunts, great-aunts, sisters) | _____ | _____ |
| Colon cancer | _____ | _____ |
| Heart attack before age 50 | _____ | _____ |
| Familial hypercholestrolemia | _____ | _____ |

List any other family illnesses that you think may influence your health:

_____

_____

III. *Your Health History*

Please check any conditions listed below that apply to you:

_____ History of rheumatic fever

_____ Heart murmur

_____ Mother took DES

_____ History of sexually transmitted disease(s)

_____ Males: history of undescended testicle(s)

_____ You or your partner had an abortion

_____ Ulcerative colitis

_____ Six or more sexual partners in the last year

_____ Six or more sexual partners (total) since starting sexual activity

List any other past illness that you have had that you think may influence your health now:

_____

_____

List any toxic substances that you are exposed to either at work, school, or home:

_____

_____

IV. *Self-Care*

|  | *Always* |  |  |  | *Never* |
|---|---|---|---|---|---|
| Do you floss your teeth daily? | 1 | 2 | 3 | 4 | 5 |
| Do you see your dentist yearly? | 1 | 2 | 3 | 4 | 5 |
| Do you use a sunscreen to prevent sunburn? | 1 | 2 | 3 | 4 | 5 |
| Do you avoid prolonged exposure to loud noises? | 1 | 2 | 3 | 4 | 5 |

When was your last tetanus shot? _____

List any current medications you take regularly (including oral contraceptives):

_____

_____

Do you know your usual blood pressure?      Yes _____      No _____

If *yes*, what is the usual reading? _____

|  |  | *Always* |  |  |  | *Never* |
|---|---|---|---|---|---|---|
| *Men:* | Do you check your testicles for lumps every three months? | 1 | 2 | 3 | 4 | 5 |
| *Women:* | Do you check your breasts for lumps each month? | 1 | 2 | 3 | 4 | 5 |

Date of last Pap smear _____

Have you ever been tested to see if you are immune to German measles?

Yes _____      No _____      Don't know _____

### V. Nutrition

How frequently do you eat foods in each of these categories? Place appropriate number beside each item:

0 = never
1 = once a month or less
2 = two or three times a month
3 = one to three times a week
4 = daily
5 = more than once a day

*Frequency*

1. Grains
   a. High-fiber (whole-wheat bread, brown rice, whole-grain cereals)                                                  _____
   b. Low-fiber (white bread, white rice, fast-cook cereals, regular crust pizza, hamburger buns)                       _____

2. Fruits and Vegetables:
   a. Vitamin C–rich (oranges, grapefruit, cantaloupe, strawberries, broccoli, cabbage, bok choy, tomato)              _____
   b. Dark green and leafy, rich in Vitamin A and folic acid (spinach, broccoli, chard, asparagus, watercress, lettuce, greens)   _____
   c. Other fruits and vegetables (carrots, corn, eggplant, peas, zucchini, peaches, apricots, potatoes)               _____

3. Dairy products
   a. Low-fat (low-fat cottage cheese, yogurt, milk)                                                                    _____
   b. Medium-fat (white cheese, 2% fat milk, 4% fat cottage cheese)                                                     _____
   c. Higher-fat (whole milk, ice cream, yellow cheese)                                                                 _____

Frequency

4. Protein
   a. Low-fat (dried beans, poultry, fish)
   b. High-fat (nuts, seeds, soybeans, high-fat meats)           ____
5. Other foods
   a. Fast foods (pizza, MacDonald's, Taco Bell, etc.)
   b. BBQ meats (hot dogs, BBQ beef, ribs, etc.)               ____
   c. High-salt foods (potato chips, fries, pickles, olives)    ____
   d. High-fat foods (avocados, sour cream, butter, sauces,
      fried foods, margarine)
   e. High-sugar foods (cakes, cookies, candy, donuts)          ____
6. Liquids
   a. Water
   b. Diet soda                                                 ____
   c. Coffee (caffeinated)                                      ____
   d. Soda (caffeinated, i.e., colas)                           ____
   e. Decaffeinated coffee or soda                              ____

*Eating habits.* Do you:

Frequency

7. Eat breakfast?                                               ____
8. Eat regular meals?                                           ____
9. Restrict your food intake for the purpose of controlling
   weight?                                                      ____
10. Binge (ingest many calories at one sitting)?               ____
11. Purge (vomiting, fasting, laxative use)?                   ____
12. Go on special diets (Scarsdale, Atkins, Cambridge, Pritikin,
    etc.)?                                                      ____
13. Add salt at the table to foods?                            ____
14. Add salt while cooking foods?                              ____
15. Is there anything you would like to change about your
    present eating habits?        Yes ____       No ____

    If *yes*, what would you change? _____

    _____

VI. *Exercise*

                                                               Yes      No

16. Do you exercise vigorously for at least 20 minutes, 3 or
    more times per week?                                       ____     ____
17. Do you include flexibility, warm-up, and cool-down
    exercises in your physical workout?                        ____     ____

|  | Yes | No |
|---|---|---|

18. Do you use part of your leisure time for participation in individual, family, or team activities that increase your level of fitness (gardening, bowling, baseball, basketball, walking, hiking, biking, etc.)?                                  ___    ___

19. What concerns do you have pertaining to physical fitness?

_____

_____

VII. *Sleep*

How often do you:

| | Always | | | | Never |
|---|---|---|---|---|---|
| 20. Fall asleep when you are ready? | 1 | 2 | 3 | 4 | 5 |
| 21. Get enough sleep? | 1 | 2 | 3 | 4 | 5 |
| 22. Wake feeling rested? | 1 | 2 | 3 | 4 | 5 |
| 23. Feel you get enough rest every day? | 1 | 2 | 3 | 4 | 5 |
| 24. Lie awake and worry? | 1 | 2 | 3 | 4 | 5 |
| 26. Get to bed later than you want or need to? | 1 | 2 | 3 | 4 | 5 |
| 26. Worry about getting enough sleep? | 1 | 2 | 3 | 4 | 5 |

VIII. *Sexuality*

27. Are you sexually active now?        Yes ___      No ___

| | Always | | | | Never |
|---|---|---|---|---|---|
| 28. Are you satisfied with your level of sexual activity or inactivity? | 1 | 2 | 3 | 4 | 5 |
| 29. Are you satisfied with your sexual relationships? | 1 | 2 | 3 | 4 | 5 |

|  | Yes | No |
|---|---|---|
| 30. If you are heterosexually active: | | |
| Do you use a contraceptive method? | ___ | ___ |
| Are you satisfied with this method? | ___ | ___ |

31. Do you have any concerns about sexuality or contraception?

_____

_____

IX. *Auto Hazards* (*Note:* The leading cause of death in young adults is auto accidents.)

|  | Yes | No |
|---|---|---|
| Do you: | | |
| 32. Drive after drinking alcohol or taking drugs? | ___ | ___ |

|  | Yes | No |
|---|---|---|
| 33. Ride with drivers who have been drinking alcohol or taking drugs? | ___ | ___ |
| 34. Tend to exceed the speed limit? | ___ | ___ |
| 35. Not wear a seat belt 90 percent of the time? | ___ | ___ |
| 36. Travel in a car or other motor vehicle over 15,000 miles/ year (average is 12,000 miles)? | ___ | ___ |

X. *Social Support*

37. Do you have one or more persons (friends, relatives, etc.) with whom you feel at ease and with whom you can discuss personal concerns, worries, or problems that you may have now or in the future?

____ I have one such person

____ I have more than one such person

____ Yes, in the past, but not at the present time

____ I would like to have a close friend

____ I do not feel the need

If you have such a person/people:

|  | A Great Deal | Moderately | Not at All |
|---|---|---|---|
| 38. How much do they make you feel liked or loved? | ___ | ___ | ___ |
| 39. How much do they make you feel respected or admired? | ___ | ___ | ___ |
| 40. How much can you confide in them? | ___ | ___ | ___ |
| 41. How much do they agree with or support your actions or thoughts? | ___ | ___ | ___ |
| 42. How much could they help if you needed to borrow $10, get a ride to the airport, or move to a new apartment? | ___ | ___ | ___ |

43. Are you satisfied with your level of social support?   Yes ___   No ___
If *no*, what would you like to improve/work on?

_____

_____

XI. *Alcohol/Tobacco/Other Drugs*

|  | Always |  |  |  | Never |
|---|---|---|---|---|---|
| 44. Do you currently drink alcohol? | 1 | 2 | 3 | 4 | 5 |

If *yes*:

|  | Always |  |  |  | Never |
|---|---|---|---|---|---|
| 45. Does drinking interfere with your schoolwork? | 1 | 2 | 3 | 4 | 5 |
| 46. Have your family or friends complained about your drinking, or suggested that you cut down on your drinking? | 1 | 2 | 3 | 4 | 5 |
| 47. Have you ever worried that alcohol plays too big a role in your life? | 1 | 2 | 3 | 4 | 5 |
| 48. Have you ever found that you could not remember what you did the night before when you were drinking? | 1 | 2 | 3 | 4 | 5 |
| 49. Do you drive a car when you know you have had too much to drink? | 1 | 2 | 3 | 4 | 5 |

50. Do you currently smoke tobacco?    Yes ____    No ____

If *yes*:

51. How much do you smoke?

____ Rarely

____ Occasionally

____ Regularly:    ____ Number of packs per day

52. How many years have you been smoking? ____

53. Do you currently use drugs (prescription or illegal)?    Yes ____    No __

If *yes*:

|  | Always |  |  |  | Never |
|---|---|---|---|---|---|
| 54. Do drugs interfere with your schoolwork? | 1 | 2 | 3 | 4 | 5 |
| 55. Have you had financial problems because you spent too much on drugs? | 1 | 2 | 3 | 4 | 5 |
| 56. Have your family or friends complained about your drug use, or suggested that you cut down on your drug use? | 1 | 2 | 3 | 4 | 5 |
| 57. Do you use drugs when you feel lonely or depressed? | 1 | 2 | 3 | 4 | 5 |
| 58. Are drugs secretly your best friend? | 1 | 2 | 3 | 4 | 5 |

XII. *School*

59. What do you like about school? _____

_____

60. Do you presently have difficulties with any of the following:

    \_\_\_\_ Choice of major             \_\_\_\_ Planning for future career

    \_\_\_\_ Procrastination              \_\_\_\_ Keeping interested in major

    \_\_\_\_ Fear of failure                  or coursework in general

    \_\_\_\_ Competition for grades      \_\_\_\_ Other (please explain): \_\_\_\_\_

    \_\_\_\_ Time management          _____

|  | Yes | No |
|---|---|---|

61. If you have needed help with an academic problem, have you found the support and help you've needed to deal with it effectively?    \_\_\_\_   \_\_\_\_

    If *yes*, where did you find such support?

        \_\_\_\_ On-campus

        \_\_\_\_ Off-campus

    If *no*, what did you do?

_____

_____

|  | Yes | No |
|---|---|---|

62. Have you had to drop any classes since you have been registered in college?    \_\_\_\_   \_\_\_\_

63. Have you had to take an incomplete?    \_\_\_\_   \_\_\_\_

64. Have you failed any classes?    \_\_\_\_   \_\_\_\_

65. If *yes* to (62–64), what do you feel to be the reasons?

_____

_____

66. How many days of class (on the average) do you miss in a quarter due to illness or just "not feeling up to it?"   \_\_\_\_

## XIII. *Stress*

67. Which of the following changes have occurred in your life in the past year? (Check all that apply.)

    \_\_\_\_ Close family member died     \_\_\_\_ Got divorced or separated

    \_\_\_\_ Moved to new residence       \_\_\_\_ Took on a lot of debt

    \_\_\_\_ Changed jobs/schools         \_\_\_\_ Got married

    \_\_\_\_ Left home                 \_\_\_\_ Close relationship ended

    \_\_\_\_ Close friend died          \_\_\_\_ Had major health problem

    \_\_\_\_ Other (please explain): _____

68. Which of these situations do you face on an *ongoing* basis?

    \_\_\_\_ Marital problems      \_\_\_\_ Meeting family demands

    \_\_\_\_ Financial problems      \_\_\_\_ Coping with physical problems

    \_\_\_\_ Sexual problems

    \_\_\_\_ Trouble with relatives/friends      \_\_\_\_ Coping with emotional problems

    \_\_\_\_ Housing problems

    \_\_\_\_ Wasting time      \_\_\_\_ Constantly facing deadlines

    \_\_\_\_ Pressure at work or school      \_\_\_\_ Having too many things to do

XIV. *Relationships*

69. Do you feel satisfied with the relationship you have with the following people:

| | Always | | | | Never |
|---|---|---|---|---|---|
| Parents | 1 | 2 | 3 | 4 | 5 |
| Male friends | 1 | 2 | 3 | 4 | 5 |
| Female friends | 1 | 2 | 3 | 4 | 5 |
| Roommate(s) | 1 | 2 | 3 | 4 | 5 |
| Lover(s) | 1 | 2 | 3 | 4 | 5 |
| Academic adviser | 1 | 2 | 3 | 4 | 5 |
| Teaching assistants | 1 | 2 | 3 | 4 | 5 |
| Professors | 1 | 2 | 3 | 4 | 5 |
| Employer/supervisor | 1 | 2 | 3 | 4 | 5 |
| Siblings | 1 | 2 | 3 | 4 | 5 |
| Children (if applicable) | 1 | 2 | 3 | 4 | 5 |
| Spouse (if applicable) | 1 | 2 | 3 | 4 | 5 |
| Other (please list): | | | | | |
| _____ | 1 | 2 | 3 | 4 | 5 |
| _____ | 1 | 2 | 3 | 4 | 5 |

70. How often do you feel satisfied with your communication with other people?    1 2 3 4 5

71. Is there anything about your relationships that you'd like to change?

_____

_____

XV. *Personal Assessment*

After completing this questionnaire:

72.  What concerns you most about your health and well-being?

_____

_____

_____

_____

73.  What advice would you give yourself to improve your health and well-being?

_____

_____

_____

_____

# APPENDIX 9.5

## Summary Health Assessment

Name _____ Date _____

Student Health ID No. _____ Interviewer _____

| | Health-Enhancing | Could Improve | Health-Negating | Comments |
|---|---|---|---|---|
| I. Health behaviors | | | | |
| Nutrition | ____ | ____ | ____ | ____ |
| Exercise | ____ | ____ | ____ | ____ |
| Sleep | ____ | ____ | ____ | ____ |
| Alcohol | ____ | ____ | ____ | ____ |
| Drugs | ____ | ____ | ____ | ____ |
| Auto hazards | ____ | ____ | ____ | ____ |
| Self-care | ____ | ____ | ____ | ____ |
| II. Psychosocial factors | | | | |
| Sexuality | ____ | ____ | ____ | ____ |
| Relationships | ____ | ____ | ____ | ____ |
| Social support | ____ | ____ | ____ | ____ |
| Stress | ____ | ____ | ____ | ____ |
| III. School Environment | | | | |

# Personal Health Assessment Summary Sheet*

IV. Risk factors from personal or family health history:

V. Recurrent health problems that may benefit from intervention:

VI. Self-assessment:

VII. Health professional assessment and recommendations:

VIII. Referrals: ___ M.D. ___ Health Ed. consultation ___ Counseling/Psych.

___ N.P. ___ Health Ed. group ___ Other

*SOURCE: Reprinted with the permission of Student Health Services, Health Education Department, University of California, Berkeley.

# APPENDIX 9.6

## Pretest, Posttest, and Evaluation Questionnaire for a Personal Health Assessment Program*

### Pretest-Posttest for Personal Health Assessment Program

I. Risk factors

Place a check in front of any of the conditions listed below that you think you are *more* likely to develop than the *average* person—because of family history, personal medical history, health habits, or any other reason.

_____ a. Heart attack

_____ b. Stroke

_____ c. High blood pressure

_____ d. Lung cancer

_____ e. Breast cancer

_____ f. Testicular cancer

_____ g. Cervical cancer (women only)

_____ h. Bladder cancer

_____ i. Colon cancer

_____ j. Skin cancer

_____ k. Other cancer

_____ l. Venereal diseases

_____ m. Unwanted pregnancy (both men and women answer)

_____ n. Loss of teeth, requiring dentures

_____ o. Suicide

_____ p. Serious injury or death from motor vehicle accident

_____ q. Serious injury or death from sports or other activities

_____ r. Work-related injury (e.g., back strain)

_____ s. Obesity

_____ t. Diabetes

_____ u. Drinking problem

_____ v. Tetanus

list: _____

II. Below is a list of suggestions for ways to improve health status. For each statement, indicate if this is advice you would give yourself.

| I would give myself this advice (Circle one for each statement): | Strongly agree | | | Strongly disagree | | Does not apply |
|---|---|---|---|---|---|---|
| a. Improve eating habits (e.g., more balanced, less sweets) | 1 | 2 | 3 | 4 | 5 | 6 |
| b. Start an exercise program | 1 | 2 | 3 | 4 | 5 | 6 |
| c. Get more sleep | 1 | 2 | 3 | 4 | 5 | 6 |
| d. Cut down or quit drinking | 1 | 2 | 3 | 4 | 5 | 6 |
| e. Cut down or quit use of drugs | 1 | 2 | 3 | 4 | 5 | 6 |
| f. Improve driving safety (e.g., wear seat belts, no speeding) | 1 | 2 | 3 | 4 | 5 | 6 |

*SOURCE: Reprinted with the permission of Student Health Services, Health Education Department, University of California, Berkeley.

## Student Feedback and Evaluation
## Personal Health Assessment Program

|  | Strongly agree |  |  | Strongly disagree |  |
|---|---|---|---|---|---|
| 1. I was able to assess my current health status. | 1 | 2 | 3 | 4 | 5 |
| 2. I was able to identify specific areas of health risk for me personally. | 1 | 2 | 3 | 4 | 5 |
| 3. I learned about aspects of my life that are health promoting. | 1 | 2 | 3 | 4 | 5 |
| 4. I learned about aspects of my life that are health negating. | 1 | 2 | 3 | 4 | 5 |
| 5. I learned ways I could change that may improve my health. | 1 | 2 | 3 | 4 | 5 |
| 6. I learned where to go for assistance to make the changes I want to make. | 1 | 2 | 3 | 4 | 5 |
| 7. I feel I have a place to go if I need more support or have questions about making changes in my health. | 1 | 2 | 3 | 4 | 5 |
| 8. I got what I expected from this program. | 1 | 2 | 3 | 4 | 5 |
| 9. I would recommend this program to a friend. | 1 | 2 | 3 | 4 | 5 |
| 10. Overall, I would rate this program as very helpful to me personally. | 1 | 2 | 3 | 4 | 5 |

*Comments: General*

What did you like best about the program?

_____

_____

_____

What did you like least?

_____

_____

_____

Suggestions:

_____

_____

_____

_____

# EXERCISES

1.  Imagine being in the following situation. You are working in a 150-bed hospital in a suburban setting. There is also a large outpatient clinic population. The hospital administrator feels that the hospital should have health promotion services to promote community relations. He wants to set up a self-administered HRA computer in the lobby. He makes this proposal at a meeting you two are having with the medical director about priorities for the next year. How would you respond in this meeting? Would you proceed with this project? Provide a rationale for your decision. If you choose to set up the system, what would your first steps be in developing a health risk assessment program?

2.  This is a role-playing situation for groups of three; the roles are health educator, client, and feedback observer. Rotate the roles among the group members for each situation. After role-playing each one, spend five to ten minutes discussing the experience and giving each other feedback.

    a. Use the sample computerized HRA feedback form in Figure 9.2 as the basis for a post-HRA discussion between a client and health educator.

    b. Complete the Healthstyle Self-Test in Appendix 9.2, and role-play a post-HRA discussion between a client and health educator.

    c. During a post-HRA discussion using the form in Figure 9.2, the client makes the following statements: "I didn't learn anything I didn't already know from this HRA." And then later on, "I don't care if my risk of dying sooner is increased; I enjoy smoking and I don't want to give it up."

# RESOURCES

Blum, Henrik. Social Perspective on Risk Reduction. *Family and Community Health Journal* (Aspen Systems), May 1980, pp. 41–64.

Henrik Blum is a professor of health planning at the University of California, Berkeley. His article presents risk reduction from two major perspectives: (1) the micro perspective, which includes the efforts individuals make to reduce their personal health risks; and (2) the macro perspective, which includes the efforts a society makes to minimize the risks to which its members are exposed. After reviewing the major forces affecting health, he contrasts the effects of micro and macro strategies for risk reduction. Although this article is a bit wordy and academic, it raises some important issues and strategies to consider in health education's challenge to balance individual lifestyle change with attention to broader environmental and social issues as a means to improve health.

Centers for Disease Control (CDC), Center for Health Promotion and Education, Atlanta, Georgia 30333. Telephone (404) 329-3415.

CDC is involved with a number of special projects related to the development of HRA, including updating epidemiological data, adapting the HRA for various target groups, and providing a clearinghouse for risk assessment information. Also, CDC has made available to the public a low-cost computerized HRA program.

*Medical Abstracts* Newsletter, Box 2170, Teaneck, New Jersey 07666.

This newsletter is published monthly at a reasonable cost and contains summaries of health-related research findings that have been recently published in medical, nursing, and psychology journals. It states its purpose as the promotion of patient-physician cooperation and patient education. It is six pages long and has sections on general medicine, heart disease, cancer, obstetrics-gynecology, pediatrics, aging, psychiatry, addictive behaviors, sexual medicine, and sports medicine. A good resource for busy people who don't have time to read numerous journals every month.

National Health Information Clearinghouse. *HRA's: An Inventory.* DHHS Publication No. 81-50163. Available free from National Health Information Clearinghouse, P.O. Box 1133, Washington, D.C. 20013. 1981.

This inventory gives information on twenty-nine health risk appraisals currently available to the public. No attempt is made to evaluate or compare the appraisals. The purpose of the guide is to identify the range of types of appraisals that are available, not to be fully inclusive. Where applicable, cost, method or analysis, specified target population, special ordering information, and a general description are provided for each listing. Also, a selected annotated bibliography is included. The inventory is a useful overview of the variety of HRA adaptations and settings that use the approach.

Sarochan, William. *Personal Health Appraisal.* New York: Wiley, 1976.

This book is designed for college students but is useful to the general public. It contains many self-assessment tools in a wide variety of areas, such as mental health, fitness, nutrition, and overall health status. Suggestions for behavior change are also provided.

# 10

## Techniques for making decisions and commitments

C LIENTS OFTEN FAIL when they take steps to improve their health. Such clients may have felt pressured by health professionals, friends, or family—or by their own high expectations. Pressure pushes clients to jump into action before considering whether the action is right for them. In this chapter we propose a decision-making approach to help clients clarify goals, identify and evaluate alternatives, and prepare for future successes and consequences. These techniques can help health educators increase the probability that their clients will succeed. This chapter as well as the next one is designed to help the educator in medical care settings implement specialized educational techniques that are capable of transferring more power and control to the client than has been possible with traditional educational interventions.

In the educational process, clients face the challenge of making decisions about their health behavior: to alter harmful behaviors and to add new, positive ones. As we discussed in Chapter 8, on educational assessment, the health educator identifies issues that influence client health behaviors and helps clients outline specific actions they can take to improve their health. The next step is to help clients make decisions about future goals and take the necessary actions to achieve those goals. How these decisions are made means the difference between success and failure.

Some of us have regularly gone on diets in our lifetime, losing weight only to regain the same pounds after a while. We all know people who began exercise programs on New Year's Day but who gave up on January 2nd. People are prompted to make such health decisions for many initial reasons. They are interested in improving their appearance; their doctor has told them to do so; their family members have been nagging them; or they want to feel better and improve the quality of their daily lives. In this chapter we express our belief that health decisions are really a series of small, systematic decisions made over time—a one-time initial decision to actually do something and then a continuing series of decisions to stay committed to that action. The probability of success is increased if clients (1) select realistic goals, (2) survey the options available to reach their goals, (3) choose options that fit their style, and (4) institute strategies to continue toward the goals.

## THE IMPORTANCE OF DECISION TRAINING

Doesn't everyone make decisions every day, mostly without help and with relatively positive results? Yes, they do. However, we are talking about two different types of decisions. One type is the kind of decision made every day: what to eat, to wear, where to go, whom to talk to, and so on. The other type of decision is a commitment either to change behavior (to stop smoking, to lose weight) or to add a behavior (to begin an exercise program, to begin taking antihypertensive medications). The latter decisions have far-reaching effects on health and the quality of life; and they also require day-by-day, perhaps moment-by-moment, recommitment to the initial goal.

For instance, consider Larke Wong. She has decided to quit smoking (Decision 1). She then decides which program she will attend to help her quit smoking (Decision 2). She joins the program and arrives at the day where the entire class gives up smoking together (Decision 3). Each day and hour thereafter, Larke fights the desire to pick up a cigarette (Decision 4,5, . . . ). Months later, she may or may not continue to decide not to smoke.

This decision process is much more complex than, say, deciding to buy a new washing machine. The health educator must recognize that a client's decision may relate to (1) disease detection practices (such as monthly breast self-exams), (2) treatment practices (such as taking medications regularly), or (3) health promotion activities (such as exercising or doing stress reduction techniques). The health educator must also recognize that the decision represents not only a commitment to a goal but also a continual process of recommitment. Moreover, decision-making skills can be learned.

There is no ideal way to make a decision. Individuals make decisions about their health in a variety of styles. It is important to help clients clarify the style that suits them best and to match clients with educational programs consistent with this style.

## ASSESSING READINESS

One of the health educator's first tasks is to judge where the client is in the decision process. Figure 10.1 describes the three steps in the assessment phase. Step 1 is determining whether a decision to make a health behavior change has actually been made. The educator can use the following questions to clarify Step 1 of the assessment phase:

- Does the client want to make a decision?
- Has the client made a decision and says so?
- Has the client apparently made a decision but seems unaware of it?
- Is the client so pulled by opposing sides as to be unable to make a decision?
- Does the client want you to make the decision?
- How much time, effort, and money is the client willing to invest in order to attain the goal?

This first task is closely related to the assessment phase of the educational process: the educator determines how committed to a goal the client already is.

The second step concerns the client's history. Because of past failures in making health changes or other types of behavior change, the client may be hesitant to try again. This information should enter into the overall assessment. Therefore, the following questions are important:

- Has the client tried to (lose weight, stop smoking, begin an exercise program, and so on)?
- Was the client successful? For how long?
- What is the client's perception of that past effort (the reasons for success or failure)?

Moreover, lack of success may prompt the client to depend on the professional for guidance. Inasmuch as health care professionals have been trained to be knowledgeable in their fields, they may succumb and

**Figure 10.1  Decision assessment**

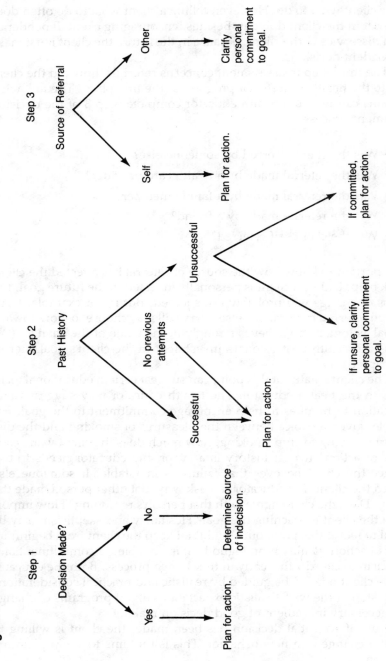

tell the client what to do. However, telling a client what to do often does not result in the client doing it. Besides, encouraging client dependency does a disservice to the client, because in the future the client must make independent decisions.

The third step in assessment concerns referrals: how did the client come to the health educator or program in the first place? The following questions can help the health educator complete Step 3 of the decision assessment process:

- Was the client referred by someone else?
- Was the referral made by a health care provider?
- Was the referral made by a family member?
- Was the referral made by a friend?
- Was the client self-referred?

It is important to know how the source of referral has affected the client to seek help. Unless a client is personally invested in the future goal, the process of change will probably not succeed. But if, for example, Jerry has been referred by someone else, Jerry still may choose to work toward the goal as long as he believes strongly in the value of the change. (We discuss the health professional's investment in the client's goal later in this chapter.)

The client's status at this point can suggest certain educational techniques to the health educator. The health educator may suggest value clarification techniques to help encourage commitment to the goal. For example, given a choice between the pleasures of smoking and the discomfort of trying to stop smoking, how much does the client value each course of action? If past history is a factor, the educator needs to ask whether the client believes that failure is inevitable. If someone else referred the client, the educator can ask why that other person made the referral. Does the client agree with that person's reasoning? How important to the client is reaching the goal? Hesitancy and skepticism may be natural to feel at this point but should not keep the client from beginning a plan of action. Reality is ambiguous; it is possible for commitment and skepticism to co-exist this early in the change process. Both the educator and the client need to be guided by realistic and practical considerations at each step of the way. Realistic expectations about programs of change are a necessary ingredient of good decision making.

Now, if an initial decision has been made, the client is willing to try out a change or a new behavior. This is the time to begin planning for action.

## CLARIFYING GOALS

Let's assume that a client has decided to embark either on modifying a habit or on beginning a new health activity. The next step is to clarify the goal. Clients may be too ambitious and want to accomplish too much all at one time; for example, lose weight, stop smoking, relieve stress. But if goals are selected that emphasize *not* doing something—such as not smoking cigarettes or not eating bread or desserts—the changes can become so severe and daily life so deprived of "goodies" that failure can be expected. Such goals only succeed in provoking a sense of frustration and failure. Therefore, the educator needs to help the client choose subgoals requiring actions that are rewarding and that work toward the desired change.

Sometimes clients state goals in general terms that need to be further refined before action is taken. If clients say they "want to feel better," their goal may really be to begin an exercise program, or to plan more nutritionally balanced meals, or to modify eating habits. Clarifying the goal helps the client look at specific ways to achieve the goal. Without that focus, action plans could ramble "all over the map." Mahoney (1979) provides a list to determine how to select a goal that will increase the likelihood of success. Successful goals have the following characteristics:

- Involve a relatively small and comfortable alteration of daily habits
- Emphasize doing something instead of not doing something
- Have the support and encouragement of important friends and family
- Are undertaken very modestly at first and then are gradually increased over time
- Have immediate and important payoff for making the change
- Are related to a change in behavior of recent development

As many as possible of these criteria should be used in goal setting. Clients should avoid large changes in their daily routine, feelings of deprivation, the subtle pressure from family and friends to continue old habits, the temptation of directing their sights to a long-term goal with little immediate payoff, and initially trying to change long-established habits. The educator is challenged to guide the client through these stages.

A strategy should be developed to achieve realistic goals. Unfortunately, a client's initial desire may be to select an action that is immediately appealing. For instance, Bob became fed up with his lack of physical energy. For months, he had noticed a sluggishness and a feeling of constant fatigue. All his muscles felt tight. It was not as easy to tie his shoelaces or get out of an easy chair as it used to be. He had heard a lot on television shows about jogging, so he decided to take up the sport. He put on an old pair of tennis shoes, his sweatshirt, and shorts and proceeded to run around the block. He carried out this plan for several days. After an exhausting short distance each day, he decided it was too much effort and too painful. After one week, he gave up jogging. Bob had made the initial decision to get more exercise, but because he hadn't chosen a program more amenable to his level of fitness, he was unable to achieve his goal of increased energy and flexibility. Besides, he had hoped for too much, too soon. A better strategy to accomplish his goal might have included a fitness evaluation, a graduated exercise plan, and appropriate conditioning, as well as warmup and cooldown exercises.

Bob's example describes a situation where initial appeal may not have been the best way to achieve a goal, even if the goal was realistic. Irving Janis and Leon Mann (1977) suggest three criteria to keep in mind when selecting an action to achieve a personal goal:

**1.** An individual's perceived state of crisis (or whether the client believes there is sufficient time to make a decision) may interfere with making a reasonable commitment to a goal. The client may believe that immediate action is necessary and may not take the time to clarify the goal and review alternatives.

**2.** It is important to delay making a commitment to an action until one has considered the alternatives available to reach the personal goal.

**3.** Anticipating future consequences and preparing for them is a critical step toward successful achievement of the goal.

Should a client want to take action immediately, the health educator's task is to clarify the client's need for prompt action. The health educator can point out alternative actions that the client had not considered, and can describe the advantages of preparing for future consequences. The educator can use the following list of questions during this step:

- What is the source of urgency?
- What does the client believe will happen if action is delayed?
- What are the benefits to be gained in delaying action?

A cautionary note is in order, though. Readiness to invest in a future goal is a fragile state, and timing is a critical element. People who are asked what prompted them to take action at this particular time may say that "the time just seemed right." The educator should examine incentives or pressures that are present and sufficient to impel the person to act. If the health educator asks the client to delay an action, he or she must do so in such a way as to maintain that initially high state of readiness while reviewing available options and preparing for future consequences.

## GENERATING OPTIONS

Let us look closer at the step of generating alternative plans of action. When people select a personal health goal, they may have a limited idea of ways to reach that goal. They may think that the only way to lose weight is to diet, rather than begin an exercise program, or a combination of the two. The technique called *brainstorming* can broaden the client's perception of alternatives. Educators can use the following guidelines when applying brainstorming techniques to the decision-making process:

**1.** Generate as many alternatives as possible.

**2.** Don't make judgments on each alternative—just get down on paper all alternatives that come to mind.

**3.** Try to be original even if the idea seems "off the wall."

**4.** Use other alternatives as springboards for new ideas.

**5.** Avoid dichotomies such as "Either I attend a class, or I don't"; instead, look for middle-of-the-road solutions.

The first two guidelines are the most important. Generating as many alternatives as possible without judgment encourages the spontaneous, creative process of generating options. The point of brainstorming is to come up with as many potential solutions as possible.

There are also other resources for generating options for actions. Clients may want to speak with friends or family members, go to the library, or read the Yellow Pages. When clients are participating in a group, the other members as well as the instructor provide additional resources and suggestions.

## PERSON-PROGRAM FIT

The next and more difficult step is to evaluate the person-program *fit*. This term describes the relationship between an educational program and a client's particular learning style. Certain conditions help achieve this relationship, such as time at which the program is offered, the program's appeal, the financial feasibility of attending the program, and whether the program is conducted in a group or is oriented to the individual.

Often the problem is not insufficient alternatives but too many! Too many alternatives can create an information overload. Clients are bombarded by the media (television, radio, newspapers, magazines) claiming the usefulness of this or that device, program, or regimen. Consumers have little means to evaluate these claims, let alone to select the most suitable program. The educator can help clients by offering them a way to evaluate options. Clients can use the following list of suggestions to evaluate their alternatives:

- What are the credentials of the person giving advice?
- Is this advisor recommended by others?
- Is the advisor in a position of gaining personally if the consumer chooses the option being offered?
- What are the participation rates of that program? How many people joined, dropped out, or succeeded?
- How long did the successful people maintain their success?
- Who leads the program? What training and credentials does the leader have?

## TECHNIQUES FOR WEIGHING OPTIONS

In order to determine which option is more likely to fit personal needs, the client must decide what elements of any option are the most important. For instance, when Jan Kelly decided she needed to deal better with stress in her life, she was concerned about several issues when she decided to attend a stress management program:

**1.** *Cost:* Jan had little flexibility in her budget, so she needed a program that did not cost very much.

**2.** *Convenience:* She had strict working hours and a commute time of thirty minutes to and from work, so she needed an evening program that was either near her place of work or near her home.

**3.** *Individualization:* She disliked the idea of participating in a stress management group; she really wanted personal instruction and counseling.

The client may also want to visit the various educational programs available, on a trial basis, simply to gather information. If clients are unsure about a self-guided program using self-instructional booklets, they may check out the booklet from the library or from a voluntary health agency and review its contents.

Six techniques that can be used to weigh the pros and cons of each option are the balance sheet, the report card, rank ordering, the practicality-probability list, the value versus utility list, and imagined conversation. By using one or more of these techniques, clients can realistically appraise the options they have devised for reaching their personal goal. If no solution seems desirable, the client may choose to generate some more alternatives.

## Balance sheet

The balance sheet method was devised by Janis and Mann (1977). The grid helps clients evaluate each option on their list, according to whether it would result in

- Tangible gains and losses for self
- Tangible gains or losses for someone else
- Approval or disapproval of self
- Approval or disapproval by others

The grid highlights the client's most important criteria. The options can then be compared to each other in light of negative and positive criteria. For example, let us look at Jan Kelly's balance sheet in Table 10.1. She had determined that cost, convenience, and an individually tailored program were the criteria that best suited her situation. Her first alternative is to join a stress reduction class offered at her local medical center. Notice the difference between tangible gains and losses, and approval or disapproval. This technique also highlights the anticipated effects on the client as well as on significant people in the client's life.

## Report card and rank ordering

The next two techniques—report card and rank ordering—are very similar except for the initial instructions. In the report card method, the client uses the key decision criteria to grade each alternative. Because one of Jan's criteria was cost, she looks at each of her options and gives an "A" to the options that are more economical, a "B" to the options that are less economical, and so on. After grading all options, the client reviews the sum total of grades to see how the options compare with each other. Table 10.2 shows an example of the report card method.

In the rank-ordering method, the client applies the key decision criteria to rank the options. The ranking proceeds from the option that

**Table 10.1   Example of how to use the balance sheet grid**

| Alternative: Join a stress reduction class at the medical center | | |
|---|---|---|
| | Positive anticipations (+) | Negative anticipations (−) |
| 1. Tangible gains (+) and losses (−) *for self* | I'll spend less money on sleeping pills if I can learn to get to sleep without pills. | The class will cost money. |
| 2. Tangible gains (+) and losses (−) *for others* | My boss will get more quality work when I'm less anxious. | I'll have less time to volunteer at the Y if I go to this class. The volunteer coordinator will lose my filing and bookkeeping skills. |
| 3. Self-approval (+) or self-disapproval (−) | I'll feel better by feeling less anxious. I feel good about choosing a class near my home. | I'll feel resentful about going to a class after work when I'm tired and want to go home. |
| 4. Social approval (+) or disapproval (−) | My boyfriend, Charlie, will like being around me more when I'm more relaxed. | If my mother finds out that I'm going to a stress reduction class, she'll start nagging me to change jobs. |

SOURCE: The Balance Sheet Grid was developed by I. L. Janis and L. Mann, *Decision-Making* (New York: Free Press, 1977), p. 407. Reprinted by permission of the Macmillan Publishing Company. Copyright © 1977 by the Free Press, a Division of Macmillan Publishing Company.

**Table 10.2   Report card example**

*Options:*   1. Join a stress class at medical center.
2. Buy and use the book *How to Beat Your Stress.*
3. Begin a regular form of exercise.

| *Cost* | | *Convenience* | | *Individualization* | |
|---|---|---|---|---|---|
| Item 1 | C | Item 1 | A | Item 1 | B |
| 2 | A | 2 | C | 2 | A |
| 3 | B | 3 | B | 3 | A |

most closely matches the desired criteria to the option that least resembles the desired criteria. After each option has been ranked, the client reviews the rank order to note those at the top and those at the bottom of the list. The client chooses to act on options that are ranked at the top. Table 10.3 shows an example of the rank-ordering method.

## Practicality-probability list

Mahoney suggests a three-step technique for narrowing the list of options to those that are *possible, probable,* and *practical.* Clients are asked to look at their list of options and

**1.** Cross out options that are simply out of the question (too difficult, complex, or bizarre).

**2.** Cross out options that are potentially possible but are least likely to succeed.

**3.** Look for options that are practical in terms of criteria the client feels are most important.

Table 10.4 shows a sample worksheet illustrating Mahoney's method.

**Table 10.3   Rank-ordering example**

*Options:*   1. Join a stress class at the medical center.
      2. Buy and use the book *How to Beat Your Stress.*
      3. Begin a regular form of exercise.

| Cost | Item | Convenience | Item | Individualization | Item |
|---|---|---|---|---|---|
| Least expensive | 2 | Most convenient | 1 | Most tailored | 2 |
| | 3 | | 3 | | 3 |
| Most expensive | 1 | Least convenient | 2 | Least tailored | 1 |

**Table 10.4   Possible, probable, practical method: Example**

*Options:*   1. Join a stress class at the medical center.
      2. Buy and use the book *How to Beat Your Stress.*
      3. Begin a regular form of exercise.

Item 1. Practical
    2. Least likely to succeed
    3. Practical

**Table 10.5    Value versus utility method: Example**

*Options:*    1. Join a stress class at the medical center.

2. Buy and use the book *How to Beat Your Stress.*

3. Begin a regular form of exercise.

Joining a stress class and getting more exercise are the most appealing.

Joining a stress class seems the most practical, knowing that I probably won't read the book anyway and will find it difficult to get more exercise.

### Value versus utility list

The fifth technique assesses options on the basis of their value versus their utility. How appealing versus how useful in reaching the goal are the options? The client selects the options that best fit these two criteria. Table 10.5 is a sample worksheet illustrating the value versus utility method.

### Imagined conversation

The sixth and final technique offered here for weighing the pros and cons of each option is to imagine having a conversation with someone who takes a different viewpoint. When clients use this method, they think about conversing with someone who is trying to persuade them to choose or dissuade them from choosing a particular option. The client keeps track of various arguments that arise favoring or not favoring options available. For example:

> I am imagining that I am talking with my boyfriend Charlie about attending a stress class at the local medical center. Charlie points out that I am usually pretty tired when I come home from work. Would I faithfully attend a class that was in the evening? Charlie believes that starting an exercise program would be more practical. He points out that I would have the flexibility to exercise in the morning before work, during my lunch hour, or in the evening. I could also choose a variety of exercises, such as doing calisthenics with the morning television exercise class or walking briskly after dinner.

### ANTICIPATING THE FUTURE

Once a solution or suitable option is selected, another step must occur before action begins. An option may well suit clients' criteria, but obstacles may arise to thwart them in achieving their goals. If one reflects, one can often think up a list of individuals or events that could interfere with success. The best way to deal with the unexpected, both positive and negative, is to prepare. Hospitalized patients who have been told beforehand what to expect from certain procedures experience much less anxiety and fewer other stress-related symptoms than do patients who experience the procedures without preparation. Anticipating and preparing for future obstacles strengthens the chances that clients will actually achieve their personal goals.

We cannot predict the future, but we can still anticipate probabilities. We can imagine scenarios that represent the potential results of a particular action. The following list describes ways to plan for the impact of client decisions:

**1.** In a setting free of interruption and conducive to contemplation, have the client imagine five scenarios that involve the plan of action. Clients should describe scenarios rich in detail and should carry each to a resolution. They should imagine what they would do, how they would feel, and how the results of their decisions would affect family, friends, and their co-workers. Clients can also write out each scenario, describing their feelings, their actions, and the effects on family and friends.

**2.** Clients may choose to have friends or family members each assume a role of a person in the scenarios developed in the preceding exercise. What issues come up in the role play? (Clients should notice unexpected feelings or effects.)

**3.** Clients can imagine themselves ten to twenty years from now telling someone about their successes or disappointments that resulted from health decisions made today. This exercise may be done alone or with the help of a family member or with friends.

The health educator can use these exercises to help clients look beyond the present decision to its effect on their future. Whether or not these scenarios actually come true, the act of preparation can build clients' confidence in their abilities to meet future challenges. Preparing for the future may also lead the client to decide not to initiate the new health behavior at this time. This process keeps clients from attempting a change for which they are not fully prepared, and thus prevents frustration and failure in the future.

## MAKING THE COMMITMENT

The client who decides to begin a plan of action is ready for the final phase of the decision-making process: commitment to a course of action.

Formal commitment can be made through the use of contracts, oral or written. The client may contract with the health professional or a friend or a family member to attend a specific number of sessions of a program or to take certain action as part of a self-directed plan. Figure 10.2 is an example of a contract to be signed by a client and by a "buddy" who has agreed to work with the client on a specific action. The contract clearly states a goal and specifies actions to reach the goal, a time frame within which the goal is to be met, and a formal commitment to the actions and time frame. Both the client and the helper sign the contract.

Continuous recommitment to the personal goal and to needed action goes beyond a final formal agreement to begin an action. Recommitment involves a series of decisions the client makes on a daily and sometimes hourly basis that contribute to continuing the action toward the goal.

### Figure 10.2

**Two-Week Self-Contract: Plan to Increase Amount of Walking**

I will increase my average daily pedometer reading by an extra ¼ mile per day, from my present 2 miles to an average of 2¼ miles per day during the two weeks of this self-contract. I will enlist the help of

_____ .

My responsibilities:
1. To focus on increasing my walking while at work, especially during my lunch hour.
2. To reward myself on each day that I reach 2¼ miles on my pedometer with 30 minutes (or more) of reading for my own enjoyment. I will forego this reward if I don't reach my walking goal.
3. To record my data in my journal at 10:00 each night.

My helper's responsibilities:
1. To walk with me, when possible, during my lunch hour and to generally support my effort to exercise more.
2. To help me review the results of this action plan in two weeks.

Date: _____    Signed: _____

Review Date: _____    Helper: _____

SOURCE: Reprinted from *The American Way of Life Need Not Be Hazardous to Your Health*, by John W. Farquhar, M.D., by permission of the publisher, W. W. Norton and Co., Inc. Copyright © 1978 by John W. Farquhar, M.D.

This process is an element in the process of sustained change, which is addressed in Chapter 12.

The following list enumerates the conditions in the clients' environment that support the decisions they have made:

## Workplace

- Are co-workers encouraging my efforts to change?
- If co-workers are not encouraging my efforts, can I solicit their help or avoid them?
- Have I removed or can I avoid "Red Flags" to unwanted habits, such as ashtrays for nonsmokers, candy machines to those who are decreasing their sugar intake?
- Do I have appealing substitutes available, such as (for nonsmokers) gum, and fruit and vegetable strips for snacks?
- Do I have visible reminders to reward myself for small successes (both *internal rewards,* such as praising or reassuring myself that I am doing a good job, and *external rewards,* such as giving myself a quarter for every one-fourth mile I walk or taking a trip to a favorite place when I lose 10 pounds)?
- Do I have rewards planned or available soon after I succeed?

## Home

- Is there a family member or friend whom I have asked to be a "buddy"?
- Are there people whom I may ask to recognize my efforts to change?
- If a family member or friend is unavailable, have I planned for other ways to be recognized and rewarded; for example, have I prepared a list of rewarding activities I will do when I have reached a personal goal?
- Have I removed or can I avoid "Red Flags" to unwanted habits; for example, high-calorie snacks for nutrition changers, ashtrays for nonsmokers?
- Have I made my home conducive to my efforts—for example, placed exercise clothing within easy access, or arranged a place in my home for quiet contemplation?
- Do I have visible reminders to reward myself for small successes?

The list can help clients evaluate whether support for the goal is available from family and friends; whether it is possible to avoid temptations, at work and home, that may interfere with achieving the goal; whether it is possible, by substituting pleasurable alternatives, to avoid feeling deprived; whether rewards for successful accomplishments are readily available; and whether the clients can arrange their homes to enhance reaching their personal goals. Gaining the support of family, friends, and co-workers, rewarding successes, and arranging the home and work settings to aid personal actions all help clients keep up their commitment.

Rather than committing to an action for a long period of time, a client may choose to contract for a trial period. If the results during the trial period are less than expected or unsatisfactory, reevaluation and renegotiation may be in order. The client may choose to return to the initial decision-making process (defining the goal, generating alternatives, weighing pros and cons, and anticipating future events).

Health educators need to be chosen carefully for their ability to support clients in the decision-making process, no matter what choice the client makes and no matter what path the client chooses to get there. Instructors must be alert to their personal investment in the client's decision. "Knowing" what a client "should" do must not interfere with the client's choices, which only the client can make. Health educators need to be flexible, supportive, and nonjudgmental.

One of the toughest situations instructors face is the client's decision to not take action. But it may be just as appropriate for one client to *not* act on a health-related decision as it is for another to act. Instructors need to be skillful at assessing readiness, and this task is not easy. It is important for instructors to be able to negotiate an agreement that is satisfying to both the client and the instructor. Should the client decide to not take action, the instructor may suggest that they reexamine the goal at a specified date in the future. In the interim, the client may be able to clarify why he or she is hesitating. The pressure is thus taken off the client to commit to an action now, thus leaving the way open when readiness is stronger.

## INSTITUTIONALIZING THE DECISION-MAKING AND COMMITMENT PROCESSES

This chapter generally views the decision-making and commitment processes from an individual perspective. And it is true that the types of decisions we are talking about (those related to health actions) are carried out by individuals. However, designing educational programs and offering opportunities for health decision making is part of the program-planning process. In order for these programs to exist, they must be supported by organizational values. We believe that the decision-making and commitment processes are so important to the success of health actions that they must be a central part of all health behavior programs. For example, many stop smoking programs devote the first session to deciding whether or not to quit smoking. Participants are guided through a value clarification process to determine how deeply they are committed to quitting. Later in the program, ways to keep from smoking and prepare for problem situations are incorporated into the sessions.

Now, it may seem difficult to justify using the time, resources, and personnel of the organization to teach techniques of decision making. Supporting a seminar in decision making or lengthening existing seminars to include decision-making techniques each requires resources that already are spread thin. But the health educator need only point to the number of clients who repeat programs or who fail to adhere to prescriptions for health behavior change, to support the need for a new approach to commitment.

Educational programs often depict health behavior change as a one-time decision. Failure to prepare the consumer for the ongoing nature of decisions and change, however, is a failure of ethics. For example, preparing for future successes and obstacles has shown to be critically important in the success, over time, of problem drinkers learning to control their drinking. Failure to prepare clients to handle future problems is like sending someone down river in a boat without a paddle. Clients rarely accomplish change without the skills they need to cope successfully with obstacles that may arise in the home and work environment. These skills are usually complex and demand practice and professional guidance. For example, the dieter may need to learn how to be assertive enough to turn down offers of second helpings. The individual who has quit smoking may need to relax rather than having a cigarette.

In summary, deciding to pursue personal health goals is a process of making decisions over time. Teaching skills in decision making as well as in preparing for problem situations increases the chances that clients will attain their personal goals. The health educator in a medical care setting is in a pivotal position to help clients learn these skills. In addition, the health educator can design programs, supervise program planning, and educate other health professionals about the importance of client readiness to act, review of options, and preparing for challenge and commitment.

This chapter has provided important groundwork for the next, which helps us understand the role of the providers in creating an environment in the medical care delivery system whereby clients can, in fact, make sound decisions on behalf of their own health.

# EXERCISES

1.  Choose a decision you were faced with recently regarding your
    health. What or who prompted you to consider your health at that
    time? Had you been faced with this type of decision before? If you
    had been, what did you do then to resolve the situation (such as
    ignore making a decision, attempt an action)? If you selected an
    action regarding your health, how would you have filled out the
    following balance sheet (Table 10.6)?

Table 10.6   The balance sheet grid

| Alternative: | Positive anticipations (+) | Negative anticipations (−) |
|---|---|---|
| 1. Tangible gains (+) and losses (−) for self | | |
| 2. Tangible gains (+) and losses (−) for others | | |
| 3. Self-approval (+) or self-disapproval (−) | | |
| 4. Social approval (+) or disapproval | | |

SOURCE: The Balance Sheet Grid was developed by I. L. Janis and L. Mann, *Decision-Making*
(New York: Free Press, 1977), p. 407. Reprinted by permission of the Macmillan Publishing
Company. Copyright © 1977 by the Free Press, a Division of Macmillan Publishing Company.

2.  Put yourself in Jan Kelly's position and think about enrolling in that
    stress class at the local medical center. Think about going to the
    class for eight weeks, once a week after work.

What is the best possible outcome(s)? How would you feel? Would this affect your actions at that time in any way? Would your success have an effect on your friends or your family? How will they respond to your success?

What is the worst possible outcome(s)? How would you feel about this? How would your actions be affected? How would these negative results affect your family and friends?

What can you do now to enhance the chances that your decision will go the way you hope? How can you prevent the negative outcomes from occurring?

3.   You are a health educator in a Planned Parenthood clinic. You are interested in incorporating techniques for decision making in your clinic setting. How would you
   a. Justify this addition to your administrator?
   b. Incorporate these techniques in actual educational programs?

# RESOURCES

AHA/CDC Health Education Project. *Strategies to Promote Self-Management of Chronic Disease.* Chicago: Center for Health Promotion, American Hospital Association, 1982.

This publication describes a step-by-step approach in encouraging self-management on the part of a client with a chronic disease. Strategies are suggested such that if "A" does not work, then the practitioner can go to "B" or "C." The authors emphasize a partnership between client and practitioner in working toward increased adherence in chronic disease management. The publication is well referenced and contains an annotated bibliography.

Coates, T. J. *Counseling Adolescents for Dietary Change.* Dallas: American Heart Association, 1982.

Coates applied behavioral principles to the counseling of adolescents on dietary changes. The publication is exemplary because the process described involves step-by-step guidelines with examples and realistic expectations. Coates takes the reader through establishing rapport between counselor and the adolescent, analyzing needs, problem solving, involving friends and family, teaching skills on how to resist pressure, starting a strategy, maintenance, and tips for the counselor.

Horan, J. J. *Counseling for Effective Decision-Making*. North Scituate, Mass.: Duxbury Press, 1979.

Written for the practitioner in counseling, this book contains an abundance of information on the process of teaching how to make decisions. The style is humorous and clear, and the book is an excellent summation of the history and collection of techniques in decision making.

Janis, I. L., and Mann, L. *Decision-Making*. New York: Free Press, 1977.

Janis and Mann have produced a book that remains a classic in the field of decision making. This book is an extensive review and compilation of research on decision making. The authors promote their theory of decision making based on people's responses to facing a decision. The response can be (1) unconflicted adherence to the original course of action, (2) unconflicted change, (3) defensive avoidance of the need for a decision, (4) hypervigilance where action is impossible, and (5) vigilance. The book makes a substantial contribution to the field by going beyond the primary decision to the state of postdecisional conflict and offers several interventions to prevent this from occurring.

Wheeler, D. D., and Janis, I. L. *A Practical Guide for Making Decisions*. New York: Free Press, 1980.

This book transforms the theory and interventions in Janis and Mann (1977) into a book for the layperson. As the title states, this book is a practical, easy-to-read guide. The authors provide additional material on consulting experts and participating in group decisions.

# 11

# The role of self-care in medical care

$S$ELF-CARE PRACTICES, or those actions individuals take on behalf of their health, have significantly affected the delivery of medical care today. As consumers take on more responsibility in health care decision making, and as practitioners encourage their clients to participate more in decision making, conflict and cooperation are natural results. In this chapter we discuss the social forces that encourage self-care, the different types of self-care actions in medical care, and the benefits of and barriers to self-care.

## HISTORY OF SELF-CARE

Although the study of self-care practices has received considerable scrutiny recently, self-care has existed for as long as humanity has existed. Long before modern physicians and hospitals existed, people were using their grandmothers' remedy for colds, as well as herbs, potions, and other remedies for most of their ailments. Families cared for their members and for their neighbors; people handed down the traditional healing methods to younger people, through generations. For the most part, ill people were cared for at home until the early 1900s.

By the turn of the century, science had made progress and medical technology had become more reliable. Infectious diseases were being brought under control through the use of modern antibiotics and improved sanitary conditions. Overall, physicians and other health care professionals had acquired more effective diagnostic and treatment tools. Since medical technology and professional training for health professionals centered in hospitals, the care of illness became localized in hospitals and clinics. Health insurance plans grew. Private insurance, employer-based insurance plans, and government-sponsored insurance enabled clients to afford medical care, which was usually offered in the medical office and in the hospital setting. The expansion, predominance of, and reimbursement for services in hospitals and clinics increased the likelihood that sick people would seek treatment at these centers rather than at home. Self-care practices continued but were no longer the treatment of choice in the middle and upper classes.

Today, there is a resurgence of self-care practices. Evolving factors in society have contributed to the more prominent role of self-care practices today:

1. A growing consumer movement
2. The women's movement
3. The inadequacy of the present medical care delivery system
4. The economics of health service delivery
5. The prevalence of chronic disease
6. Increased accessibility and visibility of self-care information and products

In the following sections, we discuss these forces and the role each plays in propelling self-care to its present importance in the medical care delivery system.

Today's consumers are speaking up and demanding more regarding the products and services they pay for; they are more willing to criticize faulty merchandise and to demand quality service. Where there is no service, consumers are coalescing into neighborhood groups (for crime prevention, for example) or acting as voting groups to acquire services.

Legislation has supported the increased participation of consumers in policy making; consumer groups have been a powerful force in increased governmental regulation of business. The Community Action Programs (to provide social services for the impoverished) established under Title II of the Economic Opportunity Act of 1964 required consumer participation on program-planning boards. The Consumer Protection Act gave consumers the right to complain about poor workmanship of manufactured products, and gave them mechanisms to seek redress, and protection against retaliation by the manufacturer.

Consumers are also taking on tasks that had been done for them, such as car and home repairs. And consumers are consulting several professionals rather than taking one expert's opinion as fact. The consumer movement has encouraged the medical care consumer to demand quality services. Consumers are expressing the desire to be partners in the delivery of health care, to be members of the health care team. Insurance plans now pay for second opinions, and consumers are suing for malpractice. Consumers are becoming more informed about their health and are willing to press for quality health services.

In particular, the women's health movement has a long history of consumer participation. As early as the 1800s women were joining together to voice complaints about what they perceived to be inadequate medical care for women. The early complaints centered on women's reproductive rights and access to birth control. In the 1960s, the center of interest expanded to include all medical services available to women. Women accused the medical care system of paternalism, of putting more faith in medical tools and science than in the feelings and perceptions of women, and of failing to include women in medical decision making. Some women began to work together to provide alternative forms of health care services. Women's clinics opened in major cities throughout the country. Women increasingly moved to educate themselves about their own bodies and to inform themselves about alternative forms of care as well as about the adverse side effects of traditional care. Women have made political attempts to influence legislation to increase women's access to information and to demand quality medical care.

Many women believe that vaginal self-exams, breast self-exams, and the diagnosis and treatment of such problems as vaginal infections can be learned and carried out satisfactorily without a health care professional. The women's health movement has influenced medical care by (1) providing self-supporting alternative care, such as is offered by feminist clinics; (2) making strides in the removal of harmful products such as the Dalcon Shield I.U.D. and diethylstilbestrol (DES), which is an often-prescribed drug to prevent miscarriages; and (3) contributing to the increased visibility of women who speak out against sexism and substandard treatment of women in many other areas of American life, such as work, education, the law, and credit.

Women's clinics that are completely layperson-controlled still exist. However, formal medical care now offers more involvement for women. Women can have a say in forms of contraception they will use, for example, and what procedures the professional will follow in doing a breast biopsy. Some medical centers provide birthing rooms to make the birth process more homelike. These rooms are a direct result of women voicing their opposition to the overmedicalization of the natural birth process.

The active involvement of women in providing alternative forms of health care, such as feminist clinics and the accompanying changes in formal medical care, has influenced other areas of health care. Improvement is evident in emergency room procedures for the treatment of rape victims, the use of nurse practitioners (who are largely women) in education and direct care, and the expansion of abortion services to include counseling.

The women's health movement has had a powerful influence on how medical care is delivered today. Both men and women now reap the benefits of consumer-oriented medical care delivery. The movement typifies the extraordinary influence consumers can have in changing systems.

## INADEQUACY OF THE MEDICAL SYSTEM

The inadequacy of the traditional medical care delivery system has several facets. Not only has the present system failed to provide consistent high-quality medical services, but it has also failed to provide services equally across racial and socioeconomic groups (Milio, 1975). Likewise, people are realizing that medical services have a minimal impact on morbidity and mortality (Dubos, 1959; Carlson, 1976). The major health problems in developed countries are primarily chronic diseases such as atherosclerosis, hypertension, and diabetes, for which there are no cures. In the context of advanced scientific knowledge, this discrepancy creates a crisis of confidence in the medical care delivery system.

Hazards related to receiving medical care—called *iatrogenic effects*—further contribute to perceptions that the system is inadequate and that dependence on the system is not in the consumer's best interest (Illich, 1976). While hospitalized for surgery, for example, patients may contract an infectious disease unrelated to their presenting condition. A procedure to test for one illness may result in negative side effects requiring additional treatment. Levin (1980) summarizes the pertinent data: according to the Office of Technology Assessment, roughly 90 percent of all medical care procedures have not undergone reasonable scientific tests of efficiency and safety; between 5 percent and 7 percent of inpatient stays result in treatment for illnesses contracted as a result of hospitalization. In teaching hospitals, the rate increases to 20 percent.

Inequitable access to services, minimal impact on morbidity, errors in medical procedures, use of untested methods, and illnesses acquired as a result of hospitalization all lead naturally to dissatisfaction with the system and to a search for alternative forms of care.

Moreover, the economics of medical service delivery have hit the consumer where it hurts—the pocketbook. According to a joint Stanford University/University of California study, the average total expense of an initial physician visit as of 1977 was over a hundred dollars. As health care costs have escalated, some people have chosen, out of a need for sheer survival, to treat themselves instead of accepting the high cost of professional care. However, the incentive to self-treat does not come solely from the individual. The medical care delivery system itself is looking for ways to lower costs. The Blue Shield Association of America and other major insurance carriers are considering self-care as a way to lower costs (Levin, 1976). The insurance industry is developing proposals whereby consumers would be reimbursed for conducting preventive practices and for achieving fewer visits to health care professionals each year. Several incentive plans are underway on a pilot basis to give employees cash rebates for using their insurance coverage less.

Chronic diseases account for 80 percent of all disease today, as opposed to 30 percent fifty years ago. The medical care delivery system was well suited to responding to acute diseases; the adaptation to meeting the needs of people with chronic conditions has been slow. Money for health care resources is spent primarily on facilities and equipment designed to treat acute illness. Health care personnel are trained to treat acute illnesses and chronic illnesses as if the dynamics were the same. But chronic diseases such as hypertension and atherosclerosis require long-term treatment and significant changes in client lifestyle. To meet these needs, staff time, institutional resources, and enlightened professional preparation are needed. Many people feel that the system undervalues these necessary shifts and has not yet met the challenges.

Professionals and consumers both recognize that promoting health and reducing risk factors for chronic diseases can contribute to healthier lives. The Surgeon General's Report, *Healthy People* (1979), outlined the importance of prevention and consumer choices in improving the health of the U.S. population. Medical journals are increasingly filled with research supporting the correlation between daily habits and future health. The increased visibility of self-care is apparent in the popular press as well. Family magazines, talk shows, and the daily paper offer information on self-care products and practices. There are also mutual aid groups, such as Mended Hearts and Alcoholics Anonymous, and organized programs available to educate people in self-care skills. The increase in media attention, the proliferation of products such as self-care "how-to" books, home test kits for taking throat cultures and testing for levels of sugar in the urine, and professional and federal recognition of the role of lifestyle in future health have been proven to be a large impetus to self-care practices in the lay population.

## INTERACTION BETWEEN SELF-CARE AND FORMAL MEDICAL CARE

What role does self-care currently play in relation to the present health care system? In the next sections, we describe examples of the interaction between self-care and the formal system. As you read, keep in mind how each example answers these questions:

**1.** What do self-care and the formal medical care system contribute to each other?

**2.** Who initiates the self-care action; who is the primary health decision maker? Where does the control lie, with the consumer or with the provider?

**3.** What barriers prevent a smooth working relationship between self-care and formal medical care?

**4.** What role might the health educator play in each example?

### Provider-taught skills

Chronic or recurring acute back pain is a significant medical problem in terms of (1) prevalence; (2) physical, emotional, and monetary cost to the patient, family, and employer; and (3) demand on the medical care system. A back patient might visit a physical therapist for this problem. Whether or not the physical therapist promotes self-care skills during the visit can affect the patient's condition, feelings about the condition, and future visits.

On one hand, the patient may passively receive sonar treatments by the therapist. The patient, suffering pain and diminished capacity, has sought the skilled touch of the expert; at best the patient experiences great relief after one or several visits and goes home until the next time relief is needed. This patient may implement certain prescribed measures at home such as buying a therapeutic mattress or taking muscle-relaxing medications. But basically the patient feels at the mercy of unpredictable and incapacitating episodes of pain and is very dependent on the physical therapist for intervention at those times.

On the other hand, the scenario can be quite different if the physical therapist helps the patient learn skills and develop confidence in the patient's own ability to take more control of the situation. The patient can be actively involved in analyzing the home or work environment and recent physical activities to discover the causes of the problem. For example, does the patient sit at a desk all day, do heavy lifting and moving, or garden on the weekends? As causes are identified, preventive measures can be taught. For example, someone who sits at a desk all day can use a cushion that will support the small of the back. The patient can be taught to recognize the warning signs of an acute episode and to respond by performing specific exercises that will keep the problem from growing. These exercises can be practiced and demonstrated by the patient in the office and then applied at home. This latter approach decreases the patient's dependence on the system for curative action and, even more importantly, increases the patient's control over the recurrence of the problem condition.

The benefits of the self-care approach can be further extended by educators who offer preventive back care classes to well people. Good examples are a class offered to nurses to teach proper technique for turning and lifting patients, or any worksite class designed to teach preventive measures to avoid injury on a specific job. A general class designed to teach the correct way to perform common daily activities such as bending, lifting, standing, and even sleeping provides skills that help participants avoid unnecessary injury and unnecessary costs to themselves or to the medical care system.

## Self-care in home care

Any home health or public health nurse will tell you that a very large part of his or her job is teaching the patient and family to perform medical self-care tasks. In this branch of the medical care system, laypeople are taught and trusted to perform tasks that in a hospital setting are usually performed strictly by health care professionals. Examples include bathing and dressing the patient, turning the patient in bed, administering medicines, and changing dressings. Patients and caregivers are taught to monitor vital signs, when to call the nurse or doctor, how to make decisions about when and how much pain medication should be taken, and how to recognize when the job is too much to handle at home any longer.

Structuring the environment to support the medical self-care program is an important feature of self-care, and one that the home care approach uniquely fosters. The health professional working in home care can help patient and family design large or small changes in the physical setting that make it easier to perform the self-care activities. For example, moving the patient's bed into a more accessible location—downstairs, perhaps—may increase the patient's mobility and participation in activities. Designing a method of storing a variety of medications and recording their use may help assure a close compliance with a sometimes complex regimen. Figure 11.1 illustrates one method of organizing the medications for a whole week, a simple chart that is used to check off each dose as it is taken. Little boxes or trays with slots for each day's pills are

**Figure 11.1    Pill organizer for one week**

|  | Mon. | Tue. | Wed. | Thur. | Fri. | Sat. | Sun. | Name of Medication |
|---|---|---|---|---|---|---|---|---|
| Morning |  |  |  |  |  |  |  |  |
|  |  |  |  |  |  |  |  |  |
|  |  |  |  |  |  |  |  |  |
| Noon |  |  |  |  |  |  |  |  |
|  |  |  |  |  |  |  |  |  |
|  |  |  |  |  |  |  |  |  |
| Evening |  |  |  |  |  |  |  |  |
|  |  |  |  |  |  |  |  |  |
|  |  |  |  |  |  |  |  |  |
| Night |  |  |  |  |  |  |  |  |
|  |  |  |  |  |  |  |  |  |

available commercially or can be devised from cartons or other household objects, such as ice cube trays or egg cartons.

The benefits of the self-care component of home care accrue to all involved. They make sick care in the more personal and familiar home environment a possible alternative to the hospital. And home care can help cut the costs of professional and institutional care.

## Self-help groups

Self-help groups are integral to the self-care phenomenon and provide one of the best arenas for patients to develop self-care attitudes and skills. As many as 500,000 of these groups may be functioning in this country (Levin and Idler, 1981). Laypeople meet in these groups to deal with the full spectrum of issues related to physical and mental health. Topics that bring them together range from addictions and chronic conditions, to recovery from acute illness or surgery; from new parents learning infant care and development, to parents of murdered children coping with this trauma and loss; from elders networking to improve nutrition and safety, to women reclaiming primary responsibility for their reproductive health care. Self-help groups are made up of patients or their family and friends, or of well people solving or preventing problems that threaten their health.

A few common denominators in these groups are of particular interest. Groups are made up of laypeople with common experiences coming together to share information and support. Although health professionals may be involved in a variety of ways, an essential feature of self-help groups is that participants usually get past the undue dependency on the medical care provider that can develop at times of illness and life crises. Group members commonly break through the sense of isolation and helplessness that seem to be generated by these difficulties. At first they depend on the group for support, but they soon learn to give support in return to others sharing similar burdens. New and often unexpected personal strengths may emerge. Somehow, even the small victories of other group members nurture hope. It is the hope that unlocks a reservoir of personal energy that helps people to work toward improving things in their own lives as much as possible.

Renewed hope and strength may be the key contributions of self-help groups. But other outgrowths are also of importance to us. When people tap their strength, self-respect and confidence emerge. When people sense that they have some control over their health, they are more willing and able to take an active role in matters that affect their health. They may also be ready to try out a more equal relationship with their physician or nurse practitioner. No longer feeling passive, dependent, resentful, and resisting, patients begin seeing their doctor or nurse practitioner more as a partner in matters pertaining to their own health. The examples of others in the group who have worked through similar problems give people the opportunity to learn and give them the confidence to try new skills in self-assertion and communication. In some cases this step may be small; perhaps for the first time a patient gains the courage to ask the doctor to explain a treatment in a way that the patient understands. Maybe the patient simply finds other ways to get that information and therefore understands what the doctor says at the next visit. Not everyone wants or is capable of the same degree of self-care responsibility. Self-help groups allow participants the freedom to learn as much self-sufficiency skills from that group experience as they want or can handle.

Let us look briefly at some of the self-help groups and how they relate to medical care. Among the most easily integrated into the medical care system and the most common are groups like Reach to Recovery, Mended Hearts, and other volunteer visitor groups. In these programs, laypeople who have recovered from a particular medical problem themselves come to the hospital to visit others undergoing the same or a similar procedure. These volunteers share their personal experiences with the patient and present a picture of regained health, providing a model for that patient's successful recovery. Cancer support groups offering a variety of educational and emotional support services are increasingly available in hospital settings. Most teach self-care skills and acquaint participants with resources in the community that are available to help with a variety of problems often associated with living with cancer. Alcoholics Anonymous and programs modeled after it have been widely accepted by providers as helpful to a significant number of patients attempting the difficult task of regaining control over addictive behaviors damaging to health.

A vast array of volunteer health agencies and disease-specific foundations offer self-help resources that individuals may use with or without the referral of their provider. The Arthritis Foundation, American Heart Association, and American Diabetes Association, to name a few, offer a wide range of self-care information and support programs.

Medical care providers demonstrate varying degrees of enthusiasm for self-help groups. Some routinely refer their patients because they see these groups as able to provide services complementary to the medical treatment required and as able to effect a change where professional services have sometimes failed to do so. Other professionals do not see the benefits of self-help groups and, as a result, fail to refer patients to these resources. In the extreme, some professionals may denigrate the role of self-help groups, seeing these groups as sources of misinformation or as provoking undue anxiety in patients. Yet a growing body of research supports the therapeutic value of social support during critical periods in individuals' lives (Berkman and Syme, 1979; Mumford, Schlesinger, and Glass, 1982).

## Consumer health library

Another potential for a mutually satisfying interaction between self-care and medical care is found in the health library or information center for consumers. Health information centers are located within hospitals or clinics or are free standing. They make available a broad range of medical and health information resources in lay language. Health libraries may house lending or reference libraries, films, pamphlets and articles, information about educational and support programs and organizations, bookstores, or any combination of these services.

A health library for consumers is an asset in a number of ways. Laypeople can take the initiative to come in and look up a topic whether or not their provider encourages them to do so. Locating such a library in a medical care setting affirms patients' rights to learn as much as they want about their health or disease. Many of the books written for consumers use the workbook format or provide decision-making algorithms. These approaches help readers to design and implement self-care actions completely on their own if they want. These actions may range from treating the flu to planning an exercise program or adopting a diet that will reduce the risk of heart disease.

This type of resource center also assists self-care efforts by providing some quality control in selecting informational materials. The profusion of health and medical information in all forms of the media may sometimes produce more confusion than understanding. It can be very helpful to have knowledgeable professionals do some screening and selection of materials. The screening process need not be so strict that only a single narrow viewpoint is allowed expression. Figure 11.2 is a sample of an evaluation form that can be submitted to a practitioner, along with an item to be evaluated. It can be helpful to keep completed

**Figure 11.2   Health improvement center evaluation for reading materials**

**Health Library Evaluation Request**

The attached item _____ is being evaluated for:

_____ General distribution to patients in the health library

_____ Distribution only on the specific request of patients in the library

_____ Inhouse reading for patients in the library

Would you please comment on the following:

_____

Accuracy of facts

_____

Style and presentation of subject matter

_____

Objections that would limit its usefulness for purposes checked above

Please rate this item (Check one):

☐ Excellent   ☐ Very good   ☐ Good
☐ Fair        ☐ Poor        ☐ Unacceptable

Your name: _____ Dept.: _____ Date: _____

SOURCE: Designed by Caren Quay, M.S., Regional Health Library Consultant, Northern California Kaiser-Permanente Medical Care Program.

forms in file for reference later when reordering materials or making recommendations to consumers or other providers.

Consumer health libraries can be seen as a benefit to busy practitioners as well as to consumers. Providers who believe in the importance of patient education do not always have the time to complete all they want to cover during a few periodic visits. These health professionals appreciate the potential for improving the educational encounter by encouraging the active partnership of their clients. Health professionals are happy to have a resource center where patients can expand on the learning that began, but couldn't be completed due to time constraints, in the office or hospital. They are grateful to be able to offer a possible avenue of assistance to that group of patients who repeatedly come in with symptoms that are real but don't require medical treatment. Clients suffering stress-related symptoms, for example, may be able to learn to manage their stress based on information available in the center. Those who come to see the doctor every time they have a cold or flu virus may be able to learn self-care strategies for those viruses as well as how to determine when it is necessary to see a physician. Figure 11.3 shows a patient referral card to a health library. This type of preprinted card makes it easy for providers to refer patients to the health library. They just give it to the client and check the books or films they want the client to ask for in the library.

### Self-care workshops

A good example of the partnership between provider and layperson is the provision of opportunities for building self-care skills among two groups in the well population. The first group is the "worried well": those individuals who come to the medical care system seeking help not usually provided by that system; for example, mental health services, stress reduction, and problems with daily living that are not sickness related. The second group comprises those with acute illness that is not amenable to medical care; such as people who come in seeking relief from the common cold or flu symptoms. A number of opportunities are provided in medical care for these members of the well population to learn self-care skills. Such opportunities can (1) lower unnecessary visits to the health care professional, (2) increase the appeal of the medical care institution, (3) decrease absenteeism and temporary disability claims among the working population, and (4) expand the partnership between provider and consumer.

Most existing opportunities to learn self-care skills are presented as a series of seminars or workshops that emphasize access to information and skill building. They may be offered at the medical care site, such

**Figure 11.3   Referral form for health library**

---

**Referral Card—Films**

St. Elizabeth Community Hospital
9:00 A.M.–5:00 P.M. Monday–Friday

Allergy-Dermatology

_____ *Acne—Why Me?* 24 min.
_____ *Allergy* (Adult) 13 min.
_____ *Asthma* 12 min.
_____ *The 3-Leaf Story of Poison Oak* 8 min.

Cancer

_____ *Effects of Drugs* 30 min.
_____ *The Role of Emotions in the Treatment of Cancer* 41 min.
_____ *Learning to Live Without Cancer* 31 min.

Eye, Ear, Nose, Throat

_____ *Contact Lenses* 16 min.
_____ *Glaucoma* 13 min.
_____ *Nerve Deafness* 17 min.
_____ *Tonsils and Adenoids* 13 min.

OB/GYN

_____ *Freedom from Pregnancy* 9 min.
_____ *Hope Is Not a Method of Contraception* 17 min.
_____ *Tubal Ligation* 4 min.

---

SOURCE: Prototype developed by Caren Quay, M.S., Regional Health Library Consultant, Northern California, Kaiser-Permanente Medical Care Program.

as in hospitals or clinics; at various work settings in industry; or in neighborhood settings, such as churches, senior citizen centers, or neighborhood recreational centers. A medical care professional may or may not be involved in the seminars. These programs focus on similar topics:

**1.** Owning and operating medical tools such as a thermometer, blood pressure cuff, or otoscope.

**2.** Preparing the home for self-care such as acquiring bandages, antiseptic cream, and over-the-counter medications (such as aspirin, cough syrup, and antihistamines).

**3.** Learning when to see a health professional; for example, when certain acute symptoms arise such as unconsciousness, profuse bleeding, or broken limbs.

**4.** Learning self-care treatment skills such as emergency first aid and care of common maladies such as colds, flu, and nausea. A commonly used method of teaching treatment is the application of an algorithm or decision-making protocol. Figure 11.4 is a sample algorithm showing how to decide if a problem requires medical attention. This self-care algorithm instructs the client to observe symptoms and to decide on the course of action.

**5.** Learning how to interact more productively with the health care professional; for example, by asking questions, being specific about

**Figure 11.4    Self-care algorithm**

---

### Should You See a Doctor for This Cold?

Symptoms indicate complications that require medical attention.

1. Is your temperature greater than 101°F?

2. Have you had a cough for over one week that is becoming worse?

3. Are you short of breath with mild exercise? Chest pains? Wheezing?

4. Has your sore throat been present more than 4 days?

5. Do you think you have a fever (temperature greater than 100°F)?

6. Have you noticed any enlarged lymph nodes?

7. Have you noticed that your tonsils are enlarged?

8. Do you have ear or facial pain?

9. Have your symptoms lasted over 4 days?

Any of Questions 1–4 ⟶ Yes ⟶ Call to get appointment for today.

No

Any of Questions 5–9 ⟶ Yes ⟶ Make appointment for another day.

No

Great! Follow suggestions for self-care. ⟶ Rest, take temperature daily, and go through questions again if there are changes in your condition.

symptoms, and watching for and reporting unexpected side effects of medications.

**6.** Learning to keep home medical records that detail immunizations, major illnesses, and family histories of certain illnesses. Figure 11.5 shows an example of a home medical record.

Some hospitals and clinics are offering self-care courses to their own employees. From an employer's standpoint, self-care skills could improve morale and decrease medical care usage and absenteeism. From an employee perspective, health care professionals can be offered the opportunity to work with fellow employees, thus providing job enrichment. Hospitals are also beginning to offer self-care workshops to local companies. Reasons for hospitals' entry into worksite programs range from community service to increasing their visibility in the community for economic reasons (attracting consumers to that health care setting when medical care is required).

Self-care seminars broaden the potential influence of the informed consumer. The greater the number of consumers who acquire and use these skills, the greater the impact on the medical care delivery system. The potential impact is derived from consumers (1) making more appropriate use of services and (2) interacting in an equitable manner with their health care providers.

**Figure 11.5  Home health care record**

| | Health Record | | | |
|---|---|---|---|---|
| Name: _____ Date of Birth: _____ Blood Type: ____ | | | | |
| Date | Immunization/ Presenting Problem | Health Care Professional | Hospital | Treatment |
| | | | | |
| | | | | |
| | | | | |

## SELF-MANAGEMENT METHODS

As a self-care approach, self-management methods give clients the skills to initiate, carry out, and maintain health actions. These skills either can be learned from a health care professional or can be self-taught. The key idea is that health decisions and health actions originate with the individual consumer, not with the health care professional. This participatory model allows clients to direct their own health care, and to use the health care professional as a consultant.

Self-management is composed of three stages. Each stage requires various skills by the layperson:

**1.** *Self-monitoring:* Being aware of personal behavior and physical signs and symptoms

**2.** *Self-evaluation:* Comparing present behavior to expectations of appropriate behavior

**3.** *Self-reinforcement:* Administering personal rewards for behavior that meets the client's expectations

These stages require that individuals be able to (1) observe their own behavior, (2) establish standards of appropriate behavior, (3) seek support from others or make the environment more conducive to the health action, (4) evaluate personal behavior, and (5) establish a reward system dependent on the appropriate health action.

The self-reward system is especially important. One payoff of self-management methods is the increased sense of personal control. This reward may result in increased self-esteem, increased motivation to continue the health action, and/or confidence to initiate other actions.

### Deterrents

Some clients find self-care frightening because they are not familiar with self-management. Kanfer (1980) outlines specific types of clients who may run into initial difficulty:

**1.** *Some clients have developed lifelong patterns of dependency on professionals.* Early sessions with such clients can offer small steps at self-management, which are gradually increased.

**2.** *Some clients are afraid of risks.* Reducing their fear of the unknown may be the first step a health educator needs to take.

**3.** *Clients who have not been rewarded for their efforts soon learn not to make efforts.* For example, if a client loses five pounds and no one notices, the frustrated client may quit trying. Lack of recognition for progress may lead, over time, to a failure to initiate any program of change. Gradual change as well as success and rewards help to increase the clients' belief in their own ability to change.

**4.** *Clients may simply lack skills.* Learning and practicing skills in the home and work settings help to overcome this obstacle.

**5.** *Clients who are rewarded for inappropriate behaviors may be reluctant to change.* For example, when a client drinks a couple of glasses of wine before a social event, becomes relaxed, and then is praised at the event for acting so calm and relaxed, it will be more difficult to give up the wine before social events. The feeling of relaxation and the praise are rewarding or increasing the likelihood of drinking wine before social events. These clients may need help in weighing the pros and cons of change.

Once the client and educator recognize and overcome these deterrents to self-management, they begin a process of goal clarification, self-monitoring, and designing a plan of personal action. (For more detail on this process, read Chapter 10, "Techniques for Making Decisions and Commitments."

## Benefits of self-care

The six examples just discussed illustrate many of the benefits to be gained by integrating self-care and medical care. These benefits accrue to both consumers and the medical care system. Let us summarize those benefits, first from the consumer viewpoint and then from the viewpoint of the medical system. Notice that although we separate the two for purposes of discussion, it is hard to separate them in fact. Often what is advantageous to consumers in many ways benefits the system, and the benefits to the care delivery system positively affect consumers.

A characteristic outcome of self-care is increased skill on the part of consumers. Whether the skill is gained in a self-care class or in an office visit, consumers come away able to do something for themselves that they were not able to do before. The resulting sense of competence is both a reward and a further incentive for assuming self-care responsibility. The ability to make a decision and initiate action gives consumers more control over their lives. The patient or caregiver in the home care situation, as well as the visitor to the consumer health library who uses the information to plan a personal health promotion regimen, both experience this sense of greater control.

The consumers' increased sense of control and competence have a positive effect on their self-esteem, which may affect their relationship with their medical care provider. Where an active role is assumed by a patient and encouraged by the provider, adherence to medical regimens and positive health outcomes can be improved (Stone, 1979). Therefore, the consumers' encounters with medical care can be enhanced by the application of self-care.

Consumers can also save money to the extent that self-care skills can help consumers avoid illness and injury or better manage a chronic condition. The consumer may save in lower insurance deductibles, premiums paid by employers may decrease, and unnecessary use rates in the medical care setting may decline.

What benefits does the medical care system derive by incorporating self-care approaches? The system certainly benefits when the satisfaction of its consumers is increased. When clients improve their adherence to medical regimens and improve their health status, provider satisfaction increases. Provider satisfaction is increased when self-care programs and services help providers be more effective in the educational component of their practices. Both the support group for the cancer patient and health library services, for example, supplement what providers can do in the short time they have with patients.

The system even benefits from the sometimes abrasive encounters it experiences with consumers who are oriented toward self-care. The women's health movement may have arisen in part out of dissatisfaction with the formal medical care system, but ultimately the exchanges between the representatives of the movement and of the system have brought some very positive changes to the formal system. In the context of a society that places such a strong emphasis on technology in medicine, the women's health movement and other self-care spokespeople have provided a needed humanizing influence.

## WHO CONTROLS CARE?

We feel that the client should control the outcome of medical treatment, and that the treatment itself should be a team action. The issue of control involves the questions "Who initiates the self-care action; who is the primary decision maker? Does control lie in the hands of the consumer or in the hands of the provider, or do both consumer and provider share in the decision making related to health care actions?" The previous examples point to a variety of working relationships between medical self-care and the formal system of health care delivery. In some cases the consumer may initiate, and in others the health care provider predominates. Figure 11.6 is a self-care professional interaction scale. The scale describes a continuum of interaction between consumers and professionals.

**Figure 11.6  Self-care/professional interaction scale**

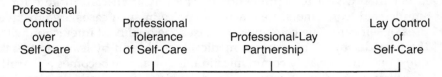

In the first category, "Professional control over self-care," a good example is some physical therapists' relationship to the patient in the treatment of back pain. As the expert, such a physical therapist maintains authority over what preventive, diagnostic, and treatment techniques he or she approves and shares with patients. Here, the patient is basically following the instructions of the professional.

"Professional tolerance of self-care" is expressed in the situation where the professional maintains some control over decision making, but the consumer initiates more actions. In our example of self-help groups, health professionals may be involved as organizers or leaders of the groups. The professional may believe in these benefits while also remaining invested in professional training as the ideal form of leadership. In addition, participation in self-help groups such as Reach to Recovery and Mended Hearts is initiated through physician referral within the hospital setting. In this example, the professional retains some control over who participates and, by referring the patient, sanctions the usefulness of such groups in the recovery process.

The consumer health library provides another example of "professional tolerance of self-care." Within a medical care setting, the review process for approving materials for the health library may be limited to the expression of only one viewpoint. Providers may tolerate the existence of the resource but might not refer their patients. Other providers may see the resource as a complement to their care.

However, the consumer health library is also an example of the next category on our interaction scale, the "professional-lay partnership." Professionals may often refer clients to the library as a means to increase the clients' involvement in care. The health library may be readily accessible in the medical care setting; providers can encourage both the well consumer and the patient to take advantage of information and tools for health actions.

Self-care workshops provide skills for the consumer to play a more active role in the professional-lay partnership. The skills in home diagnosis and treatment strengthen the consumer's ability to use professional services more appropriately. For example, consumers may diagnose a cold or fever and may decide they require rest and increased fluid intake rather than a visit to a professional. The physician can do little for a simple cold; consumers' treatment of choice in such cases are effective uses of self-care. The consumer increases the quality of interaction with the provider by keeping home medical records and by learning to ask questions and to clarify communication. Medical care becomes a sharing of information between consumer and provider. This sharing of decision making has been encouraged, for example, by the women's health movement. Today women are more active in making decisions about birth control, birth practices, and surgical procedures such as breast biopsies and hysterectomies. In a satisfying home care relationship, there is a partnership between the patient and family members and the professional. The professional gives prescriptions and makes recommendations and the family provides the treatment. A give-and-take in providing health care is possible.

Self-management techniques offer another opportunity for equitable interaction between the client and professional. In our example of the traditional physical therapist and patient, a self-management program could be initiated that would help the patient increase activity level (back exercises, regular walking) or in pain control (decreasing use of medications). The physical therapist could guide the patient through the stages of self-management by clarifying the skills required at each step. The client could select a goal (regular walking), choose a time frame (walk each day), specify the extent of activity (walk one mile), and design a reward system (for each mile walked, save one dollar toward a special trip). Clients would be responsible for monitoring the activity each day and for consistently rewarding themselves for progress. The physical therapist would be available for consultation.

As an example of "lay control of self-care," books and pamphlets on self-management techniques could be made available in the health library for a consumer who seeks help in initiating a health activity or in decreasing an undesirable habit. The consumer would check out a book on self-management and design a personal action plan. For example, the client may want to stop smoking. The client could check out the American Lung Association packet *Freedom from Smoking in 20 Days* (1980). By following its guidelines, the client would keep track of the number of cigarettes smoked daily, how progress would be recorded, and what rewards would be given for progress. The client would be responsible for all stages of the personal plan.

Women's clinics exemplify another source of "lay control of self-care." Women can teach other women how to do breast self-exams and vaginal exams, and they can run rape crisis centers for women on a peer basis.

The continuum of interaction between self-care and professional care includes a variety of relationships. The interaction ranges from professional control to lay control, with a diverse array of relationships in between. Self-care takes on different definitions in each of these settings. Sometimes one party wants more control than the other party is willing to give up. Or, conversely, one party may want the other to take on more than the other is willing. These barriers to a smooth working relationship are discussed in the next section.

## BARRIERS TO ESTABLISHING SELF-CARE

The previous examples of interactions between self-care and professional care show the different professional and consumer roles and the responsibility each takes in achieving optimum health. Given the varying degrees of receptivity to self-care on the part of clients, providers, and institutions, what is the role of health educators in medical care regarding self-care? Where do their responsibilities and loyalties lie when conflicting values, needs, and desires exist?

Health education philosophy is consistent with the principles of self-care. The following excerpts from the Code of Ethics of the Society of Public Health Education (a national professional organization of health educators) speak to this issue:

- I value the privacy, dignity, and worth of the individual, and will use skills consistent with these values.

- I will observe the principle of informed consent with respect to individuals and groups served.

- I will support change by choice, not by coercion.

- I will foster an educational environment that nurtures individual growth and development.

To assure optimum consumer-professional interaction in self-care, the health educator in medical care must weigh the individual's needs with program objectives while being aware of organizational policies toward self-care. Barriers to a cooperative relationship may become more apparent when the health educator can find the answers to the next series of questions.

### Consumer problems

The first question to ask is "What are the needs and desires of the consumers you are serving? How much do they want a role in caring for themselves?" This question is hard to answer, because there are fine lines among (1) not being involved in self-care because of a need to depend on the health professional, (2) a lack of interest or value in self-reliance, (3) a desire to get a return on one's money for services rendered, and (4) not being involved because of lack of skills in self-care. Research is being conducted to devise a scale that measures consumer receptiveness to self-care (Krantz, Baum, and Wideman, 1980; Green and Moore, 1980). However, until such a scale is perfected, the health educator must gauge receptiveness. To what extent is the client ready for self-care? The following list of questions provides a guide:

**1.** Has the client requested more involvement in health care decisions? What reservations has the client expressed: Fear of doing something wrong? Lack of skills? Feeling that care is not the client's responsibility?

**2.** Is the client willing to learn a self-care skill?

**3.** How supportive are family members and friends to self-care practices? Are they willing to learn self-care skills? Or do they consistently forget self-care training appointments and fail to follow instructions at home? Are they supporting the client's self-care skills? Do they encourage practice? Or do they make practice more difficult through criticism or failure to encourage?

**4.** Do consumers have access to self-care information?

**5.** Do consumers have the means to evaluate self-care information and products?

In some cases, especially in prepaid medical plans, consumers may feel that the institution is not giving them a fair return on their investment if professionals are encouraging self-care. Some consumers want providers to make decisions and perform all medical care tasks. They do not want home care; they want to go to the hospital. They may resent being asked to assume more responsibility, preferring to call on the health professional at every turn.

Besides wanting their money's worth of service, a closer look at this group of consumers may indicate that they are really seeking something from these visits and calls other than the necessary medical treatments. People who overuse the medical practitioner often have social or emotional needs that their caring health professional is partially meeting. Support services may offer a more satisfying and potentially more productive means of meeting those needs. The kinds of self-help groups discussed earlier in this chapter can provide one such means of support. Studies have shown that self-care classes for seniors can divert a number of visits and calls from the one-to-one provider-patient encounter into a social, health-promoting learning situation (Nelson et al., 1982). This could be a healthy alternative to overdependence on the provider. In this way, self-care can contribute to appropriate use of medical services and can benefit the consumer as well.

When tension arises, however, it is probably most often expressed by consumers desiring more self-care responsibility than the provider is ready to support. This is especially true if some of the consumer's choices include alternative treatments, such as meditation or biofeedback, with which the provider is unfamiliar.

Two factors have contributed to health professionals' reticence to embrace self-care philosophy and practice. One is that providers believe that their years of special training give them the necessary information and make them the most suited to tell patients what to do in matters of health and disease. The other is that the training or personal experience of many health professionals may have given them little opportunity to engage in the kind of educational activities or group support experiences that health educators employ to stimulate clients' personal responsibility, sense of control, and growth. Recently, the training of health care professionals has been changing dramatically to include interpersonal skill training. However, a substantial number of practicing professionals remain who were not exposed to educational techniques and communications skills.

Let us now look at some ways in which provider and patients express this resistance. We will consider the impact this resistance has on self-care and discuss possible avenues open to the health educator in dealing with the situation.

Providers sometimes feel patients are better off having *less* information; they may believe that more facts will only confuse and frighten patients and may possibly undermine the patient-doctor relationship. This attitude can affect how much a doctor will offer in the way of information as well as the doctor's level of comfort with patients attending support groups or visiting a health library, for instance. Moreover, with the proliferation of support groups and health information in the media, the physician has less control now over the information to which patients have access. The physician may be concerned with the *quality* of this information.

The health educator in the medical care setting can elicit provider support at least for the programs and information offered in that setting. The health educator can establish a procedure for engaging providers in a review of the educational materials to be distributed or used in programs. A simple evaluation form such as the one pictured in Figure 11.2 can be used to elicit providers' comments. This form is also a way to educate health practitioners about quality health education materials and increases the likelihood that they will make use of these resources in their practice when appropriate.

If patients are expressing a desire for a support group in a medical setting, and providers in general seem uninterested or concerned about the impact of that group, the health educator may be able to find one sympathetic practitioner with whom to explore the possibility. Preferably the provider is one who specializes in the topic area. That person's involvement in designing and implementing the program can allay the fears of other providers. The health educator can also establish health parameters for the group. A lay support group is not meant to replace professional medical diagnosis and treatment, but to supplement it. Providers can be invited to these groups occasionally to act as resource people to answer questions about treatment. The more personal experience providers have with support groups, the more likely they are to refer their patients to them.

The busy doctor or nurse may also be concerned about the amount of time taken by the patient who has many questions or who wants to be satisfied that a particular treatment or procedure is necessary. It is easier to keep visits brief if patients do not raise questions or debate the professional's recommendations. This problem points to another dilemma for health educators when they design self-care programs: are we providing a service to patients and consumers by teaching and encouraging self-care in an environment where such activities may not be welcomed? Certainly we must prepare consumers for realistic expectations and strategies for dealing with the reception they might encounter. For instance, role playing an encounter with an unreceptive professional may help the consumer develop effective communication skills. Teaching *assertive* questioning (as opposed to *aggressive* questioning) increases the chances for a successful experience for consumers who want to assume more responsibility in their health care.

Many practitioners believe in the value of education as part of medical care but lack the time or skills to fully educate every patient. Self-care programs and resources can help these providers in meeting their educational goals for their patients. The astute health educator will find ways to let providers experience the satisfaction available to them in being able to direct their patients to these supplementary educational resources. One way to accomplish this would be to establish a simple referral system incorporated into the provider's practice.

The health educator working in medical care has a unique opportunity to change the climate of the institution from within. This is best done in small steps by (1) broadening the base of knowledge and experience of self-care within the organization and (2) building the credibility of the program by assuring some early successes that providers can appreciate.

## Programmatic barriers

On the program-planning level, barriers to self-care may arise from three sources: the extent of support for self-care from consumers, the lack of support from health professionals, and the lack of resources. Here are some questions that you can seek answers to before you plan self-care programs:

**1.** Do the consumers in your environment request self-care programs?

**2.** Do the health professionals request self-care programs?

**3.** Have health professionals expressed the fear that self-care skills will replace the need for paid professional services? How realistic is that fear in this setting?

**4.** Are there sufficient resources to teach self-care skills? What about money? Personnel? Equipment? Space?

**5.** Are there opportunities within health education programs to practice skills and renew those skills in the future?

If the answers to these questions reveal that there is a great deal more preparation to do before self-care programs can be implemented, the educator need not give up. Rather, the answers to these questions will help the educator to put in priority order those planning strategies that will ensure the best environment and foundation for self-care activities in that organization.

## Institutional barriers

Barriers at the institutional level center around administrative attitudes, the institutional climate, and the economic incentives for the organization. Here are some questions to ask:

**1.** Do departmental protocols for treatment include self-care skills?

**2.** Is there financial support for self-care resources such as health libraries or self-care classes for employees?

**3.** What avenues exist in the organization for consumers to voice dissatisfaction with services?

**4.** What economic incentives are there for the organization to support self-care practices? Is this organization a fee-for-service system or a prepaid health plan?

Because of an excess of hospital beds in some communities and subsequent competition among hospitals, some hospitals have offered self-care and health promotion programs as a way of attracting consumers. The practice of offering programs for this purpose puts the health educator in a difficult ethical position. The professional health educator is serious about offering programs that effectively promote health and prevent disease. If the hospital is using these self-care programs primarily to attract consumers, then the implied and real expectations differ. Once again, being aware of the conflicting interests, the health educator acknowledges the limits of such services and helps ensure that expectations of consumers, providers, and administrators match the real potential of educational programs.

In summary, the first step in overcoming barriers is to be aware of them. The next step is to determine how feasible it is to overcome those barriers. In answering these questions, the health educator takes the first step.

## JOIN THE REVOLUTION

We have covered a wide range of factors, implications, and possible solutions for health educators who try to stimulate self-care in medical care settings. We think that the arenas in which the integration of self-care and medical care is taking place are among the most exciting in which to be practicing health education. There is in fact a revolution underway right now as these two large and powerful forces bump, clash, and discover new, complementary roles. The rewards of finding successful ways for the two to interact are many. The opportunity for health educators in medical care to contribute to this movement is significant and challenging.

# EXERCISES

1.  Think of the last time you made a choice between treating yourself for a health problem and seeing a health professional. What were the deciding factors that made you choose the course you did? Was the experience positive or negative? What can you learn from your own experience that can be applied to your role as a health educator who will offer self-care opportunities to others?

2.  The Over Sixty Clinic in Berkeley, California, encourages self-care in its health services for senior citizens (see Resources section).

What benefits do you think might exist for the clinic in doing so? What benefits might exist for the clients?

3.   Choose a medical care setting with which you are familiar. Select a self-care project you would like to develop in this setting. Analyze the setting for barriers to self-care. If barriers exist, suggest two solutions and describe how the solutions would help solve the problem.

# RESOURCES

Barry, P. Z., Pezzullo, S., Beery, W. L., De Friese, G. H., and Allen, W. J. *Self-Care Programs.* Chapel Hill: Health Services Research Center, University of North Carolina, 1979.

This booklet is a result of a conference held in Battle Creek, Michigan, in 1978. Experts from around the United States gathered to discuss the dimensions, expected outcomes, and risks associated with self-care; evaluation issues; possibilities for program development; and the broader implications for self-care within the context of the health system.

Berkeley Over Sixty Health Center, 1860 Alcatraz, Berkeley, California 94703. (415) 644-6060. Thomas White, Assistant Director.

The clinic was established in January 1976 by the Gray Panthers. It offers comprehensive primary care services within the context of promoting self-responsibility and positive health habits for senior citizens.

Ferguson, T. (ed.). *Medical Self-Care.* New York: Summit, 1980.

In this compendium, Ferguson has collected many articles from past issues of the journal *Medical Self-Care.* He has added new material to provide a well-rounded reader for individuals interested in taking an active self-care role in treating disease and maintaining health.

Gartner, A., and Riessman, F. *Self-Help in the Human Services.* San Francisco: Jossey-Bass, 1979.

This book provides an overview of self-help groups in the United States. Gartner and Riessman describe the different forms of self-help groups, why they succeed, their promise for the future, and inherent limitations.

Health Activation Network, P.O. Box 923, Vienna, Virginia 22180.

An organization that actively promotes the concept of skill building in the arena of self-care. HAN consults with organizations to provide courses in health activation or self-care skills.

Katz, A. H., and Bender, E. I. *The Strength in Us: Self-Help Groups in the Modern World*. New York: Franklin Watts, 1976.

This book discusses mutual aid groups in the United States and other countries. The authors trace self-help groups through history, discuss the range of purposes of self-help groups and their relationship to professionals, and propose future possibilities.

Levin, L. S., and Idler, E. L. *The Hidden Health Care System: Mediating Structures and Medicine*. Cambridge, Mass.: Ballinger, 1981.

The authors develop the premise that organized groups of individuals (the family, organized religion, volunteer organizations, neighborhoods, and ethnic and racial groups) provide an extensive nonprofessional health care system. Levin and Idler maintain that the primary providers of health care are laypeople. The future of health care will inevitably be affected by the recognition of the power in the existing network of laypeople.

Levin, L. S., Katz, A. H., and Holst, E. *Self-Care: Lay Initiatives in Health*. New York: Prodist, 1976.

This book is based on the proceedings of a symposium on "The Role of the Individual in Primary Health Care," held in Copenhagen, Denmark, August 1975. The book discusses what self-care is, its function in primary care, the potential for self-care in the future, and research issues.

*Medical Self-Care*, P. O. Box 717, Inverness, California 94937.

This bi-monthly journal is written primarily for the layperson. It contains articles, resources, and brief synopses of current medical literature pertaining to those actions individuals can take to diagnose, treat, and prevent illness and to promote a state of well-being.

Parker, P., and Dietz, L. N. *Nursing at Home*. New York: Crown, 1980.

This comprehensive handbook is for people who find themselves taking on the role of home nurse for a friend or loved one. Explanations, instructions, and illustrations address each of the many tasks the care partner will face. The authors also do a nice job of discussing the relationship between the caregiver and patient: the fears and expectations of each and a positive approach to a constructive and nurturing partnership. This book is written to increase the confidence as well as the knowledge of the lay reader.

Rees, A. M. *Developing Consumer Health Information Services*. New York: Bowker, 1982.

This resource book is for librarians and those in a position to evaluate and manage the provision of health information services and programs. It contains chapters on medical consumerism, health library programs, program development and management, and networking.

Rusek, S. B. *The Women's Health Movement*. New York: Praeger, 1978.

> Rusek describes, in a substantially referenced and detailed manner, the origins of the women's health movement, the historical relationship between providers in the health care delivery system and women, strategies for changing the system, and an overview of social movements in general. The perspective taken is that of a sociologist and feminist.

Self-Help Clearinghouse, Graduate School and University Center/CUNY, 33 West 42nd Street, Room 1206A, New York, New York 10036.

> This organization provides a central source for self-help groups from all over the United States, as well as resources in the field of self-help. Produces a monthly newsletter, *The Self-Help Reporter.*

Watson, D. L., and Tharp, R. G. *Self-Directed Behavior.* 2nd ed. Belmont, Calif.: Wadsworth, 1981.

> After discussing the principles of behavior, the authors outline the necessary steps in a program of self-determined change. They discuss specifying the problem, analyzing reinforcers, intervening evaluation, and termination of the initial plan of action. Throughout these steps, the reader is encouraged to practice the skills in the exercises at the end of each chapter. The book is written for both the practitioner and layperson.

# 12

## Maintaining changes over time

AN IMPORTANT RESPONSIBILITY of health educators is designing and offering programs that provide for the long-term maintenance of our clients' desired health behavior changes. As discussed in Chapter 11, self-care is itself a way to maintain health behavior change, because it involves the patient in his or her own treatment. In this chapter we use two case studies to examine factors that contribute to lasting change. Among the range of factors discussed are clients' personal needs, expectations, and support; program design; appropriateness for particular clients; involvement of providers; and organizational reinforcement, continuity, and motivation. The best possible way of assuring lasting change may be to foster clients' skills and confidence in their ability to deal with the dynamics that determine their state of health. Programs can be designed and institutional policies developed to help achieve these goals. By helping our clients experience a sense of control over their lives, we leave them with a touchstone for future success.

John Wright is forty-seven years old. He is married, has two children (ages nine and fourteen), and has worked for TNI Manufacturing Company for ten years. He considered himself in good health until now— but he is presently a patient in Southern Memorial Hospital, just diagnosed as a heart attack victim.

Through the recovery period at the hospital, John discusses his health with the physician, the dietitian, the physical therapist, the social worker, and his family. Having received many recommendations to alter his diet, exercise more, and to stop smoking, John vows he will make these changes to prevent another heart attack. He and his wife, Lori, attend presentations on the healthy heart at the hospital, and both acquire a number of pamphlets on different topics. Once home, John and Lori continue to attend the Healthy Heart Program, but this time the program includes seminars designed for outpatients. In addition, he joins a cardiac exercise program. Eight months later, he has been able to modify his diet, and he is walking two miles a day. However, he has not stopped smoking.

Sheila Brown is an active, healthy-looking woman of twenty-eight. For the past four years, she has been employed in a high-pressure administrative job. Because of her talents, her company has moved her rapidly up the corporate ladder. Every twelve to eighteen months she has been assigned to a new position, requiring adjustments to new working relationships, new job content, and a new working environment.

At the same time, her personal life has not been without stress; one long-term relationship has ended, and she is now involved in a new one and experiencing difficulties with it. During this period, she has experienced a wide variety of physical symptoms, ranging from sleeplessness to chronic headaches and stomach pain. On one occasion she suffered numbness in her face and arm, accompanied by dizziness. These symptoms worried her and prompted her to seek medical advice on several occasions, resulting in expensive laboratory tests and neurological work-ups, including a computer tomography (CT) scan and electroencephalogram (EEG). Each time the doctor was unable to identify a physical cause for the symptoms; he suggested that Sheila was working too hard and should try to relax. At the time of the last visit, the doctor recommended a stress management class that was offered by the local public health department as part of their new health promotion program. Sheila eagerly signed up and attended three of the four sessions. She found the class informative and learned some relaxation techniques she thought would work for her.

After the class was over, however, the stressors in her life remained unchanged. She tried to apply her new skills to manage her stress level and experienced occasional success. But she found that when she was most in need of the relaxation techniques, she was least likely to do them, or could not perform them effectively. Her symptoms continued.

## WHAT FACTORS BLOCK CHANGE?

When some people attempt to change a long-standing habit or initiate a new habit, they succeed and are able to maintain the new behavior; other people make a change but then seem to relapse to old ways. Why? Many health care professionals assume that as long as they instruct a patient or client regarding a given health habit change, and the client has understood those instructions, the change will be made. Furthermore, they give little thought to whether the change will last or how to make it last.

Many consider information the key; once it is shared, change should occur. Physicians have given out countless brochures on weight control; dietitians have given hundreds of meal plans to newly diagnosed diabetics; health educators have planned and offered numerous classes to help people make changes related to their health. Yet we continue to see patients and clients who, even with the firmest convictions, attempt a change and, not long after, find themselves in the old habit pattern. The result is, both patient and provider conclude that health education doesn't work.

Often the provider blames the client. Considerable research has been devoted to the noncompliant patient (Haynes, Taylor, and Sackett, 1979). Some of the factors studied in an attempt to understand this noncompliance include length of time between intake and appointment, sex, age, socioeconomic status, complexity of the prescribed regimen, and the communication pattern between health care provider and patient. Few definitive answers have emerged to the question of why some patients do not carry out instructions over a period of time. A number of studies point to poor communication between provider and client as a key factor in noncompliance (Stone, 1979). Other studies highlight the failure of programs to tailor approaches to individual needs, the lack of rewards in correctly carrying out the regimen, the absence of formal commitment such as a contract on the part of the provider and client, and the failure to include the client in assessing progress (Dunbar, Marshall, and Hovell, 1979).

To further complicate matters, knowledge about sustained change is weakened by poor follow-up over time. Few health care professionals can afford the luxury of following their clients' progress when the clients no longer make regular visits to the health care setting. This difficulty exists in the outpatient or industrial medicine clinic as much as in the hospital. Long-term follow-up is rarely done.

The client often feels caught in a recurring cycle. The pattern starts with the client wanting to make a change. He or she then tries to make the change by (1) following a book, (2) designing a personal self-management program, or (3) joining an organized group of some type. The client may have an initial success but eventually returns to the original habit. And then the client has feelings of failure and hopelessness, of ever being able to really change. We've all heard the joke "I've lost hundreds of pounds—the same 25 pounds over and over again!" We laugh, but the dilemma is really quite serious. This recurring theme results in a diminished sense of control over one's life and a decreased probability that this goal—or any others—will ever be realized.

Repeated failure to maintain a desired behavior affects the provision of health care, too. Expensive services might have been avoided if the client had taken early action. Practitioners become frustrated by clients who do not maintain their health-related regimens. Sustaining actions over time is also related to the economics of medical care delivery. Treatment of a preventable disease or delayed treatment of a chronic disease contribute to the rising costs of medical care. In a fee-for-service setting, each visit brings in revenue, but avoidable visits cost the client, the employer, and/or the insurance company unnecessary expense. Prepaid settings discourage unnecessary visits. If a high number of avoidable visits occur, the system is less able to care for acute illness. Thus the client and the system may both suffer from the absence of supported behavior change.

## WHO'S RESPONSIBLE FOR SUCCESS?

Where does the responsibility for maintenance lie? With the client? With the practitioner? Or with the programs offered or the settings within which those programs exist? We believe that the responsibility is shared among all these people. Lasting change is best supported where clients learn and apply principles of maintenance in the context of supportive programs and consistent institutions.

Each element in Figure 12.1 contributes to the process of supported change. In order to understand what characteristics each element brings

**Figure 12.1   Sources of support for change**

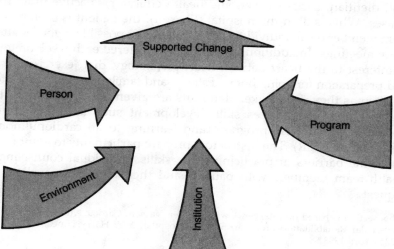

to this process, let's return to our opening case studies and take a closer look at the two health education programs in which John Wright and Sheila Brown participated. One is a program designed to help people to make lifestyle changes related to a chronic illness; the other is designed to help well people implement new health-promoting behaviors in their lives. We will give a somewhat detailed description of John and Sheila's experience with the programs. As you read these descriptions, notice what the individual clients bring, what the program offers, and how the institution contributes to supported change. At the end of each program description, you will have the opportunity to analyze the programs on these levels. Look for factors that increase or decrease John's and Sheila's chances for achieving and maintaining their personal goals.

## The Healthy Heart Program

In our first example, John had recently had a heart attack. John and his wife became involved in an educational program for heart patients at the hospital where John was a patient. Eight months after leaving the hospital, John was successful at making changes in his diet and in increasing his activity level. He has been able to maintain these two changes in health behavior. He has not quit smoking, but may be able to do so better on the basis of these two first steps. What elements in the Healthy Heart Program and within John resulted in this successful change? Let us look more closely at the Healthy Heart Program.*

The Healthy Heart Program consists of three programs; one for inpatients, one for outpatients, and one for recovered heart patients. Each member of the health care team (physician, nurse, physical therapist, dietitian, social worker, and health educator) is active in all three phases. While still in the hospital (Phase I), the patient is seen by each team member on an individual basis. Whenever possible, spouses attend these meetings. In addition, five classes are offered each week on topics of interest to the heart patient: heart physiology, diet, exercise, stress, and preparation for going home. Patients and family members may attend as often as they would like. Handouts are given out at each class. Program content emphasizes skill development such as diet planning, beginning an exercise program, and learning to do cardiopulmonary resuscitation (CPR). The instructors prepare participants to identify and overcome barriers in practicing those skills. Individual counseling by health team members with patients and their families is available on request.

*This section is based on interviews with Andrea Nassen, Cardiac Nurse Specialist, Cardiovascular Rehabilitation Program, St. Paul Hospital, 5909 Harry Hines, Dallas, Texas 75235, April 1983.

Phase II of the Healthy Heart Program is for outpatients. A block of time is set aside once a week for outpatients and their spouses to meet with team members for (1) refresher sessions on specific information or skills given while in the hospital; (2) problem-solving sessions on difficulties that the patient or a family member has encountered during this period; and (3) more indepth sessions on topics such as the recovery process, sex and intimacy, diet, exercise, cardiac emergencies, and stress. This phase lasts six weeks.

Phase III of the Healthy Heart Program is available to former heart patients and their families. A monthly evening meeting, consisting of a meal and speaker, is available at no charge. Phase III patients are contacted and reminded of upcoming meetings. At these gatherings, old acquaintances meet and share news of their recoveries, and share a meal based on Healthy Heart guidelines; they pass around pamphlets, recipes for the evening meal, and other materials; and a speaker talks on a topic of interest to the recovering heart patients. Health team members also attend this phase of the program. Figure 12.2 shows a sample menu. This menu-invitation serves as a reminder and outreach tool to program

**Figure 12.2   Invitation and menu for the Healthy Heart Program, Phase III**

YOU ARE INVITED
TO THE
HEALTHY HEART DINNER MEETING


Wednesday, October 12, 1983
Dinner—6:00 P.M.
Speaker—7:00 P.M.

Dr. Joan Liu will speak on
"Walking for Health"

\* \* \* \* \*

MENU

Baked Halibut
Carrots Almondine
Tomato and Green Bean Vinaigrette
Whole Wheat Rolls
Fruit Compote

participants, thus itself contributing to maintenance efforts. This maintenance phase continues indefinitely, and former patients and their partners come as often and as regularly as they choose.

Our heart patient, John, was told about the Healthy Heart Program by his physician the day he was released from the coronary care unit. During the next week (Phase I) while John was on the medical ward of the hospital, he and Lori met individually with the other health team members and were encouraged to attend the series of five classes on heart physiology, diet, exercise, stress, and preparing for going home. John was determined to prevent another heart attack and vowed he would change his diet, stop smoking, and get more exercise. Lori was willing to help wherever she could.

John and Lori attended the five classes and picked up useful tips on each topic. Individual sessions with each health team member helped them to decide what they could do to modify their health habits. John and Lori believed that the first thing they both could start working on was changing their eating habits. With the help of the dietitian, they designed an appetizing, practical plan. They established an educational contract with the dietitian to try this plan for four weeks. Figure 12.3 shows a sample contract.

**Figure 12.3   Sample educational contract**

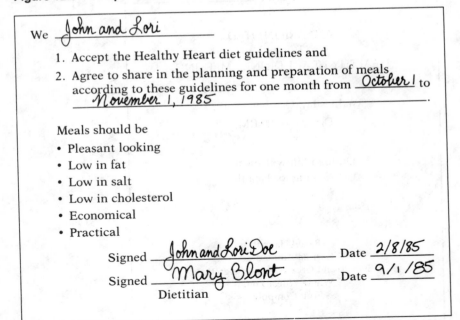

We *John and Lori*

1. Accept the Healthy Heart diet guidelines and
2. Agree to share in the planning and preparation of meals, according to these guidelines for one month from *October 1* to *November 1, 1985*.

Meals should be
- Pleasant looking
- Low in fat
- Low in salt
- Low in cholesterol
- Economical
- Practical

Signed *John and Lori Doe*          Date *2/8/85*
Signed *Mary Blont*                 Date *9/1/85*
     Dietitian

After John's release from the hospital, John and Lori began attending the Phase II part of the program once a week. One of the first problems John brought up in the group was an overwhelming feeling of frustration with changing his diet, trying to stop smoking, and getting more exercise—all at the same time. The group praised John and Lori for initiating these changes but agreed that John had taken on a lot. The group suggested that he work on one or two of the changes at a time. John decided to stick with diet changes and increasing his exercise for now and try to stop smoking at a later date, once he achieved these present goals.

Two months later, John returned to work. He and Lori began attending the monthly Phase III meetings. John saw fellow patients, his physician, and other health team members at these monthly meetings. He and Lori enjoyed the speakers, and the meals helped to give them ideas for alluring, healthy meal preparation. John knows it is important for him to stop smoking. Because he has greater confidence in his ability to take control over some of the health-related activities in his life, he is ready to make that his next goal.

Now that you know more about the Healthy Heart Program and John and Lori's participation, take a few minutes to analyze what factors in this situation contributed to John's success at making long-term lifestyle changes. Exercise 1, at the end of this chapter, can help you examine these factors, which are analyzed later in this chapter.

## The stress management class

Now let's turn our attention to a health promotion program designed for clients who are not clinically ill but who are concerned about physical symptoms and want to feel better. Sheila Brown, who had experienced symptoms of stress severe enough to warrant several doctor's visits, attended a four-week stress management class sponsored by the local public health department. Let us look in some detail at the content of this program, class by class.

The instructor introduced herself and invited participants to do the same and to share with the group what they hoped to get out of the class. The instructor gave an overview of the course, its objectives, and the kinds of activities, in class and at home, that would be employed to achieve those objectives. She showed a film on the causes and physiology of stress, and then led a discussion that clarified the differences between beneficial and harmful aspects of stress. Participants were given a simple record sheet and asked to notice and write down their stress symptoms and surrounding circumstances during the upcoming week. Figure 12.4 shows an example of the kind of stress record sheet Sheila Brown received

**Figure 12.4   Stress record**

| Symptoms of Stress | | | | |
|---|---|---|---|---|
| A one-week record from 2/8/85 to 2/15/85 | | | | |
| *Symptom* (e.g., headache, muscle tension) | *Circumstances* (What is going on? Who is around?) | *Day* | *Date* | *Time* |
| headache at back of neck | Paul practicing piano again! | Mon. | 2/9 | 6 PM |
|  |  |  |  |  |
|  |  |  |  |  |

during this first class. Exercises involving this kind of recordkeeping help people to personalize what is learned in a classroom setting and to see how new information applies to them in their everyday lives. The instructor ended the class after leading the members in a progressive relaxation exercise and encouraging the class to practice it at home at least once a day.

In the second class, participants reviewed the homework assignments together and discussed their personal experiences with the stress record sheets. The instructor lectured on the relaxation response, talked about the role of meditation in relaxation, and then taught some deep-breathing exercises. She then led the group in an autogenic relaxation exercise, a relaxation technique that involves participants in a simple form of self-suggestion or self-hypnosis. Class participants talked about the effects they felt from the exercise. The instructor advised the group to practice the relaxation exercises at home every day. She asked them to record the times they had felt deeply relaxed in the past week and to notice the surrounding circumstances. Figure 12.5 is a sample record sheet for a type of exercise designed to increase awareness of deep relaxation. Record sheets can help people identify existing skills as well as capture the results of applying new skills.

In the third class (which Sheila missed), the participants reviewed and discussed the week's assignment with each other, and the instructor

**Figure 12.5   Relaxation record**

| When? | Where? | What Was I Doing? | Surrounding Circumstances (What was going on around me? Who was there?) |
|---|---|---|---|
| Mon. 7 P.M. | home | Taking hot bath | Playing Vivaldi record; Paul out for the evening. |
| Tues. 6 A.M. | park | meditating | two Tai Chi exercisers close by (felt safe) |
| | | | |

*Times I Experienced Deep Relaxation*
A one-week record from 2/15/85 to 2/21/85

helped them evaluate the factors that contributed to their successes or failures. She introduced creative visualization—a technique of creating a mental picture of a desired state or goal. She used an audiotape to help students practice this technique in class. Then she discussed, in some detail, physical exercise and its role in stress management. Homework was as follows: participants were to examine their own activity patterns, assess possibilities for changes, and come back to the fourth class with at least one practical way they could build more physical activity into their schedules if they felt they needed more exercise.

In the fourth and final class, the homework and insights were discussed. Most of the class period was devoted to discussion and to practicing communication, assertiveness, and relationship skills. At the end of this final session, the instructor distributed a bibliography and a resource list of other, more thorough programs in stress management. She emphasized that the class should be seen as only a beginning, and encouraged the group to continue to practice and apply the skills to which they had been introduced.

Sheila attended three out of four classes. She missed the third class because it was her best friend's birthday, and she had promised to take her out to dinner. Sheila found the sessions that she did attend interesting and felt that she learned a lot. Although she felt a little embarrassed doing the relaxation exercises that the instructor led, she did notice that, at least some of the time, she was quite relaxed after doing them. This was especially true of autogenic relaxation. (Autogenic training is the process of relaxing in response to the repetition of simple sentences describing a sensation of heaviness, a feeling of warmth, and easy, natural breathing.) She resolved to practice this technique twice a day. But actually she found it extremely difficult to stop what she was doing and actually take the time to practice. The deadlines and pressures at work constituted one of her greatest sources of tension. Yet she had to meet those deadlines, and was reluctant to take even fifteen minutes to do her autogenic relaxation exercises. Also, even when she did practice, she found it harder to concentrate than when the instructor had led the exercise.

Although she missed the third class on exercise and stress, Sheila had been aware that she felt very relaxed when she did get some exercise such as tennis or swimming. But she had been unable to find and stick to any regular exercise schedule, although she kept meaning to. With her motivation once more increased, she signed up for an exercise class after work but often felt too tired to go. Instead she would go home and fall asleep on the sofa.

Some of the communication skills that she practiced in the last session helped Sheila express feelings and opinions to her boyfriend that she had previously kept to herself. She also was able to talk to her boss about her work schedule and negotiate to make some tasks less pressing. She felt encouraged by those successes and relieved to be able to be more herself in these relationships. On occasion she still held in her feelings instead of expressing them, and the resentment and anger then stayed with her and interfered with her ability to relax.

The next time Sheila was in a bookstore, she spent some time browsing through the books on stress management and some of the related topics. She bought one of the books on the resource list the instructor had distributed. The book made a lot of sense and contributed to her motivation to keep trying to improve her stress management skills. At this point, however, if Sheila had been asked about the benefits of her participation in the stress management class, she would have said that although she understood her stress better, so far she hadn't been able to get it under control to her satisfaction.

Admittedly, the long-term benefits of this single health education program look fairly limited. Without underestimating the impetus generated by the class, a health educator must ask the question "Was the maximum benefit Sheila derived from this program all that was possible?" Sheila actually took several positive steps as a result of attending this class. But in the end she felt discouraged. Were there some ways the program could have addressed the issues so that Sheila's motivation and attempts could have been more successful over time?

Before we present an analysis of the situation, do Exercise 2 at the end of the chapter, and identify the positive and negative maintenance factors that exist on the personal, program, and institutional levels.

## THE ELEMENTS OF SUSTAINED CHANGE

You probably already have some ideas on how the person, the program, and institutional policies and practices work together toward achieving the goal of lasting change. Let us compare John and Lori's Healthy Heart Program with Sheila's stress reduction class, from these three perspectives.

### On the personal level

A number of personal factors affect the success of change efforts. The questions must be asked "What or who is behind the client's request for help? Was it the doctor, an anxious spouse, or the client who felt ready for a change? And why? Is the moving force fear or hope for improving the quality of life?" Incentive may vary according to the responses to these questions. Both John and Sheila were highly motivated, but the experience of a life-threatening heart attack may have forced John to take his health behavior more seriously than did Sheila, who was basically well.

What do clients need or expect the program to do for them? What expectation of success do clients actually have? John wanted a program that could help him prevent another heart attack. Sheila needed an immediate solution to her physical distress. We do not know whether either person anticipated that changes such as they were undertaking would require constant effort over the months and years to come. Sheila lost some of her incentive to keep doing the relaxation techniques when they didn't cure her stress symptoms right away. Helping clients to form realistic expectations can be of major significance in encouraging them to stick with their efforts.

John's situation, but not Sheila's, shows the existence of social support for efforts undertaken. Lori was helping John, and the Healthy Heart Program encouraged participation by spouses. In addition, support was made available from fellow heart patients in all three phases. Sheila's stress reduction class did not help her identify or build social support for her change. Perhaps if Sheila had invited a friend or co-worker to practice relaxation techniques, or had made an educational contract with someone, she would have received some ongoing encouragement.

The physical and social environments of the client, at home and work, play an important role in sustaining change. As we saw in Sheila's situation, her fast-paced workload and frequent job changes led to a stressful work environment. No mention was made regarding her physical environment and modifications that might have helped her relax more easily. Assessing such features as noise level, privacy, or visual restfulness of surroundings might have helped Sheila identify areas needing improvement. Analyzing the home and work environments for sources of support or possible obstacles for the change help clients incorporate change into their present lifestyle. The provider may need to initiate this analysis by questioning the client about home and work settings. (For help in evaluating the environment, see the checklist in Chapter 10, p. 323.) Together they may be able to solve problems that exist. The client can then take action to create a more supportive physical environment and to ask for desired social support. Was it realistic to expect Sheila to begin doing relaxation exercises in a workday already filled to excess with obligations? Note that after he returned to work John still could get help from his health care team as he worked on incorporating his diet changes and exercise program into his day.

Another step in transferring new skills into daily routine is to design a reward system. The praise from the group members in Phase II was a type of reward for John. This recognition acknowledged his commitment to change and spurred him to keep working on his goals. John or Sheila could have set up a point system whereby they gave themselves a point for each time they performed the desired activity. A set number of points could allow John or Sheila to give themselves a preselected reward. Prearranged rewards such as material goods or pleasurable activities, as well as notice and praise from other people, help to keep personal energy and motivation high as one works toward a goal. In cases where the final goal is long-term, such as in weight loss, rewards along the way make the investment pay off more immediately.

## On the program level

One of the first questions we must ask is "Does the program fit the client's needs and expectations?" The instructor in the stress management class, for example, could have been more explicit about the limitations of the class, emphasizing that this class was only an introduction to a long learning process. Although the instructor asked what the participants' expectations were, no adjustments were made in the four sessions to meet participants' needs. The four sessions were actually fixed and non-negotiable. Sheila expected immediate relief and more personal analysis of situations and problem solving. Her expectations could not be met by this class, especially in four sessions.

Opportunities to practice new skills can be designed for class time and through homework assignments. Although Sheila's group practiced the relaxation techniques in class, the instructor always led them. Allowing participants to lead the exercises or using audio tapes and making them available for purchase could enhance implementation at home. By missing the third class, Sheila lost an opportunity to practice new skills under the guidance of the instructor. Sheila's momentum in learning and practicing stress management skills was seriously hampered. The dietitian in the Healthy Heart Program might have reviewed and revised John and Lori's meal plans with them or asked them to demonstrate choosing meals from sample menus. Homework allows clients to try out new behaviors in their routine setting. Subsequent discussion of problems encountered in doing the homework can lead to solutions to those problems, and problem solving increases the chances that the client will continue new behavior.

Assuring sustained change was a weak part of the stress management program but was beautifully illustrated in the Healthy Heart Program. To maintain a new behavior, it is very helpful to have the opportunity to renew skills and investment in the goal. Not every educational program has the luxury of offering follow-up sessions. The resource list that Sheila's instructor distributed takes on added importance in light of the limited scope of the program. Did it list other classes in the community that Sheila could use to continue her learning? In this case, the responsibility to follow up falls on Sheila. However, what is the likelihood of Sheila's following up when she is feeling generally disappointed in her lack of success with managing her stress?

Phase II and Phase III of the Healthy Heart Program, in contrast, were able to help John and Lori refine and sustain their skills. In addition, this continued contact renewed enthusiasm for healthy habits. As John felt successful in changing his diet and getting more regular exercise, he became confident that he could now undertake the challenge of trying to stop smoking. Participants in Phase I were periodically contacted and reminded of the availability of Phase II and upcoming meetings in Phase III. Including the health team members assured a continuity of philosophy from treatment through recovery and on to sustained lifestyle change. A program that includes the members of the health team provides many opportunities for sharing information in a variety of ways. For instance, in the Healthy Heart Program, opportunities arose through conversation with the health team members and through participation in classes, the problem-solving group, and the Phase III evening meetings. From the time of the heart attack to returning to normal activities, the message and contact with providers were continuous.

## On the institutional level

The philosophy of an institution guides the design of educational programs in that setting. The institution's policies provide the framework within which programs must operate. For instance, the policy framework either encourages follow-up or it doesn't. It may encourage follow-up by providing funding for support groups to maintain progress over time, or by less costly means such as phone calls or establishing support groups of laypeople. Policy might also dictate that follow-up is no longer a responsibility of the institution once the client has left the setting.

Several institutional practices in the Healthy Heart Program demonstrate commitment to supporting long-term change. These include the provision of continuous care from the hospital to the medical office, the teamwork approach to care, and the incorporation of learning experiences into the treatment provided.

Within the physician's private practice, Sheila's referral to a stress management class complemented the physician's prior admonitions to relax more. If at Sheila's next visit the practitioner had checked to see if she had attended the class and encouraged her in her efforts, Sheila might have felt greater commitment to following the stress management regimen.

Another question that must be asked in assessing the institution's commitment to or role in supporting long-term change is "Why are the institution's decision makers offering the program?" Due to a number of economic factors, hospitals, for example, may offer health education programs primarily for public relations or to attract consumers. If increasing business is the primary objective of a program, there is less likely to be attention to, and resources for, ensuring long-term outcomes.

We have referred to a number of elements on the personal, program, and institution levels that affect long-term change. Table 12.1 lists these elements for reference in assessing the likelihood of maintenance. Health educators can review these elements and identify those which require modification in a given situation. For example, if a client's expectations do not coincide with a program's purpose, the client can be referred to a more suitable program. Health team members may be alerted to the need for more follow-up to assure that participants' efforts will be supported over time.

**Table 12.1　Factors that help maintain change**

| I Client factors | II Program factors | III Institutional factors |
|---|---|---|
| • Personal needs and motivation | • Program-client fit | • Continuity of care |
| • Expectations | • Opportunities for practice | • Referral systems |
| • Support from family and friends | • Problem solving on difficulties encountered or anticipated | • Teamwork |
| • Home environment | | • Learning experiences in treatment |
| • Work environment | • Follow-up | • Incentive for maintenance |
| | • Resources available | |
| | • Including health team members | |

## IMPLICATIONS FOR HEALTH EDUCATORS

Factors associated with the individual, program, and institutional levels of health education practice all contribute to the client's ability to sustain changes in health behavior over time. Maintaining change is a complex, dynamic process as opposed to a one-time accomplishment. Rather than thinking of health-related change as a static state achieved once and for all, we must remember that it is more accurately described as movement toward improved well-being. Making and sustaining change is an uneven journey, at best. It is uneven because of wavering motivation, changes in social supports, fluctuation in stress, and the fact that what is adequate today may not be adequate tomorrow.

What does this reality imply for those of us practicing health education within a medical care setting? Our responsibility for the long-term maintenance of our client's health behavior is important but not limited. On the one hand, we are responsible to the client to increase the chances that changes will endure over time; yet we must recognize the individual's right to decide not to make or sustain the behavior change. We are expected to offer quality programs that achieve the outcome desired by our clients, yet we do not control all the factors that influence that outcome. For instance, we may not always get the resources needed to offer a top-notch program. Our institution's priorities may not correspond to our need for resources. It is also possible that perceived needs for the program differ. Health educators must respond to the needs of the client and yet must offer programs that the organization sees as beneficial; these perceptions may not be synonymous. Given these limitations, we may sometimes be offering programs that do not provide adequately for maintenance of behavior change. Is it better to offer a less than ideal program than to offer no program? In each situation, the benefits must be weighed against the drawbacks. Regardless of the course of action chosen, the limitations of short-term educational programs must be made clear to both the client and the system so that we do not set people or programs up for failure.

Above all, and in spite of the need to balance a multitude of sometimes conflicting factors in the medical care setting, we must not lose sight of our commitment to helping clients experience success in their efforts to effect changes in their health choices and behaviors. We must be aware of the complexity of the change process and must articulate this to clients, providers, and administrators. We must take into account many human and economic limitations as we seek to enhance the sense of control our clients have over their own lives. Programs and institutions serve a valuable function in guiding and supporting individuals' efforts toward health. However, people who provide programs or run institutions have neither the means nor the desire to make clients totally dependent on them for their health. And so we need to educate in order to achieve one of the most important means of ensuring successful health changes over the long term, namely, self-care. Encouraging and providing for clients' development of basic skills and confidence in health decision making and action is the key to maintaining positive health changes over time. Clients can reapply these qualities over and over again as circumstances and health requirements change. As health educators practicing in medical care, we can foster these qualities by encouraging their adoption by clients, by integrating self-care components in educational programs, and by stimulating our institutions to adopt policies that in turn stimulate self-care health decision making.

# EXERCISES

1. *The Healthy Heart Program:* List the characteristics of John's situation you believe to be responsible for his success over time, according to the following categories.
   a. *Client factors:* What about John himself and his responses contributed to success?

b. *Programmatic factors:* What factors in the Healthy Heart Program helped John change his lifestyle?

c. *Institutional factors:* How did the hospital in which John was a patient contribute to John's maintaining change over time?

Do you see any barriers to John's success in sustaining his new lifestyle? Would you change anything in the scenario to further support John's chances of success?

2. *A Stress Management Class:* List the characteristics of Sheila's situation you believe to be responsible for her lack of success, according to the following categories:

   a. *Client factors:* How did Sheila's personal approach to and involvement in the program contribute positively to long-term behavior change? What did she herself do or not do that decreased long-term effectiveness?

   b. *Programmatic factors:* What teaching methods in the program increased Sheila's chances of continuing her new skills over time? What was missing that might have helped?

   c. *Institutional factors:* In what ways did the local public health department and the physician in private practice support Sheila's resolve to make permanent changes? Can you see some possibilities for improvement in these areas?

3. You are a health educator in a neighborhood clinic. You want to offer a stop smoking program. You are aware of the difficulty of maintaining cessation and want to offer as much support as possible to those who go through your program. Make a list of two or three obstacles to permanent change that you would imagine might exist on each of the three levels we have discussed. Now suggest strategies for overcoming these obstacles.

# RESOURCES

Davidson, P. O., and Davidson, S. M. (eds.). *Behavioral Medicine: Changing Health Lifestyles.* New York: Brunner-Mazel, 1980.

The authors break new ground by compiling research in the complex arena of lifestyle changes. Their book contains chapters on topics such as weight loss and smoking cessation. A strong theme running throughout the book is the continuing difficulty of maintaining changes. They offer suggestions to increase sustained behavior change. A useful and well-written book.

Farquhar, J. *The American Way of Life Need Not Be Hazardous to Your Health.* New York: Norton, 1978.

Written by the director and founder of the Stanford Heart Disease Prevention Program, this book contains a wealth of information on changing or initiating health actions. The author skillfully weaves facts pertaining to heart disease with humorous figures, exercises, and "how-to's."

Haynes, R. B., Taylor, D. W., and Sackett, D. L. (eds.). *Compliance in Health Care.* Baltimore, Md.: Johns Hopkins University Press, 1979.

This book is one of the foremost compilations of research on compliance to date. The authors describe the critical issues in compliance and noncompliance, suggest strategies for increasing adherence to prescribed regimens, and outline research implications for the future. Well-referenced and easy-to-read.

Kanfer, E. H. Self-Management Strategies and Tactics. In A. P. Goldstein and F. H. Kanfer (eds.), *Maximizing Treatment Gains—Transfer Enhancement in Psychotherapy.* San Francisco: Academic Press, 1979.

Although this chapter was written with psychotherapeutic concerns in mind, many of the suggestions can be readily applied to health behavior change. Maintaining success over time can be enhanced by the client's active participation in defining goals, measuring and rewarding progress, and learning to solve problems when obstacles arise.

Mahoney, M. *Self-Change.* New York: Norton, 1979.

This book is written primarily for the individual who would like to resolve a personal problem or initiate actions to improve daily living. Strategies are outlined for examining the problem or goal, methodically initiating an action, and maintaining that action over time. The principles are based on current behavioral science and are written in an easy-to-read manner.

# PART FOUR

# AN INTEGRATING
# CASE STUDY

# 13

## The Data Tech case

MARLENE ANDREWS WAS watching the row houses through the train window, one by one, as they seemed to march by on that crisp December afternoon. She tried to force her thoughts to stay focused on her long-awaited Christmas holidays. But no matter how hard she tried, her mind wandered back to her meeting that morning.

Marlene Andrews is the health education coordinator for the Valley Community Hospital. The hospital is a 200-bed, nonprofit hospital that serves a small working-class community in the Northeast.

Even though Marlene was leaving for a ten-day Christmas vacation that day, she had scheduled an emergency meeting with the hospital administrator, the medical director, and the public affairs director. By January 1, Marlene was to present a proposal to the board of directors. Marlene was both excited and terrified about the implications her proposal might have for the future of health education at Valley.

Valley Hospital was the only hospital serving its community. The hospital enjoyed a very positive reputation for the quality of medical care, and especially for its aggressive community relations program. For over ten years the hospital had offered patient education services for its hospitalized patients. It offered formal educational programs for newly diagnosed diabetics, postmyocardial infarction (heart attack) patients, stroke patients, chronic obstructive lung disease patients, and new mothers on the maternity ward. The hospital also initiated outpatient educational programs to offer long-term support and follow-up for discharged patients. Valley Hospital worked closely with community agencies, such as the visiting nurses association, the public health department, the community college, and the voluntary health agencies (American Cancer

Society, American Lung Association, American Heart Association, American Red Cross, and the YMCA) to co-sponsor these programs.

In the last five years, Valley Hospital has become quite active in health promotion. The hospital sponsored an evening lecture series on nutrition, preventing back injuries, managing stress, and physical fitness. They also co-sponsored a stop smoking program with the Lung Association, and a weight loss program with Weight Watchers, Inc.

Both the outpatient patient education and health promotion programs were offered in the hospital's conference rooms and in the hospital's auditorium. It was not uncommon for several hundred people from the community to attend the lectures. The hospital attributed the popular success of the evening lecture series to their ability to identify topics of wide interest, as well as to their ability to get advance coverage of the programs in the local newspapers.

Participants in the outpatient programs paid fees to the hospital to cover the costs. This arrangement did not seem to deter the people who were intent on quitting smoking or losing weight.

For several months, Marlene had received phone calls from personnel managers of local companies asking her to bring the hospital's health education programs to their worksites. One company in particular, Data Tech, wanted the hospital to conduct back care classes for all its employees. The chief executive officer was convinced that the company could save a great deal in reduced workers' compensation claims if the workforce had one hour of back care instruction.

Marlene had been reading about hospital-sponsored employee health promotion programs for years. The Data Tech request was forcing her to decide what Valley Community Hospital's role would be in outreach efforts. She knew that the time was right to help the hospital determine its policy in regards to offering services in sites other than its own premises. There was, however, an urgency about the Data Tech request: the chief executive officer of Data Tech was married to a member of the hospital's board of trustees. Marlene knew that she would be pressured to respond affirmatively to the Data Tech request.

Marlene's professional instincts caused her to hesitate. If the hospital chose to set a precedent with Data Tech, with a categorical approach— for example, a one-hour back care seminar for employees—would this be the best way to go?

As Marlene settled back in her train seat, she began to make a list of the questions that she would have to face before she stood before the board to make her recommendations. Once you have examined the list, which follows, work through the exercises at the conclusion of the chapter.

**1.** Is the time right for Valley Community Hospital (VCH) to expand its services?

**2.** What are the potential benefits to VCH of offering employee health promotion services to employers in the community?

**3.** What are the potential risks to VCH due to offering employee health promotion services to employers in the community?

**4.** If VCH decides to offer employee health promotion outreach services, how should they be organized? Should VCH offer categorical programs on request, or should VCH provide a comprehensive employee health promotion package?

**5.** What criteria should VCH use to decide which employers to work with? Should VCH work with all companies that request service? What conditions should exist in the company before VCH agrees to come in?

**6.** How should VCH handle requests for services that have little chance of meeting employer expectations?

**7.** How will VCH know if their employee health promotion services do any good? What should VCH promise?

**8.** How should VCH bill the company for this service? Should the employer pay? Should the employees pay?

**9.** How will VCH prevent a situation where employees are invited, but no one shows up for the educational services?

**10.** To what degree should employees and management be involved in the planning of employee health promotion programs?

**11.** To what extent should employee health promotion programs include issues of worker safety and quality of work life?

**12.** How will VCH handle requests that clearly are bandaids for more severe morale or labor problems?

**13.** How will VCH control the quality of instructors and programs on other employers' premises?

**14.** Should VCH work with unions as well as work with management during the program planning? Whose programs are these?

# EXERCISES

1.  Go back to the model for health education program development that was presented in Chapter 1. Take the health education programming steps (assessment, planning, implementation, and evaluation) and follow them through the institutional level for the Data Tech case presented in this chapter. Assume the role of Marlene Andrews. Where data are missing in the case presentation, fill in the details as realistically as you can imagine them.

2.  Go back to Chapter 2, Table 2.1. Prepare a formal statement in favor of, or in opposition to, the Data Tech request for back care classes. Assume the role of Marlene Andrews, and prepare the statement as if you were going to present it to the board of trustees at the Valley Community Hospital. You may want to consult Appendix 2.3 and Appendix 2.5 in Chapter 2.

3.  Go back to Appendix 5.2 in Chapter 5. Assume that you are Marlene Andrews and that you did accept the Data Tech request on a demonstration basis. Complete the education protocol for occupation-related back injuries. Attach the teaching plan and time line.

# RESOURCES

American Hospital Association/Centers for Disease Control Health Education Project. *Hospital-Sponsored Community Health Promotion.* U.S. Department of Health and Human Services, Centers for Disease Control, Center for Health Promotion and Education, Community Program Development Division, Atlanta, Georgia. Washington, D.C.: U.S. Government Printing Office, August 1981.

> This document contains a literature review and five case studies of hospital-based health promotion programs. The five examples illustrate the types of programs and services that hospitals can develop to meet the various health needs of their communities.

Dean, D. H. Bringing Health Promotion to the Worksite: Issues, Opportunities, and a Developing Model. *Health Education Quarterly, 8*(4), Winter 1981: 359–372.

> Dean describes an employee health promotion pilot project initiated by the Kaiser-Permanente Medical Care Program in Portland, Oregon. The key

issues discussed are employee participation and how to prevent attrition over the intervention period. Dean recommends that one intensive behavior change initiative every two months is the best way to offer health promotion services to preserve employee interest and participation.

Keenan, C. Health Promotion: Hospital-Based Health Promotion Needs Solid Marketing Backup. *Hospitals, 56*(11), 1982: 92–96.

The author of this article reports that, although many hospitals have entered the health promotion market, few presently report a profit. Keenan summarizes the payoffs to hospitals for engaging in outreach employee health promotion services. Success or failure to generate revenue may be caused by the marketing strategy that the hospital adopts as part of its long-range planning efforts. A number of key marketing questions are listed in the article.

Koo, P. A. *Guide to Occupational Health and Health Promotion: Programs in Hospitals.* Nashville, Tenn.: Center for Health Studies, 1982.

This guide was written to help hospital managers identify the opportunities and benefits of hospitals offering occupational health and health promotion programs to industry. Koo presents a model for program planning that includes the following steps: (1) planning, (2) marketing, and (3) program design. Outlines for a few categorical programs are provided. The employee health promotion program sponsored by the Wellness Center at Johnson Memorial Hospital is described. Hypothetical income statements and breakeven computations are a welcome addition to the case study materials.

Parkinson, R. S., Beck, R. N., Collings, G. H., Eriksen, M., McGill, A. M., Pearson, C. E., and Ware, B. G. *Managing Health Promotion in the Workplace: Guidelines for Implementation and Evaluation.* Palo Alto, Calif.: Mayfield, 1982.

The aim of this book is to help managers in businesses and unions, as well as health professionals, to set up a health promotion program or to upgrade an existing one. The first section of the book presents guidelines for planning and implementing employee health promotion programs. The model for program planning presented in the guidelines includes the following steps: (1) assessing needs, (2) setting priorities and objectives, (3) determining organizational location, (4) implementing strategies, and (5) identifying and allocating resources. Section II provides seventeen examples of company programs. Section III includes twelve background papers on issues and approaches in worksite health promotion.

*Promoting Health.* A newsletter of the American Hospital Association, P. O. Box 96003, Chicago, Illinois 60693. $24 per year.

This newsletter is the only periodical of its kind specifically directed at professionals engaged in hospital-based health promotion activities. It is intended to help hospitals meet the challenge of moving beyond their traditional role into the broader arena of health promotion and disease prevention. The newsletter is a practical tool for use by practitioners and decision makers who are involved in developing patient education, community health education, and employee programs.

# References

Alogna, M. Assessment of Patient Knowledge and Performance. In G. Steiner and P. A. Lawrence (eds.), *Educating Diabetic Patients*. New York: Springer, 1981.

American Cancer Society Recommendations. *Cancer, 30*, 1980: 194–240.

American College of Physicians. Annual Physical Recommendations from American College of Physicians. *Annals of Internal Medicine, 95*, 1981: 729–732.

American Group Practice Association. *AGPA Patient Education Program: The Basics*. Alexandria, Va.: American Group Practice Association, 1977.

American Hospital Association. *Hospital In-Patient Education: Survey Findings and Analyses*. Chicago: American Hospital Publishing, 1978.

Anderson, S., Auquier, A., Hauck, W. W., Oakes, D., Vandaele, W., and Weisberg, H. I. *Statistical Methods for Comparative Studies: Techniques for Bias Reduction*. New York: Wiley, 1980.

Arvidson, B., Connelly, M. J., McDaid, T., Sitzman, J., Squyres, W., Van Raalte, L., Vitlar, M., and Wellenkamp, D. A Health Education Model for Ambulatory Care. *Journal of Nursing Administration*, March 1979, pp. 16–21.

Barbour, A. A Comparison of the Disease Model and the Growth Model. In S. Miller, N. Ramen, A. Barbour, M. A. Nakles, D. Garrell, and S. Miller, *Dimensions of Humanistic Medicine*. San Francisco: Institute for the Study of Humanistic Medicine, 1975.

Berkman, L. F., and Syme, S. L. Social Networks, Host Resistance and Mortality: A 9-Year Follow-Up of Alameda County Residents. *American Journal of Epidemiology, 109*, 1979: 186–204.

Berry, W., Schoenbach, V., Wagner, E., Graham, R., Karon, J., and Pezzullo, S. *Description, Analysis and Assessment of Health Hazard Appraisal Programs, Final Report*. Contract no. 233-79-3008, University of North Carolina at Chapel Hill. Prepared for National Center for Health Services Research, Hyattsville, Md. March 13, 1981. Available from Technical Information Services, Springfield, Va. Tel. 703-487-4650.

Bower, E. L. *The Process of Planning Nursing Care*. St. Louis: Mosby, 1972.

Brekon, J. *Hospital Health Education: A Guide to Program Development*. Rockville, Md.: Aspen, 1982.

Breslow, L., and Somers, A. Lifetime Health Monitoring Program: A Whole Life Plan for Well Patient Care. *Patient Care, 13*(11), 1979: 83–149.

Brown, E. R., and Margo, G. E. Health Education: Can the Reformers Be Reformed? *International Journal of Health Services, 8*(1), 1978: 3–26.

Campbell, D. T., and Stanley, J. C. *Experimental and Quasi-Experimental Designs for Research.* Chicago: Rand McNally, 1966.

Canadian Task Force on Periodic Health Examinations. The Periodic Health Examination. *Canadian Medical Association Journal, 121* 1979: 1193–1254.

Carlson, R. J. The End of Medicine. *Executive, 3,* 1976: 6.

Chapman, E. N. *Supervisor's Survival Kit: A Mid-Management Primer.* Palo Alto, Calif.: Science Research Associates, 1975.

Committee on Educational Tasks in Chronic Illness (Public Health Service, Health Resources Administration, Bureau of Health Planning and Resources Development, Division of Facilities Development). *A Model for Planning Patient Education.* HEW Publication no. (HRA)76-4028. Washington, D.C.: U.S. Government Printing Office, 1975.

Cook, T. D., and Campbell, D. T. *Quasi-Experimentation: Design and Analysis Issues for Field Settings.* Chicago: Rand McNally, 1979.

Council on Wage and Price Stability. *The Complex Puzzle of Rising Health Care Costs: Can the Private Sector Fit It Together?* Washington, D.C.: Council on Wage and Price Stability, 1976.

Cronbach, L. J., and Associates. *Toward Reform of Program Evaluation.* San Francisco: Jossey-Bass, 1980.

Davis, L. N. *Planning, Conducting and Evaluating Workshops.* Dallas: Learning Concepts, 1976.

Deeds, S. G., Hebert, B. J., and Wolle, J. M. *A Model for Patient Education Programming.* Washington, D.C.: American Public Health Association, Public Health Education Section, February 1979, pp. 22–26.

De Friese, G. H., Beery, W. L., Braham, R. M., and Barry, P. Z. *Health Promotion/ Disease Prevention in the Clinical Practice of Medicine and Dentistry.* Chapel Hill: Health Services Research Center, University of North Carolina, 1981.

De Joseph, J. Writing Educational Protocols. In W. Squyres (ed.), *Patient Education: An Inquiry into the State of the Art.* New York: Springer, 1980, pp. 45–112.

Department of Preventive Medicine and Community Health, University of Texas. *Course Syllabus on Preventive and Community Medicine.* University of Texas, Medical Branch, Department of Preventive Medicine and Community Health, Health Sciences Consortium, 200 Eastowne Drive, Suite 213, Chapel Hill, NC 27514.

Dickelman, N. L., and Broadwell, M. M. *The New Hospital Supervisor.* Reading, Mass.: Addison-Wesley, 1977.

D'Onofrio, C. N. Evaluating Patient Education Programs, Politics, and a Proposal for Practitioners. In W. Squyres (ed.), *Patient Education: An Inquiry into the State of the Art.* New York: Springer, 1980.

Dubos, R. *Mirage of Health.* New York: Harper, 1959.

Dunbar, J. M., Marshall, G. D., and Hovell, M. F. Behavioral Strategies for Improving Compliance. In R. B. Haynes, D. W. Taylor, and D. L. Sackett (eds.), *Compliance in Health Care.* Baltimore, Md.: Johns Hopkins University Press, 1979.

Eddy, W. B., and Warner, B. W. (eds.). *Behavioral Science and the Manager's Role.* San Diego, Calif.: University Associates, 1980.

Fitz-Gibbon, C. T., and Morris, L. L., *How to Design a Program Evaluation.* Beverly Hills, Calif.: Sage, 1978.

Flanagan, J. A Research Approach to Improving Our Quality of Life. *American Psychologist,* February 1978, pp. 138–148.

Frame, P. S., and Carlson, S. J. A Critical Review of Periodic Health Screening Using Specific Screening Criteria. *Journal of Family Practice, 2,* 1975: 29–36, 123–129, 189–194, 283–289.

Freedman, C. R. *Teaching Patients: A Practical Handbook for the Health Professional.* San Diego, Calif.: Courseware, 1978.

*Freedom from Smoking in 20 Days.* American Lung Association, 295 27th Street, Oakland, CA 94612. 1980.

Green, K. E., and Moore, S. H. Attitudes Toward Self-Care. *Medical Care, 18*(8), 1980.

Green, L. W. How to Evaluate Health Promotion. *Hospitals, 53,* October 1, 1979: 106–108.

Green, L. W. National Policy in the Promotion of Health. Keynote address for the Tenth International Conference on Health Education, London, England, 1979. American Hospital Association. *Implementing Patient Education in Hospitals.* Chicago: American Hospital Publishing, 1979.

Green, L. W., Kreuter, M. W., Deeds, S. G., and Partridge, K. B. *Health Education Planning: A Diagnostic Approach.* Palo Alto, Calif.: Mayfield, 1980.

Green, L. W., Wang, V. L., Deeds, S., Fisher, A., Windsor, R., Bennett, A., and Rogers, C. Guidelines for Health Education in Maternal and Child Health. *International Journal of Health Education,* supplement, 21(3), July–September 1978. Whole issue.

Haynes, R. B., Taylor, D. W., and Sackett, D. L. (eds.). *Compliance in Health Care.* Baltimore, Md.: Johns Hopkins University Press, 1979.

Health Education, Student Health Services, University of California at Berkeley. *Picture of Health Workbook.* Berkeley: Health Education, Student Health Services, University of California.

Hecht, R. *Guide to Media Program Development.* Stanford, Calif.: Division of Instructional Media, Stanford University School of Medicine, 1978.

Holmes, T. H., and Rahe, R. H. The Social Adjustment Rating Scale. *Journal of Psychosomatic Research, 11,* 1967: 213–218.

Hulley, S. B., Rosenman, R. H., Bawol, R. D., and Brand, R. J. Epidemiology as a Guide to Clinical Decisions: The Association Between Triglycerides and Coronary Heart Disease. *New England Journal of Medicine, 302* (25), 1980: 1383–1389.

Illich, I. *Medical Nemesis: The Expropriation of Health.* New York: Pantheon, 1976.

Ingals, J. D. *A Trainer's Guide to Andragogy.* Waltham, Mass.: Data Education, 1973.

Janis, I. L. *The Contours of Fear.* New York: Wiley, 1968, pp. 166–224.

Janis, I. L., and Mann, L. *Decision-Making*. New York: Free Press, 1977.

Joint Commission on Accreditation of Hospitals. *Accreditation Manual for Hospitals*. Chicago: Joint Commission on Accreditation of Hospitals, 1976.

Kanfer, F. H. Self-Management Methods. In F. H. Kanfer and A. P. Goldstein (eds.), *Helping People Change*. New York: Pergamon Press, 1980.

Kirscht, J. P. Patient Education and Blood Pressure Control in the Long Run. *American Journal of Public Health*, 73(2), February 1983: 134–135.

Knowles, M. *The Adult Learner: A Neglected Species*. Houston, Texas: Gulf, 1978.

Krantz, D., Baum, S. A., and Wideman, M. V. Assessment of Preferences for Self-Treatment and Information in Health Care. *Journal of Personality and Social Psychology*, 39(5), 1980: 977–990.

Levin, L. S. The Layperson as the Primary Health Care Practitioner. *Public Health Reports*, 91(3), 1976: 206–210.

Levin, L. S. Self-Medication: The Social Perspective. In *Self-Medication: The New Era . . . A Symposium*. Washington, D.C.: Proprietary Association, 1980.

Levin, L. S., and Idler, E. L. *The Hidden Health Care System: Mediating Structures and Medicine*. Cambridge, Mass.: Ballinger, 1981.

Leventhal, H. Fear Communications in the Acceptance of Preventive Health Practices. *Bulletin of the New York Academy of Medicine*, 41, 1965: 1144.

Mager, R. F. *Preparing Instructional Objectives*. Belmont, Calif.: Fearon, 1975.

Mahoney, M. J. *Self-Change: Strategies for Solving Personal Problems*. New York: Norton, 1979.

Mazzuca, S. A. Does Patient Education in Chronic Disease Have Therapeutic Value? *Journal of Chronic Diseases*, 35(7), 1982: 521–529.

Milio, N. *The Care of Health in Communities: Access for Outcasts*. New York: Macmillan, 1975.

Miller, S., Ramen, N., Barbour, A., Nakles, M. A., Garrell, D., and Miller, S. *Dimensions of Humanistic Medicine*. San Francisco: Institute for the Study of Humanistic Medicine, 1975.

Morisky, D. E., Levine, D. M., Green, L. W., Shapiro, S., Russell, P., and Smith, C. R. Five-Year Blood Pressure Control and Mortality Following Health Education of Hypertensive Patients. *American Journal of Public Health*, 73(2), February 1983: 153–162.

Mullen, P. D., and Zapka, J. E. (eds.). Guidelines for Health Promotion and Education Services in HMOs. Washington, D.C.: U.S. Government Printing Office, 1982.

Mumford, E., Schlesinger, H. J., and Glass, G. V. The Effects of Psychological Intervention on Recovery from Surgery and Heart Attacks. *American Journal of Public Health*, 72(2), 1982: 141–151.

Neidhardt, E. J., Conry, R. F., and Weinstein, M. S. *Autogenic Methods*. Vancouver, British Columbia: Western Center Health Group, 1982.

Nelson, E. C. Roberts, E. Simmons, J., and Mason, N. *Final Report to Administration on Aging. Self-Care for Seniors: A Community-Based Education Program*. Hanover, N.H.: Dartmouth Medical School, 1982.

Patton, M. Q. *Qualitative Evaluation Methods.* Beverly Hills, Calif.: Sage, 1980.

Pfeiffer, J., and Jones, J. (eds.). *Handbook of Structured Experiences for Human Relations Training,* vols. 1–5. La Jolla, Calif.: University Associates Publishers and Consultants, 1975.

Robbins, L., and Hall, J. *How to Practice Prospective Medicine.* Indianapolis: Methodist Hospital of Indiana, 1970.

Rosenstock, I. R. Historical Origins of the Health Belief Model. *Health Education Monographs,* 2(4), 1974: 328–335.

Ross, H. S., and Mico, P. R. *Theory and Practice in Health Education.* Palo Alto, Calif.: Mayfield, 1980.

Rossi, P. H., and Freeman, H. E. *Evaluation: A Systematic Approach.* 2nd ed. Beverly Hills, Calif.: Sage, 1982.

Shortell, S. M., and Richardson, W. C. *Health Program Evaluation.* St. Louis: Mosby, 1978.

Squyres, W. D. The Professional Health Educator in HMOs: Implications for Training and Our Future in Medical Care. *Health Education Quarterly,* 9(1), Spring 1982: 67–80.

Stone, G. Patient Compliance and the Role of the Expert. *Journal of Social Issues,* 35(1), 1979: 34–59.

Suchman, E. A. *Evaluative Research: Principles and Practice in Public Service and Social Action Programs.* New York: Russell Sage Foundation, 1967.

Surgeon General (U.S. Department of Health, Education, and Welfare; Public Health Service; Office of the Assistant Secretary for Health and Surgeon General). *Healthy People: The Surgeon General's Report on Health Promotion and Disease Prevention.* Washington, D.C.: U.S. Government Printing Office, 1979.

Task Force on Patient Education, President's Committee on Health Education: *Health Education Monographs,* 2(1), Spring 1974: 1–10.

Tufo, H. M., Bouchard, R. E., Rubin, A. S., Twitchell, J. C., Van Buren, H. C., and Bedard, L. Problem-Oriented Approach to Practice. *Journal of the American Medical Association,* 238(6), August 8, 1977: 502–505.

U.S. Department of Health, Education, and Welfare; Public Health Service; Office of the Assistant Secretary for Health. *Proceedings of the National Conference on Health Promotion Programs in Occupational Settings.* Washington, D.C.: U.S. Government Printing Office, 1979.

Weed, L. L. Medical Records That Guide and Teach. *New England Journal of Medicine,* 278, 1968: 593.

Weiss, C. H. *Evaluation Research: Methods of Assessing Program Effectiveness.* Englewood Cliffs, N.J.: Prentice-Hall, 1972.

Weiss, C. H. Where Politics and Evaluation Research Meet. *Evaluation,* 1(3), 1973: 37–45.

# Index

**Note:** Italicized page numbers refer to resource listings.

American Group Practice

on formalization of educational
functions, 101, 102
American Heart Association, 86, 338,
380 .
American Hospital Association, *157,
257*
on responsibility for health
education, 38–40, 45–48
support of patient education by, 29,
49–55
survey of education departments
by, 100
*American Journal of Public Health*, 199
American Lung Association, 348, 380
American Medical Association, *58*
on planned patient education,
42–44
professional standards of, 53
American Nurses' Association, *3, 58*
professional standards of, 53–54
American Psychological
Association, *3*
American Public Health Association,
*2*, 86
American Red Cross, 380
American Society for Healthcare Edu-
cation and Training, 41
American Society for Health, Man-
power, Education and Training, *2*
American Society for Training and
Development, 86
American Society of Hospital Phar-
macists, *58*
professional standards of, 55
*The American Way of Life Need Not Be
Hazardous to Your Health*, 376
Anderson, S., 195, 196
Andrews, Marlene, 379–80
Anemia, preventive procedure with,
280 (table)
Anxiety in assessment of mortality
risk, 264
Appointments, assessment, 276, 277,
281
"An Approach to the Diagnosis and

Treatment of Problems of Health
Behavior," *258*
Arthritis, 170
The Arthritis Foundation, 338
Assessment, 141–42, 148–49
of administration support, 134–35
building support for, 243
client level of, 230–35
by clients, 193
of educational goals, 128, 130
expanding role of, 244–45
extra-physiological dimensions of,
221
goals of, 222–23
of group learning needs, 78
of health risks, 260–82
identification of behavioral influences in, 229–30, 250
as intervention, 223, 230–38
in introduction of new programs,
97, 98 (table), 380–82
medical v. educational, 221, 222,
239–42
misconceptions about, 242–43
of need for direct service,
96 (table), 96–97
in program development,
10–11 (table)
programmatic level of, 235–38
of prospects for decision-making,
310–12
by providers, 193–94
quality of, 223–25
techniques of, 225–28
Association for Hospital Medical
Education, 53
Association for the Advancement of
Health Education, *3*
Atherosclerosis, 332, 333
Attendance sheet, 194, 206–7
Autogenic relaxation, 366, 368
Autonomy in clinical decisions, 127.
*See also* Self-assessment; Self-care

Back care class
teaching methods for, 163 & table
worksite, 380–82

Proposal for introduction of new program, 103, 104 (table)
Prospective medicine, assessment of mortality risk by, 260–61
Proteinuria, preventive procedure with, 280 (table)
Protocols
  and accountability, 137–38
  for client behavior change, 138–40
  codification of standards in, 127
  flexibility in, 137–38
  guidance of action plans by, 127–28
  sample, 141–47
  sample, filled-in, 148–54
  self-diagnostic, 342 & Fig.
  writing of, 135–37
Providers. *See also* Personnel
  assessment model of, 239–42
  autonomy of, 127
  and client adherence, 360, 361
  and consumer information resources, 339–40
  contribution of, to sustained behavior change, 362–74 *passim*
  definition of, 1
  and difficult clients, 243–44
  and educational fallacies, 242–43
  guidance of, by protocols, 127–28
  health educators as, 69–70, 72 (table), 77–78
  in home care, 335–36
  importance of evaluation to, 188–89
  interdisciplinary coalitions of, 243
  involvement of, in evaluation, 189–91
  involvement of, in planning, 122 & table
  partnership of, with client, 223, 225, 238, 239, 241–42, 244, 337, 340, 342–43, 345–49
  priorities of, in program development, 117, 119–20
  promotion of behavioral change by, 138–40
  resistance to self-care by, 351–54

role of, in health risk appraisal, 271–72
satisfaction of, 193–94, 346
self-care workshops for, 343
and staffing requirements, 192
and support groups, 337, 338
teaching of self-management skills by, 334–35
view of program effectiveness by, 183, 185 (table)
*Psychological Theories and Human Learning: Kongor's Report, 258*
Public health, objectives of, 19–21
Public opinion as factor in program evaluation, 184, 185 (table)

Qualitative data, 198–200
*Qualitative Evaluation Methods, 217*
Quality assurance standards, 121, 223–25, 235–38
Quality of life. *See also* Lifestyle
  as factor in assessment, 240–41
  and therapeutic options, 128, 130
Quantitative data, 198–200
Questioning skills, 226–28
Questionnaires, assessment, 225–26, 246–49
  identification of risk factors with, 261–64 *passim*, 274–77 *passim*, 283–87, 291–301
  for instructors, 236, 251–53

Random assignment, 196–97, 199–200
Rank-ordering technique, 317, 319 & table 10.3
Rape, 332, 348
Reach to Recovery, 337, 347
*Recording Nutritional Information in Medical Records, 55*
Redman, B. K., *126*
Rees, A. M., *180, 356*
Referrals
  and budgetary constraints, 203
  and decision-making control, 347
  documentation of, 193

Wong, Larke, 309
Workshops
  and client control, 347–48
  instructor-training, 79, 236–38,
    251–55
  self-care, 340–43
Wright, John, 358–59, 362–65,
  369–72
Wright, Lori, 358–59, 364–65, 369,
  371

"Writing Educational Protocols," *158*

Young Men's Christian Association
  (YMCA), 380

Zander, K. S., *159*
Zealous practitioners, 103